Narrating Patienthood

Lexington Studies in Health Communication

Series Editors: Leandra H. Hernández and Kari Nixon

National and international governments have recognized the importance of widespread, timely, and effective health communication, as research shows that accurate, patient-centered, and culturally competent health communication can improve patient and community health-care outcomes. This interdisciplinary series examines the role of health communication in society and is receptive to manuscripts and edited volumes that use a variety of theoretical, methodological, interdisciplinary, and intersectional approaches. We invite contributions on a variety of health communication topics including but not limited to health communication in a digital age; race, gender, ethnicity, class, physical abilities, and health communication; critical approaches to health communication; feminisms and health communication; LGBTQIA health; interpersonal health communication perspectives; rhetorical approaches to health communication; organizational approaches to health communication; health campaigns, media effects, and health communication; multicultural approaches to health communication; and international health communication. This series is open to contributions from scholars representing communication, women's and gender studies, public health, health education, discursive analyses of medical rhetoric, and other disciplines whose work interrogates and explores these topics. Successful proposals will be accessible to an interdisciplinary audience, advance our understanding of contemporary approaches to health communication, and enrich our conversations about the importance of health communication in today's health landscape.

Recent Titles in This Series

Challenging Reproductive Control and Gendered Violence in the Americas: Intersectionality, Power, and Struggles for Rights, by Leandra Hinojosa Hernández and Sarah De Los Santos Upton

Politics, Propaganda, and Public Health: A Case Study in Health Communication and Public Trust, by Laura Crosswell and Lance Porter

Communication and Feminist Perspectives on Ovarian Cancer, by Dinah Tetteh

Narrating Patienthood

Engaging Diverse Voices on Health, Communication, and the Patient Experience

Edited by
Peter M. Kellett

LEXINGTON BOOKS
Lanham • Boulder • New York • London

Published by Lexington Books
An imprint of The Rowman & Littlefield Publishing Group, Inc.
4501 Forbes Boulevard, Suite 200, Lanham, Maryland 20706
www.rowman.com

6 Tinworth Street, London SE11 5AL, United Kingdom

British Library Cataloguing in Publication Information Available

Library of Congress Cataloging-in-Publication Data

Names: Kellett, Peter M., editor.
Title: Narrating patienthood : engaging diverse voices on deeper cultural health
   narratives / edited by Peter M. Kellett.
Description: Lanham : Lexington Books, [2019] | Series: Lexington studies in health
   communication | Includes bibliographical references and index.
Identifiers: LCCN 2018046663 (print) | LCCN 2018047623 (ebook) |
   ISBN 9781498585545 (Electronic) | ISBN 9781498585538 (cloth)
Subjects: LCSH: Communication in medicine. | Physician and patient. |
   Narration (Rhetoric) | Hospitals—Sociological aspects.
Classification: LCC R118 (ebook) | LCC R118 .N366 2019 (print) |
   DDC 610.69/6—dc23
LC record available at https://lccn.loc.gov/2018046663

Printed in the United States of America

Contents

Acknowledgments

I would like to thank Hema and Zola for all their support throughout the writing of this book, and for helping me to keep a healthy life-work balance in everyday life. My own story would be a much duller one without you both. Thanks to all the scholars of health involved in this book (and those not involved) who focus on collecting and exploring the experiences of patients everywhere. It is an important work, as it enables us to try to make the world around us fairer and healthier. Special thanks to all the patients who contributed narratives from their lives that made this book possible. I would also like to include a special acknowledgment here to all the chapter authors who served double duty as both researcher and patient. Writing from your own lives is a much-appreciated form of invitational bravery. Finally, I would like to acknowledge the enormous impact that Walter Fisher has made through his work to those of us who do narrative scholarship in the field of communication. He passed as this book was nearing completion.

Introduction

Through the recent process of writing my own story of heath communication and disease, *Patienthood and Communication: A Personal Narrative of Eye Disease and Vision Loss* (2017), I became acutely aware of several "truths" of my own experience and its narration. Across the five years documented in my story I had to learn how to become an empowered, self-advocating patient. It was not easy, and I had to unlearn a lot of personal, familial, and cultural conditioning to get there. The better I got at this, though, the better my health care. I also learned that my story—my patienthood narrative—was not just a form of representation for my experience, but was also fully a *speech act*—albeit a long one. It could *do things* like encourage others to tell their stories, advocate for better information for fellow patients, and actively help in some small way to shape the discourse and level of understanding around the disease I have (MacTel), and that I share with my identical twin brother, David. I became aware that who I was, where (and when) I lived, and how I expressed myself made a difference. I am a white, middle-aged, (fairly) artic-ulate, (as of now) able-bodied, middle-class, straight, male with reasonably good health insurance, a rare eye disease, and an encouraging and protective spouse. I also happen to live where I am surrounded by three major research hospitals with substantial ophthalmology departments. Others, I knew, would likely have very different experiences with this disease (and other diseases/ illnesses) based on who they were and where (and when) they lived. I also learned that various *forms* of communication (both face-to-face, and online), and *contexts* of communication (intrapersonal, relational, organizational, familial, and so on) were, and remain, central to how I navigate, construct, make sense of, and reduce the uncertainty of, my illness experience. I am a relational partner, a friend, a family member, a patient with ongoing doctor-patient relationships, and a communication professor, with an eye disease that affects vision. Each and all these aspects interconnect, as they do for others in different and important ways. But what to make of all this in a broader context of the experiential, and scholarly world beyond myself and my disease? And, so, this book.

I wanted to hear the experiences of others undergoing parallel or perhaps even quite different struggles with, and around, "truths" like these. Specifically, I wanted to collect, in narrative form, a broad range of health communication experiences that enable us to examine and address more closely the following questions: (1) How do patient narratives provide the means for, and illustrate the development of, self-empowerment as patients, increased understanding of multiple stakeholders involved in the care process, advocacy and even activism on behalf of patients, and more effective communication as a basis for better care? (2) How do various identities (such as race, class, gender, sexuality, and disability) intersect with, and impact, people's narrated experiences of patienthood? and (3) How do people in various patienthood processes and experiences describe communication as central to those experiences? These three key questions, and related issues, became the central concerns of the three parts of this book.

Part I (Voicing, Empowering, Advocating) begins with two chapters that illustrate the power of narrative accounts of patienthood experiences to inform various publics (Reznik), and to advocate for patients in a variety of important ways (Hoffmann-Longtin & Hayden). The succeeding two chapters present more personal accounts of the power and importance of patient narratives. Chapter 3 (Orbe) shares the long-term development of his self-understanding and empowerment as a patient, for example, in interactions with health-care providers as well as orientations to accessing health care as a patient. Chapter 4 (Daugherty & Young) provides a much-needed global/advocacy perspective in asking us how telling the stories of (and for) others (here the poor of war-torn Syria) is an important and impactful part of health communication scholarship and practice.

Part II (Differences That Matter) includes chapters that centrally examine cultural differences and identities in how they impact health behavior, access, and broader issues of inequity and communication. Chapter 5 (Dillon & Basu) illustrates how race can impact how African Americans think about and access/engage in end-of-life care and the dying process. Chapter 6 (Meluch) vividly shows how the health-care process and experience of one woman is impacted by socioeconomic (class) factors. It illustrates how care providers and patients are impacted by economic status differences. Chapter 7 (Hintz & Venetis) explores how culturally grounded assumptions about gender mitigates the diagnostic and treatment process in ways that can negatively impact women and their lives. Chapter 8 (Brown) foregrounds sexual identity, as it can variously impact the health-care process and related communication, by exploring heath care through the voice of a queer patient. Finally, this part is completed by chapter 9 (Johnson), which is a moving account of how disability impacts health communication and care. None of these chapters claim to speak for or represent whole segments of our population yet, together, they do provide an interesting and provocative account of how differences matter in health communication.

Part III (Intersections of Communication and the Personal, Relational, Professional, and Cultural) expands and illustrates the discussion by providing detailed narrative accounts of various, and very different, health-care and related communication experiences. Chapter 10 (Spieldenner et al.) shows us how the researcher and the topic of the research become deeply intertwined, and how the persona of the "Community Researcher" takes form as patient and researcher fuse together. Chapters 11 (Yamasaki) and 12 (Archiopoli) illustrate the important and fascinating world of online narration and support, where an organic relationship between the personal and public, as well as internal (decision-making, etc.) and external aspects of narrative and narration occurs. They evoke the important issues of representation, relationships, and narrative sharing experiences. Chapter 13 (Castle & Kellas) takes us into the world of Lupus—showing us the important contribution to our understanding of patienthood of examining the typical plot archetypes of patients with Lupus. Chapter 14 (Ohs) takes us through four birth experiences of the author that richly illustrate the need to understand what the effective communication of care means in context, and the importance of the culture of care provider settings, in the birthing experience. Deconstructing dominant cultural narratives, this chapter also powerfully illustrates the intersection and blending of researcher and patient identities. Blending medical and familial identities, chapter 15 closes the book with an intriguing comparison of two cases that have the writer (Dastidar) also approaching patienthood as both doctor/researcher in examining one narrative case (Dax) and sister in examining the second narrative case (Shuvo). Medical, familial, and cultural contexts of the lives of two different patients are compared.

Looking across the parts and chapters of this book, one of the most rewarding aspects of this project was, for me, seeing the rich variety of approaches to what it means to do narrative health research. Some chapters shared autoethnographic narratives. Others report on work that involves collecting the personal narratives of others, both singular and in multiples. Some chapters explore diachronic narratives—tracing changes such as growth as a patient across time. Others examine specific aspects or content of narratives synchronically, such as plotlines or themes as they illustrate or forward particular theories. Interestingly, still others took narrative in a broader discursive and cultural sense of collectively held accounts (metanarratives), rather than as the speech acts of individuals. Others approach narrative as something implied behind, and tying together, a set of facts. For these scholars, hidden narratives—the story behind the story/stories—can be skillfully revealed. Finally, of note, it is wonderful to read narratives of health and illness written by colleagues. Several chapter authors took the brave step in sharing from their own lives, and in doing so, finding ways to balance professional and personal dimensions of self. Given this rich variety of narrative work in this volume we, as readers and scholars, are engaged by different articulations of narrative research and patient narration.

The studies in this volume, taken collectively, bring together and help to extend and apply some key ongoing conversations in narrative approaches to health communication. Several of the chapters help to push forward our understanding of cultural and intercultural (and inter-identity) communication competence as a crucial line of inquiry and practice. Several chapters directly address and show the development of patient self-empowerment. The lived reality of inequity, diversity, and difference, and some of the major gaps in understanding that manifest systemically from these factors in health care are richly illustrated. Other key concepts that appear throughout the book are the communicative workings of stigma, sense-making, uncertainty reduction, and patienthood. Crucially throughout the book, chapter authors ground their work in, and make substantial contributions to, the narrative frameworks developed by Frank (illness narratives), Charon (narrative medicine), and others. We owe a great deal theoretically and practically to these scholars as we all try to make the world fairer and healthier.

With the variety and interest of the narrative studies included in this volume, comes limitations. Of note is the reliance on stories that largely originate in the United States. Much could be done in subsequent research to compare and contrast patient narratives of people more globally. Similarly, much could be done to examine patient experiences across the lifespan. How do illnesses and health issues have long-term impacts on people's life stories? How do people's life stories impact the illness experience? There is much work yet to be done in examining the ever-changing reality and impact of technology and our online lives on our health narratives. Finally, there is much work to be done in examining the impact of contemporary world dynamics—war, displacement, the refugee experiences of many on narrations of health and illness. With these nods to the limits of this current work, we glace toward future possibilities for work that explore how and why people narrate their patienthood as they do.

REFERENCE

Kellett, Peter M. (2017). *Patienthood and communication: A personal narrative of eye disease and vision loss.* New York, NY: Peter Lang.

Part I

NARRATING PATIENTHOOD: VOICING, EMPOWERING, ADVOCATING

Chapter 1

Narratives of Patient Experience

Benefits for Multiple Audiences

Rachel M. Reznik

On the first day of my job as a research assistant, interviewing patients living with HIV, I sat anxiously waiting for the first patient in a small, bureaucratic office. He arrived in baggy jeans, a t-shirt, and a jacket. Now that my interviewee was here in person—a living, physical presence—my anxiousness quickly transformed into nervousness. What if I did not ask the right questions? What if I made a mistake? As I awkwardly started the interview process, and asked him questions about his illness and treatment, my nerves faded away. He was talking with great ease. He was telling me his story and wanted to be heard. Something simple but significant had occurred: the ease and fluency communicated themselves to me; and the desire to be heard called to a desire to hear. It was my privilege to listen.

Narratives provide a compelling way for those experiencing a health issue or illness to share their experience. Narratives are important, as one's life story, "which every person constructs by weaving together the variety of events and experiences that make up life into a balanced entity," can be interrupted by events such as illness which appear to put that experiential thread at risk (Overberg, Alpay, Verhoef, & Zwetsloot-Schonk, 2007, p. 937). However, these stories also afford benefits to other audiences, as they can foster social support for others experiencing the same or similar issues; and can open an avenue for providers to improve care, and for students to learn about patients' experience of illness and health care.

Put simply, narratives are "stories with a teller, a listener, a time course, a plot, and a point" (Charon, 2006, p. 3). Central to Charon's definition is a listener, referring to other patients, lay caregivers, professional caregivers, providers, and medical students. Common interest in narrative across a broad range of disciplines in the later part of the twentieth century "emphasizes its importance in expressing and structuring discourse, identity, and experience"

(Spencer, 2017, p. 374). Narratives involve people making meaning by interpreting and articulating connections between "countless seemingly unconnected experiences, beliefs, attitudes, and understandings, and so on" (p. 33) and are "informed by and reveal the contexts within which their relevant understandings are formed and acted upon" (Babrow, Kline & Rawlins, 2005, pp. 37–38). As Peter Kellett (2017) relates in his personal narrative of eye disease and loss of vision, a narrative may include an account of a patient's internal processes, such as their thoughts and feelings, as well as addressing external processes such as their communication and behaviors, and the context of those processes.

THE IMPACT OF UNCERTAINTY AND STIGMA

While it can be difficult for patients to disclose their stories to others, there are several benefits to doing so, including a way to share the stress, engage in sense-making, and connect with others who may be more knowledgeable than the patient regarding their condition (Kellett, 2017). In the sharing process, such patients may also gain a greater level of self-understanding and enhance their sense of self-esteem (Herxheimer & Ziebland, 2003). Sharing one's personal health-related story is a means of reducing the shame individuals may feel about their health condition or status, and of encouraging greater inclusivity (Davis & Quinlan, 2017). Narratives can help create "hopeful communication" and even bring humor into otherwise very serious situations which might be fraught with uncertainty, emotional upheaval, and a fear of loss of one's identity (Kellett, 2017). This might be especially important for those facing terminal or life-altering health conditions. Significant health events may create a climate of uncertainty not only for patients but also their families, and some of those events may result in stigma as well. The following section explores the impact of both concepts on narratives for patients themselves, their fellow patients, and their loved ones, and addresses the reciprocal relationship between narrative and experience.

According to Brashers (2001), "uncertainty exists when details of situations are ambiguous, complex, unpredictable, or probabilistic; when information is unavailable or inconsistent; and when people feel insecure in their own state of knowledge or the state of knowledge in general" (p. 478), and it is a core feature of both acute and chronic illnesses (Brashers et al., 2000). Uncertainty management theory (UMT) helps explain the process by which individuals experience, appraise, and respond to uncertainty around health information (Brashers, 2001). According to UMT, appraisals about the meaning of uncertainty need not be negative, and indeed reducing uncertainty is not the only goal individuals have; they may want to maintain levels of uncertainty or even increase their uncertainty if certainty is believed likely to result in psychological distress (Brashers et al., 2000). One way that individuals manage their uncertainty (e.g., increase, decrease, or maintain it at the same level) is by seeking information from others, or by avoiding information, thus either stimulating or constraining communication (Brashers et al., 2000).

These varied communication responses have implications for story tellers and story listeners alike. Kellett (2017) describes a conversation in which his struggles were shared with a neighbor: the neighbor's response, recounting how someone had been finally cured, after receiving holistic Eastern medicine, of a condition which had hitherto stumped experts in Western biomedicine, induced feelings of uncertainty or "new ambiguity" within him. Hearing others' stories can play a role in uncertainty management as these narratives might have the effect of reducing uncertainty, or they might, alternatively, increase uncertainty. This uncertainty also extends to patients' loved ones. Some people in this category reported avoiding health information as a way to resist the possibility of overexposure to such information, and not be reminded about another's health issues too frequently, or to maintain privacy boundaries and keep their distance from details deemed by the listener to be too private or intimate (Barbour, Rintamaki, Ramsey, & Brashers, 2012). Avoiding information makes it possible for people to remain hopeful and optimistic in cases where what they eschew is likely to be disconfirming information (Rains & Tukachinsky, 2015).

Another response to uncertainty is to seek out new information. For those with either acute or chronic illness, information may be sought to understand the diagnosis, make treatment decisions, and help make predictions about the prognosis (Brashers, Goldsmith, & Hsieh, 2002). Thus, illness narratives are not only beneficial for the story tellers themselves, but also for fellow patients who are facing the same or similar situations and seeking insight into their conditions, as these narratives may serve as examples of how to complement, edit, and orient one's own life story (Overberg et al., 2007). People report that they want to read narratives about topics which they are experiencing in a negative way, thinking about, or directly suffering from themselves, thereby using other patients' stories to further cultivate and nurture their own story into a balanced, meaningful narrative (Overberg et al., 2007). Narratives are sought out to gain practical information about how to cope with emotions, understand how the illness will impact one's daily life, and realistically anticipate what physical discomforts are likely to come with the illness (Overberg et al., 2007).

In addition to uncertainty around their symptoms and prognosis, people may also feel uncertainty about the stigma associated with their illness (Checton, Greene, Magsamen-Conrad & Venetis, 2012). Irving Goffman (1963) described stigma as "an attribute that is deeply discrediting" (p. 3). Stigma has also been described as the disgrace that is linked with particular circumstances, characteristics, traits, or behaviors (Scambler, 1984). Rintamaki and Brashers (2010) conceptualize stigma as the "negative attitudes held about individuals who are perceived to possess a trait deemed negative by the community at large, as well as those with whom these individuals are associated" (p. 157). The experience of "normal" group membership might be jeopardized or rendered very different for individuals who are thus stigmatized.

Many health issues are associated with some degree of stigma, including mental illness, alcohol- and substance-abuse disorders, human immunodeficiency virus and acquired immune deficiency syndrome, chronic obstructive pulmonary disease, cancer, and neurological conditions. Diseases are often stigmatizing to the extent that they are accompanied by mental or physical limitations (Burgener & Berger, 2008). Having a stigmatizing illness may predispose a person both to feelings of shame (Goffman, 1963; Scambler, 1984), and to potentially being treated differently by able-bodied people (Braithwaite, 1991). Stigma can negatively impact individuals' self-worth and their well-being (Davis & Quinlan, 2017). As well as shame, further consequences of stigma may include financial insecurity, and social rejection and isolation (Fife & Wright, 2000).

Indeed, a problem facing some stigmatized individuals is that their social interactions are disrupted by the repercussions of their conditions (Albrecht, Walker, & Levy, 1982). These diminished social networks and the concomitant lack of social support can hamper stigmatized individuals' ability to find value and significance in their lives (Rintamaki & Brashers, 2010). However, stigmatized individuals are not merely reactive victims; they act in vigilant and strategic ways to protect themselves during social interactions (Rintamaki & Brashers, 2010). This could translate to a decision not to disclose one's story as a means of self-protection or, conversely, could result in the choice actively to tell one's story as a means of education and advocacy (Rintamaki & Brashers, 2010).

The literature on stigma in chronic disease indicates that stigmatization, originating from self or others, is widespread, emotionally detrimental, and liable to affect both quality of life and health-maintenance behaviors. To understand how stigma affects social interaction, the cognitions and behaviors of both the stigmatizers and the stigmatized need to be examined (Rintamaki & Brashers, 2010). First, to understand how stigma guides social interaction, one must investigate the cognitive processes that stigmatizers engage in. These processes include categorization arising from a need for group protection, which in turn leads the stigmatizers to view the stigmatized primarily through a stigmatizing lens. Thus, a question for communication scholars should be: "Does a category such as illness or disability narratives risk perpetuating a reductive pathologizing lens?" (Spencer, 2017, p. 377). As individuals tend to express their attitudes during social interaction, stigmatizers could in such terms either avoid or discriminate against the stigmatized individuals. This could lead to individuals' narratives or stories not being heard. Additionally, those who experience stigma engage in a variety of cognitive processes to help them cope with their stigmatized status and may intentionally communicate their status to others. Individuals whose stigmatizing conditions are not clear, or known to others, constantly deal with dialectical tensions such as "to display or not to display; to tell or not to tell; to let on or not to let on; to lie or not to lie" (Goffman, 1963, p. 42).

People manage stigma in numerous different ways (Davis & Quinlan, 2017). One way involves associating with others who share the same stigmatizing condition (Goffman, 1963). This is analogous to the kind of information seeking, from patients with similar narratives, which was discussed earlier in this chapter. Sharing narratives can help people with stigmatizing conditions recognize and understand that they are not alone. Narratives can serve as a vehicle to connect and heal and may minimize stigma while increasing inclusivity (Davis & Quinlan, 2017).

However, there may also be complications around sharing one's story, as disclosing a stigmatized status has the potential to incur negative outcomes, such as social ostracism. Consequently, people living with stigmatizing diseases may choose to conceal their status which can, in turn, prevent social networking or impair their access to beneficial resources (Rintamaki & Brashers, 2010). Disclosure can be advantageous because concealing central aspects of one's self, such as one's marginalized identity, can over time lead to negative health consequences (McKenna & Bargh, 1998). However, some with stigmatized conditions reported that they chose to avoid seeking health information due to concerns about how they would be perceived (Barbour et al., 2012). The Internet may afford a means of alleviating some of these stigma concerns.

THE ROLE OF ONLINE NARRATIVES

Electronic media provides another way for patients to share their stories (Christiansen, 2011). Individuals' health and the symptoms of their condition are generally not the impediments to participating in computer-mediated communication that they may sometimes be in face-to-face encounters (Campbell et al., 2001). The Internet supplies a diverse assortment of resources for people seeking health information, including online support groups, blogs (Rains & Tukachinsky, 2015), and databases containing patient experiences (Giesler et al., 2017); indeed, an immense number of illness stories can now be found online (Overberg et al., 2017).

The ability to connect with other patients who have experienced a similar event can be very empowering (Kellett, 2017). Online narratives offer a way for individuals to tell their stories and receive social support from a variety of folks (including friends, family, coworkers, people undergoing the same health issue or a similar one, and even strangers), and are also a good means of expressing emotions (Harris, Cleary, & Stanton, 2015). Narratives shared on illness-related blogs have not only abetted information exchange and social support, but also facilitated emotional catharsis (Keim-Malpass & Steeves, 2012), and are thought to encourage emotional connections and empathic responses from audiences (Yu, Taverner, & Madden, 2011). Using positive words in online narratives is related to an increase in positive mood six months later, while, perhaps somewhat surprisingly, using negative emotion words has been associated with being less depressed (Harris et al., 2015). For newly diagnosed patients, online narratives can be a valuable resource, while the process of sharing information can be fulfilling in itself and may actively foster connection with other patients (Kellett, 2017). Indeed, motivations to visit online health support groups include giving support to others as well as forming new relationships (Chung, 2014).

From the perspective of loved ones, it can sometimes be difficult to know how to react to patients (Kellett, 2017), and online narratives may contribute constructively to this process. Patients and their partners experience illness differently (Checton et al., 2012). In several contexts, the Internet is said to encourage deeper social connectedness among individuals (Rainie & Kobut, 2000). Visitors, including mostly friends and family members, to websites recounting women's narratives about their experiences with cancer reported that the websites were useful in providing updates on physical and mental states, and helpful in making the visitors feel closer to the participants (Harris et al., 2015). Thus, online narratives have represented a way for visitors both to receive health information, and emotionally connect with patients.

Online narratives may also be a means of eroding some of the barriers normally associated with face-to-face communication; and there are specific benefits to gaining support via the Internet. Online support groups can be a promising avenue for members to share their stories as they may, in so doing, glean benefits such as emotional validation, routes to new information, and cathartic experiences (Greer, 2000), presumably through participating in self-disclosure and intimate communication (Walstrom, 2000). Indeed, going to an online support group to share one's story can be especially beneficial, in that online participants have engaged in more emotional support and self-disclosure than is typically the case in face-to-face groups (Perron, 2002). Additional benefits include decreased loneliness (Fogel, Albert, Schnabel, Ditkoff, & Neugut, 2002) and the opportunity for members to find acceptance (McKenna & Bargh, 1998). These benefits can be particularly important for individuals who are very ill, as all-consuming illnesses may entail reduced social involvement and a narrowly limited sense of self (Charmaz, 1991). Further benefits of online social support groups which may be of notable use to ill individuals include the avoidance of time-pressure, by being able to respond and contribute at one's own convenience (Perron, 2002); the acquisition of a sense of autonomy; and the experience of comfort or relief in the disclosure of stigmatizing and potentially embarrassing information due to the relative anonymity provided by the Internet (Walstrom, 2000).

Databases of patient experiences are another way for narratives to be shared online. The international research network DIPEx (Database of Individual Patients' Experiences) presents online narratives of people's experiences with health issues and illness which are collected in a systematic and rigorous manner (Giesler et al., 2017). Healthtalkonline.org (HTO) is an Internet database produced via a partnership with DIPEx and HERG (the Health Experience Research Group, part of the Nuffield Department of Primary Care Health Sciences at the University of Oxford), offering a large number of patient stories assembled to benefit other patients, health care professionals, and researchers (Herxheimer & Ziebland, 2003). The material for the website is created by qualitative researchers at HERG. For each condition or topic studied, a maximum variation sample of patients or caregivers is interviewed, and the result to date is a collection of 3,500 interviews on over 85 health issues and conditions (healthtalkonline.org). Users of the site can watch and listen to the patients' stories or read transcripts from the interviews. In addition to viewing patient narratives, individuals can read carefully researched summaries of the themes that emerged from the interviews in the context of current clinical evidence and best practices. HTO covers a wide range of health conditions and their treatments, and records patients' experience of their impact on daily lives, interpersonal relationships with loved ones, colleagues, and caregivers, and interactions with health-care professionals. These insights into the patients' interactions are a source of useful information not only for other patients experiencing similar health conditions, and their loved ones, but also as a training tool for health-care professionals.

Nonetheless, it must be kept in mind that electronic platforms might not be conducive to sharing one's stories. For example, warmly affirming stories (e.g., cat videos) and harshly polarized ones (e.g., political opinions) work better on Facebook than do awkwardly personal health disclosures (Kellett, 2017). While many women had a positive experience overall in telling their stories on a website, some women reported several barriers to using online tools to document their narratives, including time pressures, not feeling comfortable with computers or lacking easy access to a computer, trouble accessing the website itself, physical difficulties that prevented them from going online, and receiving fewer visitor comments than they had expected

(Harris et al., 2015). Additionally, while narratives in these contexts can indeed influence individuals' attitudes and health behaviors, they may be less useful at transmitting objective information, and may sometimes be misleading (McQueen, Arnold, & Baltes, 2015). And young people who share their stories online have particular concerns, including feeling embarrassed, facing criticism or bullying from others, and safety-related issues (Yu et al., 2011). Internet-based interventions generally have modest engagement by participants; but with that said, even brief engagement can produce positive outcomes (Harris et al., 2015).

USE OF NARRATIVES IN THE CLINICAL SETTING

As much as there is a benefit to story-telling, there is also a benefit to "story-listening" by health professionals (Ziebland, 2013). To that end, narrative medicine, calling for health-care professionals to listen carefully to, empathetically engage with, and reflect on patients' stories is recommended as an ideal standard as a compassionate and effective way to practice medicine (Charon, 2001, 2006). Narrative-based medicine involves dedicated attention to what patients say and how they say it, and representation of patients' experiences—sometimes with the intent of sharing this with the patients themselves—in the cause of increasing affiliation (with patients, other health professionals, and institutions) (Charon, 2005). Story-telling is used as an instrument to facilitate patients' emotional expression regarding their feelings, concerns, and reservations about their illness (Fioretti et al., 2016). The approach of narrative-based medicine, whereby clinicians elicit and listen to patients' stories in a medical encounter, is undertaken to increase accuracy about diagnosis, improve treatments, and build stronger relationships between patients and health-care professionals (Ziebland, 2013). Additionally, this approach results in decreased levels of pain, stress, and alienation, and an increase in levels of well-being, confidence, and cooperation regarding the illness (Fioretti et al., 2016). From the perspective of clinicians, understanding patients' stories and experiences has developed mutual understanding; and interviews were found to be "fascinating, encouraging, and comforting" (Ziebland, 2013, p. 278).

USE OF NARRATIVES IN MEDICAL EDUCATION

Regarding medical education, individuals' ability to learn is enhanced when they hear patients' stories. Patients themselves recognize the value of using stories as a teaching resource, as well as to help health-care professionals understand the social effects and consequences of health conditions, and how these conditions influence people's day-to-day experiences (Yu et al., 2011). Patient stories thus have the dual benefit of empowering those patients themselves and assisting students in learning (Gidman, 2013). Within that context, patients are increasingly being encouraged to take an active role in health-care education and to bring their voices into the learning process (Jha, Quinton, Bekker, & Roberts, 2009); and using patient experience is one way to enable patient voices to be heard in the curriculum (Kumagai, 2008).

Although patients report wanting to read the text of narratives from other patients (Overberg et al., 2007), there appear to be advantages associated with digital recordings of patient narratives for health-care students. Hearing a patient's words evokes stronger emotions than merely reading the words of a transcribed narrative, and generates empathetic responses (Field & Ziebland, 2008). Listening to digital stories allows for reflection and for the student to contextualize patients' experiences in relation to their daily lives and significant relationships (Christiansen, 2011). Students reported that watching video stories of real patients made them more interested (Brown & Macintosh, 2006; Kommalage & Senadheera, 2012), increased their motivation to learn (Brown & Macintosh, 2006), and helped with knowledge acquisition and the understanding of patients' problems (Kommalage & Senadheera, 2012). Indeed, students reported that they gained a "patient perspective" and hence a deeper understanding of an illness from viewing online narratives (Powell, Scott, Scott, & Jones, 2013). Capturing patients' experiences on video and film allows for themes and issues to emerge that might not otherwise arise in a clinical encounter (Christopher & Makoul, 2004). Specifically, students can be exposed to problematic and sensitive topics (Powell et al., 2013). Patients can be encouraged to be both positive and negative while telling their stories (Callahan, 2012) but may be less inclined to respond in these ways in a face-to-face medical encounter.

A 2008 study conducted by researchers at HERG found that several medical tutors (i.e., professors and other teachers at the university) use the site Healthcareonline.org in their teaching (Field & Ziebland, 2008). HTO was used with students studying for a spectrum of health professions, and training as doctors, nurses, midwives, pharmacists, clinical psychologists, occupational therapists, and medical sociologists (Field & Ziebland, 2008). Five site characteristics made the website particularly useful, namely: a wide array of illness and health conditions, many interviews per condition, patient authenticity, choice of interview format (written, audio, and video), and the high quality of the research underlying HTO. Tutors reported using HTO to engage and stimulate students with the wide-ranging experiences of patients from diverse backgrounds, reflecting the variety they would likely encounter in practice. Clips were embedded in lectures to provide information about various conditions or to demonstrate a lived patient experience. Tutors also used HTO to make concepts and theories relevant, to demonstrate diverse patient perspectives on illness, symptoms, and decision-making, to appeal to the varied learning styles of students, and to develop new teaching methods.

E-learning (e.g., the use of websites or DVDs) encourages student-centered learning in medical education by empowering students to become actively involved, to participate, and to take responsibility for the learning process (Thakore & McMahon, 2006). However, while many educators report using electronic narratives in their teaching, there is a paucity of research to explicate in detail what it is that students garner from these narratives, and how it might impact their learning (Field & Ziebland, 2008). One recent study involving patients' video experiences found that students who viewed video clips from patients describing a medical procedure went on to perform better in a medical exam, and showed greater confidence with communication, compared to students who viewed a module of a doctor discussing case histories and describing the medical procedure (Snow, Crocker, Talbot, Moore, & Salisbury, 2016).

CONCLUSION

Narratives constitute an important means for individuals who are experiencing a health issue or illness—from a variety of perspectives relative to that situation—to share their experiences, generate social support for others encountering the same issues, and establish an engaging way for clinicians and students to learn about patient experience of illness and health care. These are some of the key ways in which narratives can facilitate better health communication.

REFERENCES

Albrecht, G. L., Walker, V. G., & Levy, J. A. (1982). Social distance from the stigmatized: A test of two theories. *Social Science & Medicine, 16,* 1319–1327. doi: 10.1016/0277-9536(82)90027-2.

Babrow, A. S., Kline, K. N., & Rawlins, W. K. (2005). Narrating problems and problematizing narratives: Linking problematic integration and narrative theory in telling stories about our health. In L. M. Harter, P. M. Japp, & C. S. Beck (Eds.) *Narratives, health, and healing: Communication, research and practice* (pp. 31–52). Mahwah, NJ: Lawrence Erlbaum.

Barbour, J. A., Rintamaki, L. S., Ramsey, J. A., & Brashers, D. E. (2012). Avoiding health information. *Journal of Health Communication, 17,* 212–229. doi: 10.1080/10810730.2011.585691.

Brashers, D. E. (2001). Communication and uncertainty management. *Journal of Communication, 51,* 477–497. doi: 10.1111/j.1460-2466.2001.tb02892.x.

Brashers, D. E., Goldsmith, D. J., & Hsieh, E. (2002). Information seeking and avoiding in health contexts. *Human Communication Research, 28,* 258–271. doi: 10.1111/j.1468-2958.2002.tb00807.x.

Brashers, D. E., Neidig, J. L., Haas, S. M., Dobbs, L. K., Cardillo, L. W., & Russell, J. A. (2000). Communication in the management of uncertainty: The case of persons living with HIV or AIDS. *Communication Monographs, 67,* 63–84. doi: 10.1080/03637750009376495.

Brown, I., & Macintosh, M. (2006). Involving patients with coronary heart disease in developing e-learning assets for primary care nurses. *Nurse Education in Practice, 6,* 237–242. doi: 10.1016/j.nepr.2006.01.007.

Burgener, S. C., & Berger, B. (2008). Measuring perceived stigma in persons with progressive neurological disease. Alzheimer's dementia and Parkinson's disease. *Dementia, 7,* 31–53. doi: 10.1177/1471301207085366.

Callahan, C. (2012). Recording patient stories as an aid to training and service improvement. *Nursing Management, 19,* 20–22. doi: 10.7748/nm2012.12.19.8.20.c9445.

Campbell, K. M., Meier, A., Carr, C., Enga, Z., James, A. S., Reedy, J., & Zheng, B. (2001). Health behavior changes after colon cancer: A comparison of findings from face-to-face and on-line focus groups. *Family Community Health, 24,* 88–103.

Charmaz, K. (1991). Immersion in illness. In K. Charmaz (Ed.), *Good days, bad days: The self in chronic illness and time* (pp. 73–104). Rutgers University Press.

Charon, R. (2001). Narrative medicine: A model for empathy, reflection, profession, and trust. *Journal of the American Medical Association, 286,* 1897–1902. doi: 10.1001/jama.286.15.1897.

Charon, R. (2005). Narrative medicine: Attention, representation, affiliation. *Narrative, 13,* 261–270.

Charon, R. (2006). *Narrative medicine: Honoring the stories of illness.* Oxford: Oxford University Press.

Checton, M. G., Greene, K., Magsamen-Conrad, K., & Venetis, M. K. (2012). Patients' and partners' perspectives of chronic illness and its management. *Families, Systems, & Health, 30,* 114–129. doi: 10.1037/a0028598.

Christiansen, A. (2011). Storytelling and professional learning: A phenomenographic study of students' experience of patient digital stories in nurse education. *Nurse Education Today, 31,* 289–293. doi: 10.1016/j.nedt.2010.10.006.

Christopher, K., & Makoul, G. (2004). Patient narrative videos: Learning from the illness experience. In P. Twohig & V. Kalitzkus (Eds.), *Interdisciplinary perspectives on health, illness, and disease* (pp. 137–147). Amsterdam: Rodopi.

Chung, J. E. (2014). Social networking in online support groups for health: How online social networking benefits patients. *Journal of Health Communication, 19,* 639–659. doi: 10.1080/10810730.2012.757396.

Davis, C. S., & Quinlan, M. M. (2017). Communicating stigma and acceptance. In J. Yamasaki, P. Geist-Martin, & B. F. Sharf (Eds.), *Storied health and illness. Communicating personal, cultural, & political complexities* (pp. 191–220). Illinois: Waveland.

Field, K., & Ziebland, S. (2008). Beyond the Textbook: A preliminary analysis of the uses made of the DIPEx website in healthcare education. Retrieved in December 2013 from the World Wide Web. http://healthtalkonline.org/learning-and-teaching.

Fife, B. L., & Wright, E. R. (2000). The dimensionality of stigma: A comparison of its impact on the self of persons with HIV/AIDS and cancer. *Journal of Health and Social Behavior, 14,* 50–67. doi: 10.2307/2676360.

Fioretti, C., Mazzocco, K., Riva, S., Oliveri, S., Masiero, M., & Pravettoni, G. (2016). Research studies on patients' illness experience using the Narrative Medicine approach: A systematic review. *British Medical Journal Open, 6,* e011220. doi: 10.1136/bmjopen-2016-011220.

Fogel, J., Albert, S. M., Schnabel, F., Ditkoff, B. A., & Neugut, A. I. (2002). Internet use and social support in women with breast cancer. *Health Psychology, 21,* 398–404. doi: 10.1037/0278-6133.21.4.398.

Gidman, J. (2013). Listening to stories: Valuing knowledge from patient experience. *Nurse Education in Practice, 13,* 192–196. doi: 10.1016/j.nepr.2012.09.006.

Giesler, J. M., Keller, B., Repke, T., Leonhart, R., Weis, J., Muckelbauer, R., Müller-Nordhorn, J., Lucius-Hoene, G., & Holmber, C. (2017). Effect of a website that presents patients' experiences on self-efficacy and patient competence of colorectal cancer patients: Web-based randomized controlled trial. *Journal of Medical Internet Research, 19,* e334. doi: 10.2196/jmir.7639.

Goffman, E. (1963). *Stigma. Notes on the management of spoiled identity.* New York: Simon & Schuster.

Greer, B. G. (2000). Psychological and support functions of an e-mail mailing list for persons with cerebral palsy. *CyberPsychology and Behavior, 3,* 221–235. doi: 10.1089/109493100316085.

Harris, L. N., Cleary, E. H., & Stanton, A. L. (2015). Project connect online: User and visitor experiences of an Internet-based intervention for women with breast cancer. *Psycho-Oncology, 24,* 1145–1151. doi: 10.1002/pon3734.

Herxheimer, A., & Ziebland, S. (2003). DIPEx: Fresh insights for medical practice. *Journal of the Royal Society of Medicine, 96,* 209–210.

Jha, V., Quinton, N. D., Bekker, H. L., & Roberts, T. E. (2009). What educators and students really think about using patients as teachers in medical education: A qualitative study. *Medical Education, 43,* 449–456. doi: 10.1111/j.1365-2923.2009.03355.x.

Keim-Malpass, J., & Steeves, R. H. (2012). Talking with death at a diner: Young women's online narratives of cancer. *Oncology Nursing Forum, 39,* 373–378. doi: 10.1188/12.ONF.373-378.

Kellett, P. M. (2017). *Patienthood and communication. A personal narrative of eye disease and vision loss.* New York: Peter Lang.

Kommalage, M., & Senadheera, C. (2012). Using video to introduce clinical materials. *Clinical Teacher, 9,* 248–252. doi: 10.1111/j.1743-498X.2012.00559.x.

Kumagai, A. K. (2008). A conceptual framework for use of illness narratives in medical education. *Academic Medicine, 83,* 653–658. doi: 10.1097/ACM.0b013e3181782e17.

McKenna, K. Y. A., & Bargh, J. A. (1998). Coming out in the age of the Internet: Identity "demarginalization" through virtual group participation. *Journal of Personality and Social Psychology, 75,* 681–694. doi: 10.1037/0022-3514.75.3.681.

McQueen, A., Arnold, L. D., & Baltes, M. (2015). Characterizing online narratives about colonoscopy experiences: Comparing colon cancer "screeners" versus "survivors." *Journal of Health Communication, 20,* 958–968. doi: 10.1080/10810730.2015.1018606.

Overberg, R. I., Alpay, L. L., Verhoef, J., & Zwetsloot-Schonk, J. H. M. (2007). Illness stories on the Internet: What do breast cancer patients want at the end of treatment? *Psycho-Oncology, 16,* 937–944. doi: 10.1002/pon.1157.

Perron, B. (2002). Online support for caregivers of people with a mental illness. *Psychiatric Rehabilitation Journal, 26,* 70–77. doi: 10.2975/26.2002.70.77.

Powell, S., Scott, J., Scott, L., & Jones, D. (2013). An online narrative archive of patient experiences to support the education of physiotherapy and social work students in North East England: An evaluation study. *Education for Health, 26,* 25–31. doi: 10.4103/1357-6283.112797.

Rainie, L., & Kobut, A. (2000). *Tracking online life: How women use the Internet to cultivate relationships with family and friends.* Washington, DC: Pew Internet & American Life Project: Online life report. Retrieved on May 18, 2018 from the World Wide Web. [Available on-line: http://www.pewinternet.org/2000/05/10/tracking-online-life-how-women-use-the-internet-to-cultivate-relationships-with-family-and-friends/].

Rains, S. A., & Tukachinsky, R. (2015). An examination of the relationships among uncertainty, appraisal, and information-seeking behavior proposed in uncertainty management theory. *Health Communication, 30,* 339–349. doi: 10.1080/10410236.2013.858285.

Rintamaki, L. S., & Brashers, D. E. (2010). Stigma and intergroup communication. In H. Giles, S. Reid, & J. Harwood (Eds.), *The dynamics of intergroup communication* (pp. 155–166). New York: Peter Lang.

Scambler, G. (1984). Perceiving and coping with stigmatizing illness. In R. Fitzpatrick, J. Hinton, S. Newman, G. Scambler, & J. Thompson (Eds.), *The experience of illness* (pp. 203–226). London: Tavistock Publications.

Snow, R., Crocker, J., Talbot, K., Moore, J., & Salisbury, H. (2016). Does hearing the patient perspective improve consultation skills in examinations? An exploratory randomized controlled trial in medical undergraduate education. *Medical Teacher, 38,* 1229–1235. doi: 10.1080/0142159X.2016.1210109.

Spencer, D. (2017). Narrative medicine. In M. Solomon, J. R. Simon, & H. Kincaid (Eds.), *The Routledge companion to philosophy of medicine* (pp. 372–382). New York: Routledge.

Thakore, H., & McMahon, T. (2006). Virtually there: e-learning in medical education. *Clinical Teacher, 3,* 225–228. doi: 10.1111/j.1743-498X.2006.00114x.

Walstrom, M. K. (2000). "You know, who's the thinnest?": Combating surveillance and creating safety in coping with eating disorders online. *CyberPsychology and Behavior, 3,* 761–783. doi: 10.1089/10949310050191755.

Yu, J., Taverner, N., & Madden, K. (2011). Young people's views on sharing health-related stories on the Internet. *Health and Social Care in the Community, 19,* 326–334. doi: 10.1111/j.1365-2524.2010.00987.x.

Ziebland, S. (2013). Narrative interviewing. In S. Ziebland, A. Coulter, J. D. Calabrese, & L. Locock (Eds.), *Understanding and using health experience. Improving patient care* (pp. 38–48). Oxford: Oxford University Press.

Chapter 2

From Stories to Discoveries

Patients' Narratives as Advocacy in Biomedical Research

Krista Hoffmann-Longtin and Adam Hayden

Biomedical researchers are trained to use positivistic approaches to develop efficacious treatments and pursue cures for illness and disease. Accordingly, they may rarely engage persons living with the disease in the development of research questions and protocols (Sacristán et al., 2015). Just as patient narratives can create therapeutic partnerships in delivery of treatment (DasGupta & Charon, 2004), they offer value to the research process to emphasize the person with the disease, rather than the disease, in isolation. In this chapter, we are interested in the role of patient stories as tools for influencing the biomedical research process (Greenhalgh, 2009; Panofsky, 2011). Applying Ellingson's (2009) approach to crystallization, we explore intersections in the literature on patient advocacy, our own narratives, and those from biomedical researchers and patients. We seek to uncover the value and implications of involving not only patients but also patients' *stories* (Hyden, 1997) in creating an agenda for research in healthcare.

ENGAGING WITH A PATIENT NARRATIVE: AN EXEMPLAR

Adam

Shuffling along, parallel to the buffet table, displaying gait instability and balancing a ceramic catering plate with my left hand, plagued by neuropathy and weakness, I steadied myself before hooking my cane over my left arm to grasp tongs in my functional right hand and serve myself salad. Feeling comfortable in my otherness, I shrugged when the diner before me offered

to assist with assembling my meal. Whether motivated by pity, aid, or effi-
ciency, she smiled with pursed lips and a sideways glance, lifted my plate
from the table, and proceeded down the line. Although "patients included"
is a recent and flashy biomedical conference trend, advances in biomedical
research inclusivity remain passive and permissive rather than active and
enabling.

The facilitator began the closing session by eliciting from the audience,
"the most innovative developments you heard about or saw during the conference." Augmented virtual reality microscopy was a crowd favorite. Participants continued, "gene editing!" another, "liquid biopsy!" Indeed, next
followed structured "share outs" from prescribed topics to advertise all that
we learned about genomics, biomarkers, and immunotherapies.

I wondered how this might be so: I was attending this conference by
selection for a special scholarship and concomitant designation indicative
of my role as a science-literate patient advocate. Though I knew only those
twenty-five or thirty others, I spoke with directly over the course of several
days, ostensibly the program that evening, mandatory for those attending on
scholarship, comprised a majority audience of others like me: other patients.
Yet not a word was spoken about the bedside. Not a topic for share out. Not
a single line was explicitly drawn between research innovation and patient
experience. A buffet table of scientific expertise and a burden placed on the
consumer to navigate, serving as a barrier to access.

Krista

I read Adam's narrative, and immediately felt the dialectical tension he
describes. Maybe the conference participants were more excited about the
scientific researchers? Can you fault them? They are researchers, after all. At
the same time, reading Adam's story puts me in the room. His point is made
more salient by his metaphor—the inaccessible buffet of food and research
findings. Adam was hungry for participation, just as the researchers were
hungry for new discoveries. Reading this story, for me, as a scholar of communication, reminds me of the power of the narrative—how (re)storying the
conversation of Adam's role at the biomedical research conference brought
to the fore the isolation that patients potentially feel when asked to participate
without an acknowledgment of their ways of knowing (Pearce, 1989).

With the two brief narratives above, we seek to illustrate our entry points
in this topic—as a person living with brain cancer and philosopher of science,
and a teacher and researcher of communication in academic medicine. In this
chapter, we seek to use a mix of our own narratives and literature review to
illumine lessons at the intersection of biomedical research and patient narratives which are, at best, left implicit, and at worst, neglected. Our method is

patterned after the theoretical framework we espouse: first, advance a patient narrative, and second, interrogate its role in biomedical research advocacy.

Biomedical researchers are usually trained to use positivistic approaches to develop efficacious treatments and pursue cures for illness and disease. Accordingly, they rarely engage persons living with the disease in the development of research questions and protocols (Caron-Flinterman, Broerse, & Bunders, 2007; Sacristán et al., 2015). Just as patient narratives can create therapeutic partnerships in delivery of treatment (DasGupta & Charon, 2004), they offer value to the research process to emphasize the person with the disease, rather than the disease, in isolation (Greenhalgh, 2009; Panofsky, 2011). Applying Ellingson's (2009) approach to qualitative crystallization, we explore intersections in the literature on patient narratives in advocacy, our own narratives, and those from biomedical researchers and patients. We seek to uncover the meaning of involving not only patients, but more specifically patients' stories. As Hyden (1997) argues, "Patients' narratives give voice to suffering in a way that lies outside the domain of the biomedical voice" (p. 49). We offer strategies to close this gap and identify a role for narrative in creating an agenda for research in healthcare.

The roadmap for this chapter is as follows. In the first section, we discuss the extant research on patient involvement and narrative in the context of biomedical research, and explain our methodological approach. Next, we investigate the topic of expertise by considering the interplay of experiences and credibility as each informs the roles ascribed to "patients" and "researchers." We extend the conversation about experiences to promote narrative as a tool to introduce a non-positivistic way of knowing that undermines the presupposed objectivity of science. We survey limitations of our piece. Finally, we offer concluding remarks. It is our aim to consider carefully the role of narrative, expertise, different ways of knowing in the pursuit of biomedical research, and ultimately health communication and healing.

PATIENT PARTICIPATION IN BIOMEDICAL RESEARCH

An investigation of the historical relationship between biomedical researchers and patients is helpful to better understand how patient narratives can inform the biomedical research process. Over the past forty years, there has been a shift in discourse from understanding patients as subjects (merely one of many tools required to conduct biomedical research) to important participants in (and even powerful drivers of) biomedical research. This shift can be attributed to both scientific and social influences (Caron-Flinterman et al., 2007; Solomon, 2016). As scientific problems have become more complex and connected to social forces (such as social determinants of health), scientists have sought to include more lived experiences of patients in the research process. Additionally, the public has increasingly demanded the applicability of scientific discovery to lay people's and patients' lives.

Scientists and scholars tend to use two primary arguments for including patients in the research process (beyond serving as subjects). The first argument is regarding improvement of the science itself. Since patients have a type of experiential knowledge, their expertise can serve as a foil to the professional and objective work of scientists, thus creating a more complete research outcome (Entwistle et al., 1998). Alternatively, Collins and Evans (2002) contend that partnerships with patients in the biomedical research process enhances the moral and political legitimacy of the research, since they are ultimately the beneficiaries of this information.

Though recognized in the clinic, "health care can be delivered more effectively and efficiently if patients are full partners in the process" (Holman & Lorig, 2000, p. 527), the movement to involve more patients in the biomedical research process in the United States is a relatively new phenomenon. In 2003, Zerhouni, a former director of the National Institutes of Health (NIH), argued for a shift in clinical research to include more patients, specifically via community-based physicians and organizations. While no mention of patient narrative is present, the author clearly advocates for privileging patient voices in the research process, mentioning "new models of cooperation between NIH and patient advocacy alliances" (p. 64). However, bridging the gap between patients and researchers is a hard-won process. Reporting for *Nature News* five years later, Butler (2008) questioned what the NIH had done to encourage the values they espoused. He explained,

> Over the past 30 or so years, the ecosystems of basic and clinical research have diverged. The pharmaceutical industry, which for many years was expected to carry discoveries across the divide, is now hard pushed to do so. The abyss left behind is sometimes labelled the "valley of death"—and neither basic researchers, busy with discoveries, nor physicians, busy with patients, are keen to venture there. (p. 841)

As illustrated by this report, simply giving a mandate for scientists, clinicians, and patients to communicate more effectively and creating "networks" (Zerouni, 2003) were not enough to bridge the gap between these communities. With this example, it is important to note that disciplinary boundaries often shape the way that scholars understand a phenomenon. In the case of Zerouni's (2003) mandate and Butler's (2008) critique, these perspectives are legitimized in the biomedical research community, in part because of their affiliation with the NIH and the journal *Nature*. Despite Butler's (2008) critique, some scholars contend that biomedical researchers and patients have seen some successful partnerships.

Caron-Flinterman and colleagues (2007) classified three categories of patient participation in biomedical research. They include (1) the lobbying of patient organizations, (2) ad hoc use of patients' ideas and demands through intermediaries, and (3) inclusion of patient representatives in existing decision-making groups (as described in Adam's story above). Although their study was conducted in the Netherlands, Caron-Flinterman et al. (2007) argue that their literature searches and participants give a "reasonable impression" of the landscape globally (p. 347). Wehling et al. (2015) also address issues of typology, arguing that, although classification holds value, the level of diversity in disciplines and approaches may limit social scientists' abilities to define the experiences of researchers' and patients' partnerships.

More recent work by Kaye and colleagues (2012) acknowledges that current biomedical research models fail to adequately include the perspectives of patients and research participants. The authors propose that new technology can facilitate participant-centered initiatives (PCIs), defined as "tools, programs and projects that empower participants to engage in the research process using IT" (p. 4). They further argue that using PCIs through technology, such as patients sharing of data in social media and apps, can encourage ongoing interactions between participants and researchers. As Kaye et al. explain, this approach "can result in research that demonstrates high standards of research integrity but also an involvement by patients and participants that is more active and richer than more conventional approaches" (p. 5).

Imbedded in the models described above is a dialogic space between patients and biomedical researchers, where, in some cases, patient narratives are shared directly to the researchers and, in other cases, are shared via an intermediary (i.e., a researcher or physician sharing a patient's story on behalf of the patient, or more recently, an app sharing data with a researcher in which the researcher constructs the story of a patient's illness via the data received). In any case, narrative is at the center of the interaction. It is the primary tool patients must engage with biomedical researchers. However, as illustrated by Wehling et al. (2015), patients, researchers, and physicians each approach their interactions with illness and the storying of illness quite differently. One specific area where these epistemological differences manifest is in the context of objectivity. Writes Murphy et al. (2016), "the reality of patients is never directly encountered by a clinician, or anyone else, but is revealed gradually through the stories they tell" (p. 103). Murphy and colleagues (2016) remind us, "accumulating information about a patient is thus a hermeneutic exercise" (p. 103).

The Problem with Objectivity

Biomedical researchers, even more so than physicians, are trained to privilege the perspective of objectivity. Randomized controlled trials are the so-called gold standard of biomedical research, where the goal is to eliminate bias and control for as many variables as possible. When it is impossible to control for a variable, researchers treat this as a limitation of their work, caveating and listing these at the end of their studies. Conversely, most physicians acknowledge that the practice of medicine is both a science and an art (Charon, 2006; Greenhalgh, 1999; Solomon, 2016). Although many clinicians work within the paradigm of evidence-based medicine, Solomon (2016) notes that this term, itself, is political and subjective in nature. At best, the term can give epidemiologic data about a disease, but fails to offer much solace to patients who do not fit into the standard narrative of a particular disease. Narrative researchers move even further away from the objective paradigm. As Chase (2003) explains, "[narrative] researchers develop meaning out of, and some sense of order in, the material they studied; they develop their own voice(s) as they construct others' voices and realities" (p. 657). The dialectic tension between objective and subjective are inherent in Japp and Japp's (2005) investigation of the narratives of biologically invisible diseases. As they explain, "the pervasive hegemony of the biomedical model of disease limits the stories patients tell as much as it does physician's practices" (p. 122).

It is expected that these tensions may introduce significant worries for biomedical researchers for whom empirical evidence is the purported norm by which science progresses, and it is only through these evidence-based methods that a proper objectivity toward a subject or domain of investigation is maintained. Though, the philosophy of science has long advanced the position that all observation is theory-laden (Hanson, 1958). More plainly, any observation or experimental design is selected with theory in mind. Theory selection itself is a social act. Philosophers of science Bertolaso and Sterpetti (2017) remind readers of the epistemic subjectivity of theory selection, favoring plausibility accounts replete with subjectivity rather than probabilistic accounts. When available evidence fails to adjudicate between rival theories, researchers employ so-called theoretical virtues to advance the preferred theory. Peter Lipton (2003) develops a robust account of theoretical virtues and their role in identifying scientific theories which are the most likely to be at least approximately true.

Thus, the lines distinguishing subjectivity from objectivity in research are blurred, and clinging to the notion of purely objective science is unhelpful, particularly for patients and clinicians who experience the messiness of disease daily. Patient narratives should not be rejected out of hand for fear of their socially constructed nature. To move beyond the question of legitimacy of patient narrative in the understanding of biomedical research, it is useful to delve into the notion and definition of expertise.

Who Is an Expert?

When considering the role of patients and patient narratives in biomedical research, expertise becomes a significant area of contention. In the traditional biomedical model of medicine (as embodied by most biomedical researchers), patient experience is often defined as "lay knowledge," implying that it is epistemologically inferior to the expertise of researchers (Wehling, Viehover, & Koenen, 2015). This perspective is situated in the larger grand narrative of the biomedical model (Epstein, 1995; Japp & Japp, 2005; Morris, 1998), where the primary actor is the researcher using science and technology to discover and cure the patient. In this context, patients are objects of study upon which science is acted, rather than participants or cocreators of the outcome.

We suggest this model is mistaken on two accounts. First, the transactional model of care seeks to cure, assuming an acute intervention, which is poorly suited for the management of chronic illness (Carel, 2008; Holman & Lorig, 2000). Second, viewing patients as end users, or more crudely, "consumers" and "customers," fails to notice that clinicians, for their part, are similarly caught up in the biomedical model, treating patients in the clinic or at the bedside as mere "providers" (Montori, 2017, p. 79ff.) This model leaves little space for inclusion of the patient narrative. Clinician narratives further punctuate the loss of autonomy experienced by both "providers" and "consumers" of health care.

When patients have engaged with biomedical researchers, the language of biomedicine is privileged. Epstein's (1995) participants in the AIDS treatment movement described this as learning a foreign language. His participants noted that, once they had access to the language of biomedicine, they could access and influence the institutions. In other words, "Once they could converse comfortably about viral assays and reverse transcription and cytokine regulation and epitope mapping, activists increasingly discovered that researchers felt compelled, by their own norms of discourse and behavior, to consider activist arguments on their merits" (Epstein, 1995, p. 419). As Wehling and colleagues (2015) explain, it is in this space where the definition of expertise becomes most murky. The authors state, "to what extent and in what circumstances is patients' knowledge complementary to and instrumental for scientific knowledge production, and how far is it opposed to it, contesting its background assumptions and conceptual approaches and transforming the latter?" (p. 5). Shapin (1990) notes that the constitution of the expert/lay divide is defined by the question of who possesses cultural competence; thus, asking researchers to posit what a space for productive exchange of experience and ideas between biomedical researchers and patients might look like.

As mentioned earlier, Japp and Japp's (2005) discussion of legitimacy of patients' experiences offer a grim description of the current space for conversation. Because patient narratives are told within the social and political context of the grand narrative of biomedicine, patients are simultaneously constrained and enabled when telling their stories. Technical rationality is privileged, leaving patients who do not fit into the traditional narrative often feeling lost and delegitimized. In this postmodern perspective, counternarratives emerge from patients who question the dichotomy between illness and cured, seeking a space of demedicalization of their experiences (Harter, Japp, & Beck, 2005). Pearce's work (1989) on coordinated management of meaning is potentially helpful here, to both biomedical researchers and patients, to explain how these tensions have been created. As the author contends, each communicative community holds its own set of resources and practices that are often not easily accessible to those outside the group. When this happens, conflict emerges and conversation can often devolve. As Pearce (1989) explains,

> In speaking to those who logics of meaning and action are similar to their own, persons use a sophisticated vocabulary, acknowledge the dignity and honor of those who disagree with them, and usually are able to put together well-coordinated episodes. However, when speaking to someone from another group, the form of discourse attenuates quickly. A simplified vocabulary is used; the personalities and motives of the other are posed in a desiccated vocabulary of human purposes; taunts and condemnations replace argument and evidence; and one's own reasoning and life experiences are protected from exposure and anticipated criticism. (pp. 43–44)

Because one communicative community's (biomedical researchers) resources and practices have been traditionally privileged, it is no surprise that the narratives of another community (patients) have been generally seen as unhelpful. Conversational actors constantly co-construct the meaning of communication as they communicate, and as such, particular roles have been reified. For biomedical researchers, it is the role of expert, as defined above. In the case of patients, the sick role has emerged as another dominant narrative.

NARRATIVE ENGAGEMENT CONTINUED

Following the July 2017 brain cancer diagnosis of American high-profile political figure Senator John McCain, public awareness spread concerning the aggressive and deadly cancer, glioblastoma, usually abbreviated as its medical moniker "GBM." This devastating disease corners patients with no available curative treatment, left to confront a limited life expectancy and generally poor quality of life. Living with GBM requires patients to endure side effects from cytotoxic cancer therapeutics and neurological disorders stemming from tumor invasion and neurosurgical removal of the primary brain tumor—the first step in the standard of care protocol.

Adam

I received a GBM diagnosis in June 2016, one year prior to Mr. McCain's. For this reason, beyond the sympathetic reaction shared by many, I paid close attention to media coverage surrounding the health communication tactics and information dissemination of this rare and difficult to understand disease. That month was especially hot. My family vacationed with close friends near a lake in Southern Indiana, a day's trip from our home. Seeking refuge from the heat and taking active steps to manage my seizures, I chose not to join in a planned trip to a nearby amusement park. I spent much of the morning comfortably in a rocking chair set on the shaded porch of our rented cabin, reading. I decided to retreat inside to lie down when I heard the familiar tone of a smartphone notification. News broke of Mr. McCain's diagnosis. Several friends and acquaintances reached out to notify me.

Carel (2008), a philosophy scholar living with a chronic illness, provides an extensive phenomenological account of the illness. The author contrasts the philosophical treatment of the illness experience as a foil to the "natural-istic" model of illness and disease paradigmatic of the biomedical research community. Carel (2008) situates illness in a social context, describing illness as problematic in at least two ways. First, illness punctuates the ill person's inability to control how others view them, and second, all social interactions are placed in the shadow cast by illness. On Carel's view, it is not surprising that associations between McCain's diagnosis and my illness immediately presented themselves to others, prompting outreach. As I wrote in an open letter to McCain (Hayden, 2017), there is little McCain and I share in social position or common interest, yet each is now connected by a specific disease. That connection in isolation is connection enough to reshape my social posi-tion as a peer of McCain's, a position unlikely to emerge without the social implications of becoming ill. Indeed, Carel evokes Parsons's (1951) account of this feature of illness: the sick role.

In a sociological rather than philosophical context, Parsons (1951) empha-sized features of disease (later echoed by Carel (2008). Parsons contrasts biological processes of illness from sociological considerations. His novel construction of illness described the "sick role" as a "deviant role," that is, failing in some way to fulfill the institutionally defined expectations of one or more of the roles in which the individual is implicated in the society" (p. 452). In my letter to McCain, I contrast his age, storied persona as Vietnam prisoner of war, and notable history serving in the American Senate, with my youth, young fatherhood, and nonpolitical background. McCain and I are deviant in our illness; we share a sick role, in so far as we are each rendered weak and vulnerable by disease, failing our implicated societal roles. McCain fails his implicated role as battle-tested, strong, and courageous political leader. I fail my implicated role, as a young person, nearly fifty years McCain's junior, expressing the vitality as a father with very young children.

Krista

I remember reading Adam's letter to Senator McCain when it came out. As a publication venue, *STAT* is a "big get" for those of us in the communicating science and health world. I was proud to say I knew him. How sad is that? That I was proud to have a friend doing such amazing and high-profile work, because of a terrible diagnosis. In reading this again, I can see how I fall into these patterns. Communicatively, I work hard to identify Adam as a scholar and philosopher first, a "sick person" second. I often wonder if this matters discursively. Since we travel in many of the same circles, I worry (maybe I shouldn't?) about Adam being known as "the guy with the brain tumor," essentializing his identity into his diagnosis. Largely speaking, this is always a concern of mine for anyone living outside the dominant narrative. How do we honor these stories without constantly othering? And how, as an educator of current and future biomedical researchers, do I teach people how to do (or not do) this?

Parsons (1951) and Carel (2008) each distinguish two paradigms of illness: one, naturalistic (positivistic, reductionist, or biological), and the other, sociological or phenomenological. Features of the illness experience fail to be captured by a purely empiricist account of disease. The issue, then, expressed recently by Wehling and colleagues (2015) is to define how best to relate patient knowledge—the "sick role," or phenomenological—to scientific knowledge—positivistic. In violating these sick roles, both McCain and Hayden create a counter-story to the master narrative of the biomedical construction of illness, identifying them as whole people who, alongside their identity within the GBM community, still assert their identities as fathers and professionals (Japp & Japp, 2005). This introduction of additional lenses moves the reader to see the storyteller as more than just a "sick person."

With these perspectives in mind, we offer narrative as a strategic tool to move biomedical researchers away from the biomedical construction of illness, viewing patient narratives as both a tool to inform research and an epistemological lens to understand the diseases they study in a new way. If we understand illness as codified through discourse, even in the context of biomedical research, introducing the illness experience into the research community could change the research questions.

REIMAGINING THE ROLE OF
NARRATIVE AND STORYTELLING

Scholars of health communication, sociology, medicine, public health, and other disciplines have considered the role of patient narratives as a tool for conducting or informing research. Some (such as Borkan, Quirk, & Sullivan, 1991) use the gathering of patient narratives as a research methodology or narrative inquiry (Chase, 2003) to consider the relationship between patient perceptions and health outcomes. Psychiatrist and narrative theorist Adler (2012) notes a critical role for narrative as tool for patient agency, or in Adler's words, "autonomy, achievement, mastery, and ability to influence the course of his or her life" (p. 368). As this volume and other researchers (Charon, 2006; Epstein, 1993; Harter, Japp, & Beck, 2005; Wehling et al., 2015) extol, narrative is a critical tool in redefining the roles of patients and those who treat them.

However, many of these scholars acknowledge that narratives do not exist only in the context of the interpersonal relationship between the storyteller and the listener (physician, biomedical researcher, or otherwise). For example, Japp, Harter, and Beck (2005) examine the role of narrative in constructing and co-constructing the ontological meaning of health and disease. As they explain,

> Personal narratives become the building blocks of public knowledge. More and more, mediated and public dialogue, from legislative testimony to newscasts to public health promotion, rely on individual stories to embody problems, shape arguments, and engage emotions, as well as to persuade, evaluate, reward, and punish. (p. 3)

This quotation and the work of others (Epstein, 1995; Japp & Japp, 2005) illustrate the extent to which patient narratives are not only an object for researchers to analyze. Rather, the narratives, themselves, shape and are shaped by the research context in which they are collected and told.

The role of narrative in biomedical research and patient care is subject to critique. Some scholars contend that narratives in medical research can be "susceptible to the narrative fallacy (i.e., causal hypotheses are too readily constructed from sequences of events) and to the influence of constraining politically dominant narratives" (Segal, 2007, p. 290). Harter and colleagues (2005) echo this concern, reminding their readers that "narratives are shaped within certain beliefs and value systems, and serve to reinforce or challenge those systems as they are constituted in social interaction" (p. 23). Thus, examining the context, as well as the narrative, is an important part of understanding its potential for influence. A further, related, concern notes that narratives are constructed with an audience in mind, and the audience, or listener, is active in meaning-making as co-creators (Pearce, 1989; Spencer, 2016). Given the importance of narrative context, here, we reconsider the role of objectivity and subjectivity in the narrative relationship between biomedical researchers and patients.

In the mid-1990s, Epstein, a sociologist with a focus on science and technology, closely examined the role of AIDS activists in driving the agenda for biomedical research, specifically the testing of new pharmaceutical treatments. Epstein's (1995) work illustrates the complicated role of narrative in the relationship between biomedical researchers and patients. The author posits that, although AIDS activists could use their lived experience to influence the research process, they could not fully reject the biomedical model of their disease because of their need to know which treatments were most efficacious. Citing Richards's (1991) argument for more relativism in the biomedical research process, Epstein explains, "the activist critique of the randomized clinical trial unseats that methodology from the pinnacle on which it is sometimes placed, but it also assumes a greater role for such trials than analysts such as Richards would recommend" (p. 425). While Epstein considers this a departure between the views of researchers and patients, we see this as a potential place of common ground.

As much as objectivity has a place in the lab and the testing of hypotheses, subjectivity is inherent to biomedical researcher's decisions to choose what to study. Most researchers enter into a field of study because they are excited about the possibility of curing a disease or helping patients. This is an emotional or subjective act. Many research societies invite patients (like Adam) to their meetings to tell the stories of their experiences. More than ever, researchers are asked to pursue funding from private foundations often started by family members or those with complex diseases themselves. Thus, patients' stories are already present in the minds of researchers when they pursue a research question.

Patient narratives can be a tool to help biomedical researchers see beyond the "reductionist lens" of randomized clinical trials (Caron-Flinterman et al., 2007). The role of narrative in the biomedical research process does not have to be an either-or assumption. After all, the messiness of the narrative can potentially inform the way in which we approach researching illnesses, which are (almost by definition) also messy in their constitution. Cancer doesn't appear with the same symptoms for every patient; different cancers behave differently, and we still don't know why; the way in which cancer affects patients' lives is unique for each person and each family member.

Most patients would not advocate for biomedical researchers to fully dispose of the scientific methodology they use to test treatments (Epstein, 1995). Rather, they would prefer to see treatments tested within the context of real life. We envision a space where biomedical researchers invite the patient experience more fully into their thinking about scientific questions. Dahlstrom's (2014) work on the use of narrative in science communication with lay audiences offers a paradigm that, when combined with Pearce and Cronen's (1980) coordinated management of meaning, could create the dialogic space we seek to create between researchers and patients.

Taking a social scientific approach, Dahlstrom (2014) argues that narrative could be a particularly useful tool in explaining complex scientific concepts to lay audiences. The author combines extant research about narrative, science communication, and media to illustrate that narrative content about scientific topics is more likely to be remembered and shared by consumers. Dahlstrom (2014) concludes his exploration with a call for research on communicating scientific concepts that are "beyond the human scale" (p. 13618); phenomena which are beyond our perceivable reality, for example, things "as large as climate change, as small as parts per billion, or as distant as 10,000 y away" (p. 13618). However, for biomedical researchers, the lived experience of disease is, potentially, beyond their scale. If they have not lived with the illness themselves, it is a struggle for researchers to fully know or understand the experiences of patients living with the diseases they hope to cure. Empathy and inquiry are invited through story. Pearce and Cronen (1980) advance the concept of narrative between groups, arguing that, if we are coordinating meeting with one another, we must seek to understand the stories that constitute our experiences. As Pearce (1989) explains, we must first recognize our communication as fundamentally part of our own group, if we are to understand the experiences of others. Then, we must strive for a form of communication that values the other: a form called "cosmopolitan communication." The author states that "tolerance for difference liberates cosmopolitan communicators to care about and take steps to find out about worldviews other than their own" (p. 193). Combining these two perspectives, we envision a dialogic community where both biomedical researchers and patients open themselves to the resources and practices of their speech communities. Narrative is a tool that can help biomedical researchers adjust the scale of illness, seeing patients as part of the process required for knowing a disease, in all its forms.

CONCLUSION

In this chapter, we sought to identify a gap in biomedical research: namely, the absence of the patient voice, vis-à-vis patients' narratives, or their stories.

In doing so, we argue that closing this gap offers a fruitful tactic to improve biomedical research by placing the researcher and the research product in dialogue with the consumer, in this case, a patient. Incorporating patients' narratives into the research process introduces an uncomfortable dialectical tension between the purported objectivity of scientific methodology, on the one hand, and the subjective, interpretive work of telling and hearing stories, on the other. We hope to diffuse this tension by pointing to the ineliminable epistemic subjectivity of scientific experimental design and observation. In other words, researchers need not fear the specter of subjectivity; they need only to understand it.

Ultimately, this chapter offers an extended dialogue in support of the central thesis that inquiry is best practiced with a pluralistic attitude toward expertise; call this lay or experiential knowledge, as some authors have, or phenomenological or sociological, as expressed by others. Independent of which term of art is preferred, eliciting patients' narratives, specifically in the context of biomedical research, is an effective means of considering different ways of knowing.

Raising the patient voice in a new setting is not without controversy. The deviancy of patient narratives is punctuated by Carel (2008) and Parsons's (1951) emphasis on the sick role. One limitation of this piece is its tacit promotion of such deviancy. The argument in this chapter, if accepted, is a critique of the dominant paradigm in biomedical research, communicated best through a meta-narrative framed by positivistic assumptions.

Wehling and colleagues (2015) raise a concern articulated by Blume (2010), which is germane: patients only gain credibility insofar as their demands are compatible with fundamental assumptions of medical science. A similar concern is raised by medical students as it relates to the incorporation of humanities in medical education. These discussions are inextricably linked. Without compatibility with dominant background assumptions, narratives may appear uninformed, if not hostile. Shapiro and colleagues (2009) report a complaint raised by a medical student, critiquing a required humanities course in his medical school curriculum. As Shapiro et al. (2009) relate, "this young man and students like him feel a sense of grievance: it's unfair to be evaluated in an area they hadn't expected to be part of their curriculum" (p. 193). The students' reaction to humanities content mirrors that of biomedical researchers. In both contexts, the primary focus of the dominant narrative is the science, rather than the human.

Whether addressing students, clinicians, or researchers, confronting an accepted paradigm is often met with a hostile and defensive posture, creating the us-them mentality described in Pearce's (1989) work. In support of our deviance from the dominant paradigm and support of a new dialogic space for biomedical researchers and patients, we repeat a lesson explicated by Murphy and colleagues (2016), "patients always present an illness ... this process is not disinterested but includes perspectives, values, and commitments. A presentation is always motivated and expresses an angle or disposition. Nothing can remove symptoms from these entanglements, even the most sophisticated laboratory tests" (p. 104). As illustrated by these examples, biomedical research benefits from incorporating diverse angles or dispositions, learned through attention to patients' narratives.

REFERENCES

Adler, J. M. (2012). Living into the story: Agency and coherence in a longitudinal study of narrative identity development and mental health over the course of psychotherapy. *Journal of Personality and Social Psychology, 102*(2), 367–389.

Bertolaso, M., & Sterpetti, F. (2017). Evidence amalgamation, plausibility, and cancer research. *Synthese*, 1–39. doi: 10.1007/s11229-017-1591-9.

Blume, S. (2010). *The artificial ear: Cochlear implants and the culture of deafness.* New Brunswick, NJ: Rutgers University Press.

Borkan, J. M., Quirk, M., & Sullivan, M. (1991). Finding meaning after the fall: Injury narratives from elderly hip fracture patients. *Social Science & Medicine, 33*(8), 947–957.

Butler, D. (2008). Translational research: Crossing the valley of death. *Nature News, 453*(7197), 840–842. doi: 10.1038/453840a.

Carel, H. (2008). *Illness: The cry of the flesh.* Buckinghamshire, UK: Acumen.

Caron-Flinterman, J. F., Broerse, J. E., & Bunders, J. F. (2007). Patient partnership in decision-making on biomedical research: Changing the network. *Science, Technology, & Human Values, 32*(3), 339–368.

Charon, R. (2006). *Narrative medicine: Honoring the stories of illness.* New York, NY: Oxford University Press.

Chase, S. E. (2003). Narrative inquiry: Multiple lenses, approaches, voices. In J. A. Holstein & J. F. Gubrium (Eds.), *Inside interviewing: New lenses, new concerns* (pp. 651–679). Thousand Oaks, CA: Sage.

Collins, H. M., & Evans, R. (2002). The third wave of science studies: Studies of expertise and experience. *Social Studies of Science, 32*(2), 235–296.

Dahlstrom, M. F. (2014). Using narratives and storytelling to communicate science with nonexpert audiences. *Proceedings of the National Academy of Sciences, 111*(Supplement 4), 13614–13620.

DasGupta, S., & Charon, R. (2004). Personal illness narratives: Using reflective writing to teach empathy. *Academic Medicine, 79*(4), 351–356.

Ellingson, L. L. (2009). *Engaging crystallization in qualitative research: An introduction.* Thousand Oaks, CA: Sage.

Entwistle, V. A., Renfrew, M. J., Yearley, S., Forrester, J., & Lamon, T. (1998). Lay perspectives: Advantages for health research. *British Medical Journal, 316*(7129), 463–466.

Epstein, S. (1995). The construction of lay expertise: AIDS activism and the forging of credibility in the reform of clinical trials. *Science, Technology, & Human Values, 20*(4), 408–437.

Greenhalgh, T. (1999). Narrative based medicine in an evidence based world. *British Medical Journal, 318*, 323–325.

Greenhalgh, T. (2009). Chronic illness: Beyond the expert patient. *BMJ: British Medical Journal, 338*(7695), 629–631.

Harter, L. M., Japp, P. M., & Beck, C. S. (2005). Vital problematics of narrative theorizing. In L. M. Harter, P. M. Japp, & C. S. Beck (Eds.), *Narratives, health, and healing: Communication theory, research, and practice* (pp. 7–29). Mahwah, NJ: Lawrence Erlbaum Associates.

Hanson, N. R. (1958). *Patterns of discovery: An inquiry into the conceptual foundations of science.* Cambridge, UK: University of Cambridge Press.

Hayden, A. (July 26, 2017). Dear Sen. McCain: Here's what I've learned from living with glioblastoma. *STAT.* Retrieved from: https://www.statnews.com/2017/07/26/john-mccain-glioblastoma-advice/.

Holman, H., & Lorig, K. (2000). Patients as partners in managing chronic disease: Partnership is a prerequisite for effective and efficient health care. *BMJ: British Medical Journal, 320*(7234), 526.

Hyden, L. C. (1997). Illness and narrative. *Sociology of Health & Illness, 19*(1), 48–69.

Japp, P. M., & Japp, D. K. (2005). Desperately seeking legitimacy: Narratives of a biomedically invisible disease. In L. M. Harter, P. M. Japp, & C. S. Beck (Eds.), *Narratives, health, and healing: Communication theory, research, and practice* (pp. 107–130). Mahwah, NJ: Lawrence Erlbaum Associates.

Japp, P. M., Harter, L. M., & Beck, C. S. (2005). Overview of narrative and health communication theorizing. In L. M. Harter, P. M. Japp, & C. S. Beck (Eds.), *Narratives, health, and healing: Communication theory, research, and practice* (pp. 1–6). Mahwah, NJ: Lawrence Erlbaum Associates.

Kaye, J., Curren, L., Anderson, N., Edwards, K., Fullerton, S. M., Kanellopoulou, N., ... & Taylor, P. L. (2012). From patients to partners: Participant-centric initiatives in biomedical research. *Nature Reviews Genetics, 13*(5), 371.

Lipton, P. (2003). *Inference to the best explanation,* 2nd ed. New York, NY: Routledge.

Montori, V. (2017). *Why we revolt.* Rochester, MN: The Patient Revolution.

Morris, D. B. (1998). *Illness and culture in the postmodern age.* Berkeley, CA: University of California Press.

Murphy, J., Choi, J. M., & Cadeiras, M. (2016). The role of clinical records in narrative medicine: A discourse of message. *The Permanente Journal, 20*(2), 103–108.

Nordin, I. (2000). Expert and non-expert knowledge in medical practice. *Medicine, Health Careand Philosophy, 3*(3), 297–304.

Panofsky, A. (2011). Generating sociability to drive science: Patient advocacy organizations and genetics research. *Social Studies of Science, 41*(1), 31–57. doi: 10.1177/0306312710385852.

Parsons, T. (1951). Illness and the role of the physician: A sociological perspective. *American Journal of Orthopsychiatry, 21*(3), 452–460.

Pearce, W. B. (1989). *Communication and the human condition*. Carbondale, IL: Southern Illinois University Press.

Pearce, W. B., & Cronen, V. (1980). Communication, action, and meaning: The creation of social realities. New York, NY: Praeger.

Richards, E. (1991). *Vitamin C and cancer: Medicine or politics?* New York, NY: St. Martin.

Sacristán, J. A., Aguarón, A., Avendaño-Solá, C., Garrido, P., Carrión, J., Gutiérrez, A., ... & Flores, A. (2016). Patient involvement in clinical research: Why, when, and how. *Patient Preference and Adherence, 10*, 631–640.

Segal, J. (2007). Breast cancer narratives as public rhetoric: Genre itself and the maintenance of ignorance. *Linguistics and the Human Sciences, 3*, 3–23.

Shapin, S. (1990). Science and the public. In R. C. Olby, G. N. Cantor, J. R. R. Christie, & M. J. S. Hodge (Eds.), *Companion to the history of modern science* (pp. 990–1007). London, UK: Routledge.

Shapiro, J., Coulehan, J., Wear, D., et al. (2009). Medical humanities and their discontents: Definitions, critiques, and their implications. *Academic Medicine, 84*(2), 192–198.

Solomon, M. (2016). On ways of knowing in medicine. *Canadian Medical Association Journal, 188*(4), 289–290. doi: 10.1503/cmaj.150673.

Spencer, D. (2016). Narrative medicine. In M. Solomon, J. Simon, & H. Kincaid (Eds.), *The Routledge companion to philosophy of medicine* (pp. 372–382). New York, NY: Routledge.

Wehling, P., Viehover, W., & Koenen, S. (2015). Patient associations, health social movements, and the public shaping of biomedical research: An introduction. In P. Wehling, W. Viehover, & S. Koenen (Eds.), *The public shaping of medical research: Patient associations, health movements, and biomedicine* (pp. 1–15). New York, NY: Routledge.

Zerhouni, E. (2003). The NIH roadmap. *Science, 302*(5642), 63–72. doi: 10.1126/science.1091867.

Chapter 3

Cultural Communication Competency as a Two-Way Street

My Journey from Medical Avoidance to Patient Self-Advocacy

Mark P. Orbe

This chapter offers an autoethnographic account of my lived experiences as a patient. Utilizing a layered account approach (Ronai, 1995) that explores communication along the interpersonal←→intercultural continuum (Boylorn & Orbe, 2014), I present narratives from across my lifespan that demonstrate how my patient experiences have been informed by race, class, age, and gender. These patient experiences include limited health-care interactions as a youth recipient of government assisted health care, reluctant doctor-patient visits as an adult with "good insurance," and instances of racial discrimination at the hands of various health-care professionals (Chapman, Kaatz, & Carnes, 2013). A significant portion of the chapter focuses on how my work creating and facilitating cultural communication competency professional development workshops over the past more than ten years has transformed how I perceive, enact, and evaluate my interactions with doctors and other health-care practitioners.

***

I have always been a pretty healthy guy. Other than the day after I was born, I have never spent a night in the hospital. I have never had any broken bones. No major illnesses. Other than seeing an eye doctor for glasses, I don't have a single memory of seeing a doctor for any health issue as a child. I also don't have any memories of visiting a dentist before I was in my late teens and needed a root canal (not the best way to get an introduction to dentistry). My family received various forms of government assistance while I was growing up, and although some health benefits were also available through my father's employer, I don't recall ever having a family doctor. We would make do with over-the-counter medicine and different home remedies. In the most extreme cases, family members would visit the emergency room. Preventive medicine was unheard of, something of a luxury that was not a consideration given our financial situation.

The first time that my spouse told me that she made a doctor's appointment for our first child, I immediately asked what was wrong. Her quick response was, "Nothing, it's a well-care visit." Despite her very logical explanation, I remained critical and suspicious. Going to see a doctor when nothing was wrong seemed exactly like the type of "medical scam" that my father believed was part of doctors' attempts to make more and more money—something that resulted in a clear distrust of doctors and the medical community as a whole.

***

Medical doctors and other health-care practitioners in the United States serve an increasingly diverse patient population, one whose racial and ethnic diversity will see people of color becoming a majority in the next couple of decades (Rust et al., 2006). Within this context, national studies (e.g., Institute of Medicine, 2002) have revealed that in addition to issues of access, health-care disparities are associated with lack of knowledge of diverse cultures and the inability of health-care professionals to recognize how their own biases, prejudices, and stereotypical beliefs can negatively impact their ability to serve others. This acknowledgment has prompted a surge in initiatives and the recognition that being able to communicate with patients, families, communities, and fellow professionals in a culturally competent manner is crucial in reducing health disparities and promoting enhanced health and wellness (Gebbie, Rosenstock, & Hernandez, 2003; Goode, Dunne, & Bronheim, 2006). According to a joint expert panel convened by the Association of American Medical Colleges and the Association of Schools of Public Health in 2012, "an evolving multiracial, multicultural, and multilingual society makes strengthening the cultural competence of the health workforce even more imperative" (Expert Panel, 2012, p. 3).

My initial foray into the work of cultural communication competency was not predetermined or planned, it occurred after I was referred to a top administrator at a large Midwestern U.S. college of medicine. She was looking for someone who could come in and teach a culture and communication class specifically for first and second year medical students. Consequently, in 2005–2006, I was hired as a Visiting Professor to teach a course on "Physician-Patient Communication in a Multicultural Society." Based on the overwhelming success of the seminar, I was then asked to create a twenty-hour professional development certificate in cultural competency to be delivered each year to first- and second-year medical students. Beginning in 2006 and continuing to the present, I have facilitated workshops with over a thousand medical students at five different campuses. In addition, I have had the opportunity to deliver keynote speeches and present workshops on cultural competency to health-care practitioners at state, regional, and national conferences.

***

In the late 1980s, I gained my first "big boy job" as a student affairs college administrator. One of the perks of this employment was benefits, such as good health insurance. Given the family lessons learned about doctors, however, I never used my health benefits. I didn't obtain a primary physician, schedule any "well visits," or take advantage of chiropractic visits like many of my colleagues. The one exception was an instance when I sprained my ankle while playing a pick-up basketball game. I found a local health center that could schedule me in, and went to get it looked at. As the doctor was contemplating the various possibilities for a quick healing for my ankle, he asked me what type of insurance I had. Without hesitation, and much thought, I answered with the first thing that came to mind: Medicaid. The doctor quickly looked at me with a quizzical look, and responded: "You don't have Medicaid, that's for poor people." After a quick glance at my chart, he informed me, "You have Blue Cross/Blue Shields. That's much better."

***

Being in the delivery room while my spouse gave birth to our first child was life changing. No exaggeration. It transformed the ways in which I saw my spouse, my child, and my own positionality in a world filled with life←→death, purpose, love, and responsibility. Our first child (aka "my dissertation baby") was born during the third year of my doctoral program. Despite the advice of colleagues who suggested that we drive over an hour to a "big city hospital," we opted for the convenience and proximity of the local (rural, overwhelmingly white) hospital. The birth went off without a hitch— so says the spouse not actually giving birth. Our only "rookie mistake" was going to the hospital as soon as my spouse's water broke. We ended up waiting in the hospital for more than twenty hours before our baby was born.

Approximately twenty months later we found ourselves in the hospital to deliver our second child. This time we were in an adjacent Midwestern state where we could choose between several different local, yet more cosmopolitan, hospitals. We ended up choosing an award-winning hospital with high national rankings on several key attributes. Our second beautiful baby girl was born less than an hour after arriving to the hospital and with no health complications. The issues began shortly thereafter. Our children are multi-racial with maternal grandparents who are of African, European, and Native descent, and paternal grandparents who are of Asian and European descent. Accordingly, we insisted that their birth certificates reflect this reality, something evidently to which that hospital staff was not accustomed. After speaking with several individuals—nurses, doctors, and administrators—who provided their own "logic" about how our daughter's race should be recorded officially, the issue was finally settled when I vowed to write a letter explaining our preference.

At this point, my mother-in-law had arrived in town and she brought our oldest daughter with her to accompany us home. With no specific reasoning, our check-out time continued to be extended until we had been waiting for over an hour. I went to inquire about what was going on, and shortly after, a middle-aged white nurse came in to begin discharge procedures. Immediately, I sensed that something was "off." The woman was curt, conde-scending, disrespectful, and rude. My spouse has always served as a "racial perception check" for me; I consult her—usually nonverbally—to determine if I am overreacting to different public interactions where race seems to fac-tor in to how we are being treated. In this particular instance, I looked at her and she immediately shook her head affirmatively. I then expressed my con-cerns to the nurse directly: "Please do not interact with my spouse and I in a disrespectful manner. It is not acceptable." The nurse's immediate response was to become more disrespectful, so much so that I requested that she leave our room and be replaced by someone else. A hospital administrator quickly came to our room to address our concerns. Shortly thereafter, another nurse completed the check-out procedure and we were free to head home, but not before we were visited by another upper-level hospital administrator and a patient advocate who wanted to get our perceptions of the situation. I shared with them that I get it. Nurses, like others in this stressful line of work, are overworked. Maybe she was having a bad day, I offered. However, in the end, I couldn't shake the fact that her condescending, disrespectful attitude was informed by the racial dynamics of this small, southern town. In the end, I wrote two letters—one regarding the multiracial birth certificate designation, and one complaining about the nurse's interactions with us—both of which were several pages long.

***

According to Tervalon and Murray-Garcia (1998), traditional approaches to cultural competency have embraced a "detached mastery ... of a finite body of knowledge" (p. 117), something that has focused on engaging others, but not oneself. Given this, Tervalon and Murray-Garcia advocate for promoting cultural humility in place of cultural competency. Cultural humility is defined through four elements: (1) A lifelong commitment to self-reflection and self-critique, (2) A constant awareness of, and search, for that which we do not know; (3) A recognition of societal power imbalances, and (4) A commitment to developing institutional accountability regarding diversity, inclusion, and equity. While cultural competency can develop a false case of security for health-care practitioners, cultural humility advocates for lifelong learners who focus equally on what they do, and do not, know during their interactions with others.

A few communication scholars, especially those working with health-related issues, have adopted cultural humility in their scholarly work. In a recent dialogue about key concepts in intercultural communication, John Oetzel made the distinction between cultural competence and cultural humility:

> Cultural competence is akin to an ideal state, something to which we should constantly strive. It is not conceptualized as something that a person has, or does not have; instead it is something that is in constant development and achieved through learning, practice, and reflection. (Quoted in Alexander et al., 2014).

He went on to describe how he was first introduced to the concept and how he especially appreciated "its focus on self-reflection, growth, and desire to learn and critique oneself" (p. 14). Oetzel's describes cultural humility as "part attitude and part ability ... It is the desire to approach an (inter)cultural encounter with respect toward the other and their worldview, and the chance to learn about her/him and yourself" (p. 15). Like Oetzel, I have always conceptualized cultural humility as an integral part of cultural competency, not something that represents an oppositional stance as described by Tervalon and Murray-Garcia (1998). This approach is consistent with an understanding that cultural competency, as currently defined, is more of a dynamic ongoing process rather than an accomplishment or event. As such, the focus for health-care professionals has to be on "*becoming* culturally competent rather than *being* culturally competent" (Campinha-Bacote, 2003, italics in original, p. 14).

***

I teach, and learn, best through stories. They can serve as a bridge between complex ideas and real-life applications. In many instances, I draw from my own personal life narrative to retell stories that drive key points home for students (and participants in my professional development workshops). As such, my personhood/patienthood is woven through the cultural competency curriculum that I deliver disallowing any chance for "detached mastery." Much of the passion that I bring to these educational settings is grounded in the health realities informed by race, class, and gender. I strive to centralize cultural humility within cultural competency work, so that health-care practitioners see the inherent value of learning about self as much as learning about the Other. The process of *becoming* competent in this context has simultaneously meant humbling myself through a reflection of my own (in) competency as a patient.

***

When I first started facilitating cultural competency workshops with medical students, I didn't have a primary physician. In fact, I hadn't been to a doctor in over ten years. My philosophy has always been to practice a healthy lifestyle so that you didn't need to see a doctor. Since I was relatively healthy, there was no need to see a doctor. Shortly after our third child was born, approximately four years after his oldest sister, my spouse and I made the decision that I should get what became referred to as my "nip and tuck"—an effective form of birth control for men. I consulted with a doctor and successfully completed the out-patient procedure. I then returned to my normal health "regimen" for close to a decade. In other words, I focused on healthy behaviors and didn't see a doctor.

This mindset was interrupted one day when I experienced my first health crisis. I was sitting on the couch one evening, mindlessly watching television, when I shifted my sitting position and felt a small pain in my groin area. After investigating, I located a hard mass the size of a pea in my left testicle. Sensitive to touch, I continued to play around with this newfound discovery over the next few days and found that any pain or irritation occur only sporadically. Some days I wouldn't notice it at all, but others the dull pain would exist for a while. This prompted a heightened need for understanding, so I turned to the Internet with a hope for self-diagnosis and suggestions for healing. Initially, I believed that the mass could be a build-up of fluid caused by my previous "nip and tuck." Unfortunately, I couldn't find any evidence to support that explanation. Thus, my personal research left me with only one regrettable conclusion: testicular cancer.

After mulling on this self-diagnosis for a while, I called a local medical center and scheduled an appointment with the doctor who had the earliest available appointment. My mind was fixated on the worse-case scenario possible and I began to imagine an ugly battle with cancer, eventual death, and all the negative implications for my family that came with that. When the appointment finally arrived, I was on edge and found myself sitting in my underwear on the examination table waiting for the doctor to confirm my self-diagnosed death sentence. All the vitals, and other health measures, taken by the nurse practitioner reflected a healthy body. But medical uncertainty remained as I waited for some time for the doctor to see me. Again, my mind ran wildly with all sorts of worst-case scenarios. Then the doctor walked in. Shortly after introducing himself, my older white male doctor who I had never met before, started to ask me questions: How long since I had noticed the mass? Where was it located? Had it changed in shape, size, and so on? Was it painful? If so, how badly? I struggled to answer his questions in a way that seemed knowledgeable, articulate, and self-aware. As I rambled through my responses to his questions, and he began to examine me, I thought that I should share my theory that the mass might be a result of my out-patient surgery. Not wanting to sound ignorant, I made the decision not to call it my "nip and tuck."

Me: Doctor, I did wonder if this might be the result of a hysterectomy that I had when I was in my early 30s...
Doctor: [With a puzzled look] You did not have a hysterectomy.
Me: [Rambling with quick speech] No, I actually did. I know it doesn't seem true because I'm so young, but my wife and I had three children really quickly and we didn't want any more children and my procedure would be so much easier than my wife having her tubes tied ... so we decided that it was what was best for our family—
Doctor: You did not have a hysterectomy. You had a vasectomy. Only women have a hysterectomy. You had a vasectomy.
Me: [In my own head] Damnnit, man! I should have just called it a "nip and tuck!" He must think that I am an idiot ... How quickly can I get out of here???]

After a brief examination, the doctor confidently concluded that the mass was not cancerous, and recommended a second opinion from a specialist, who confirmed his diagnosis.

***

For years, I reluctantly visited doctors only when it was necessary. Part of this was due to my own ignorance about health issues, and an inability to articulate my own health-related experiences and needs effectively to health-care providers. According to Hernandez (2016), this serves as a barrier to maximized patienthood. Unfortunately, physicians' perceptions of under-represented group members exacerbate a heightened power differential that does little to erase this barrier (van Ryn & Burke, 2000), and may in fact, perpetuate health-care disparities (Chapman, Kaatz, & Carnes, 2013). For instance, Purnell et al. (2018) surveyed 1,220 practicing physicians about their perceptions of their organization's cultural competence climate and their skills and behaviors targeting patient-centered care for culturally and socially diverse patients. Less than half of providers reported engaging in behaviors to address cultural and social barriers more than 75 percent of the time. Providers who reported moderate or major structural problems were more likely to report low skillfulness in identifying patient mistrust, how well patients read and write English, and socioeconomic barriers than providers who reported only small or no structural problems.

***

When it comes to health and well-being, I believe in the power of self-care, self-awareness, and self-empowerment. For me, health is informed by the holy trinity of diet, exercise, and sleep. Watching what you eat and drink (moderation is a good rule, I think), being sure to engage in cardiovascular exercises several times a week, and adhering to a regimented sleep schedule of seven to eight hours each night are the keys to a healthy life. If I start to feel like sickness is attempting to manifest in my body [Note the language: I never claim sickness by saying things like, "I think I'm getting sick.], I go on the offensive and drink lots of water, eat vitamin-rich foods, make sure that I'm rested, and if needed, start to take Airborne twice a day.

Over the past several years, nurses and doctors consistently have commented on my good health. In fact, just last year one nurse shared that she had labeled me "an overachiever" as soon as she had looked at my chart. My healthy lifestyle has afforded me great leeway with my doctors. However, as soon as they take my family history, their demeanor immediately shifts. Making healthy choices was not the norm for my family members, and consequently, many did not live past their fifties or sixties. My family never discussed health issues openly and honestly. Consequently, I do not know the details of parents' and grandparents' deaths, beyond vaguely whispered utterances of taboo topics such as cancer, heart attacks, and aneurysms. I do know that hypertension, stress, and high blood pressure were all contributing factors to health problems and early deaths but I know very little of the specifics. This frustrates doctors who inevitably want a more detailed family history because they firmly believe that genetics are more important than my personal health regimen.

At the urging of my medical students, I have faithfully had an annual check-up for the past ten years. Typically, the results are desirable—with one exception: border-line high cholesterol levels. One older white male doctor strongly encouraged that I get on medication, and take one pill a day for the rest of my life, and explained that then I wouldn't have to worry about it. He offered his personal support for the pill which he had been taking for quite some time, but I was adamant that I would not accept this without exploring other options. He reluctantly agreed, and I made some key adjustments (e.g., adopting a more plant-based diet and avoiding high cholesterol foods like processed meat and cheeses) that consistently keep me just below the dangerous threshold of high cholesterol. Just in case, I've also gone on a forty-five-day super clean diet immediately prior to each annual check-up. So far, so good.

***

Patient-centered communication occurs when physicians situate the patient at the heart of the medical encounter. This approach contrasts traditional approaches where the doctor is the expert, and the patient as the consumer of their expertise. Instead, cultural communication competency fosters doctor's understanding as to how patients' lived experiences, personal desires, needs, and sense-making of their own illnesses should factor into the ultimate diagnosis (Epstein et al., 2005). This approach is central to my professional development workshops, however, engaging in this autoethnographic project has prompted a series of probing questions: What type of training is provided to patients in maximizing their competency when interacting with health-care practitioners? How can we facilitate greater patienthood agency? Is this a positive move, or are we then placing too much of the responsibility on the patient rather than the doctor?

***

The first two primary physicians that I had were older white men in their seventies. They were chosen because they were part of a health center within walking distance of my home. The first doctor was the only doctor taking new patients when I inquired, so it was a logical choice. I only saw him a couple of times for my annual visits before he retired, and recommended my second primary physician—evidently there were close colleagues who were very similar in their approach to medicine and doctor-patient interactions. Like his predecessor, I never really jelled with this doctor and the service at the health center seemed to get progressively worse every year I visited them. During what would become my final visit, I was left in the examination room for close to an hour with no explanation after the nurse did her preliminary work with me. After I got dressed and complained to the front desk, I left without being seen by the doctor. Then I decided that it was time for me to take some responsibility, assume some agency, and find a new doctor.

I immediately began a lengthy process of soliciting recommendations from colleagues and friends, conducting some intense online research, and making some inquiries with local medical centers. I was determined to find a younger doctor that I could relate to, and develop the type of relationship that I was advocating for with my medical students. While I received several excellent leads for a new doctor, I quickly learned that the best primary physicians either were not taking patients or had lengthy waiting lists with several obstacles to maneuver. Despite numerous set-backs, I continued to actively search for a physician and adopted a new strategy: Locate new physicians who were in the process of starting their practice and get on their schedule quickly! My current doctor is a young D.O. who was knowledgeable, welcoming, personable, respectful of my health practices, and willing to be more assertive in his recommendations when necessary. Rather than power-laden instructions from expert to novice, our interactions are more like a mutually-informed discussion between respectful partners. This was the case when I asked for his recommendations on vaccines needed for a trip to India. He shared his personal recommendations from a long, long list provided by the university travel nurse and took the time to explain the rationale for each recommendation. In the end, I decided against any vaccines and he accepted my decision. Personally, I like him, and he has told me that he appreciates my efforts to make his job easy.

***

I would like to believe that my cultural communication competency work with thousands of medical students and health-care practitioners over the past more than ten years has made a difference in shifting a medical world where health disparities are the norm. When I have any doubts, I pull up saved emails from current doctors who have written to me to tell me what a difference my workshops have meant in their professional interactions. One thing that I know for sure, however, is that my work with medical students has made a difference in *my life as a patient*. They have caused me to reevaluate my socialized perceptions of health, illness, medicine, and the medical community and to embrace a greater sense of agency in my interactions with nurses and doctors. Consequently, I bring a greater sense of understanding, responsibility and empowerment to my role as patient. In a way, my cultural communication competency work *with* medical students simultaneously has informed a sense of cultural communication competence *for me as a patient*. As I worked to transform others, I was also transformed. Go figure. Now I'm left wondering why the focus on cultural competency has been on doctors and nurses, why not also empower patients with some of the same lessons? In the end, this may be the key to true transformation of the health-care system.

REFERENCES

Alexander, B. K., Arasarathnam, L. A., Avant-Mier, R., Durhan, A., Flores, L., Leeds-Hurwitz, W., Mendoza, S. L., Oetzel, J., Osland, J., Tsuda, Y., & Yin, J. (2014). Defining and communicating what "intercultural" and "intercultural communication" means to us. *Journal of International and Intercultural Communication, 27*(1), 14–37. doi: 10.1080.17513057.2014.869524.

Berlin, E. A., & Fowkes, W. C. (1983). A teaching framework for cross-cultural health care: Application in family practice. *Western Journal of Medicine, 139*(6), 934–938.

Boylorn, R. M., & Orbe, M. P. (2014). *Critical autoethnography: Intersecting cultural identities in everyday life*. Walnut Creek: Left Coast Press.

Campinha-Bacote, J. (2003). *The process of cultural competence in the delivery of healthcare services* (4th edition). Cincinnati, OH: Transcultural C.A.R.E. Associates.

Chapman, E. N., Kaatz, A., & Carnes, M. (2013). Physicians and implicit bias: How doctors may unwittingly perpetuate health care disparities. *Journal of General Internal Medicine, 28*(11), 1504–1510. doi: 10.1007/s11606-013-2441-1.

Chin, P. (2005). Chinese. In J. G. Lipson & S. L. Dibble (Eds.), *Culture & clinical care* (pp. 98–108). San Francisco, CA: University of San Francisco Nursing Press.

Cross, T., Bazron, B., Dennis, K., & Issac, M. (1989). *Toward a culturally competent system of care*. Washington, DC: CASSP Technical Assistance Center at Georgetown University Child Development Center.

Epstein, R. M., Franks, P., Fiscella, K., Shields, C. G., Meldrum, S. C., Kravitz, R. L., & Duberstein, P. R. (2005). Measuring patient-centered communication in patient-physician consultations: Theoretical and practical issues. *Social Science & Medicine, 61*(7), 1516–1528. doi: 10.1016/j.socscimed.2005.02.001.

Expert Panel on Cultural Competence Education for Students in Medicine and Public Health. (2012). *Cultural competence education for students in medicine and public health: Report of an expert panel.* Washington, DC: Association of American Medical Colleges and Association of Schools of Public Health.

Gebbie, K., Rosenstock, L., & Hernandez, L. M. (Eds.). (2003). *Who will keep the public healthy? Educating public health professions for the 21st century.* Washington, DC: National Academies Press.

Goode, T. D., Dunne, M. C., & Bronheim, S. M. (2006). *The evidence base for cultural and linguistic competency in health care*. New York: The Commonwealth Fund.

Hernandez, L. H. (2016). "My doctor ruined my entire birthing experience:" A qualitative analysis of Mexican-American women's birth struggles with health care provides. In E. S. Gilchrist-Petty & S. D. Long (Eds.), *Contexts of the dark side of communication* (pp. 151–162). New York: Peter Lang.

Hurtado, S., Milem, J., Clayton-Pederson, A., & Allen, W. (1998). Enhancing campus climates for racial/ethnic diversity: Educational policy and practice. *The Review of Higher Education, 21*(3), 279–302.

Hurtado, S., Milem, J., Clayton-Pedersen, A., & Allen, W. (1999). Enacting diverse learning environments: Improving the campus climate for racial/ethnic diversity in higher education. *ASHE-ERIC Higher Education Reports Series, 26*(8). San Francisco: Jossey Bass Publishers.

Institute of Medicine. (2002). *Unequal treatment: Understanding racial and ethnic disparities in health care.* Washington, DC: National Academy Press.

Lie, D., Elizabeth Lee-Rey MD, M. P. H., Gomez, A., Bereknyei, S., & Braddock III, C. (2011). Does cultural competency training of health professionals improve patient outcomes? A systematic review and proposed algorithm for future research. *Journal of General Internal Medicine, 26*(3), 317–325. doi: 10.1007/s11606-010-1529-0.

Lipson, J. G., & Dibble, S. L. (Eds.). (2005). *Culture & clinical care.* San Francisco, CA: University of San Francisco Nursing Press.

Mutha, S., Allen, C., & Welch, M. (2002). *Toward culturally competent care: A toolbox for teaching communication strategies.* San Francisco, CA: Center for Health Professions, University of California.

Orbe, M. (August, 2015). *Centralizing communication scholarship in cultural competency education: Theoretically grounded praxis for health care practitioners.* Paper presented at the biennial meeting of the World Communication Association, Lisbon, Portugal.

Purnell, T. S., Marshall, J. K., Olorundare, I., Stewart, R. W., Sisson, S., Gibbs, B., Feldman, L. S., Bertram, A., Green, A. R., & Cooper, L. A. (2018). Provider perceptions of the organization's cultural competence climate and their skills and behaviors targeting patient-centered care for socially at-risk populations. *Journal of Health Care Poor Underserved, 29*(1), 481–496. doi: 10.1353/hpu.2018.0032.

Ronai, C. R. (1995). Multiple reflections of child sex abuse: An argument for a layered account. *Journal of Contemporary Ethnography, 23*(4), 395–426. doi: 10.1177/089124195023004001.

Rosenberg, E., Richard, C., Lussier, M.-T., & Abdool, S. N. (2006). Intercultural communication competence in family medicine: Lessons from the field. *Patient Education and Counseling, 61*, 236–245. doi: 10.1016/j.pec.2005.04.002.

Rust, G., et al. (2006). A CRASH-course in cultural competence. *Ethnicity & Disease, 16*(3), 29–36.

Tervalon, M., & Murray-Garcia, J. (1998). Cultural humility versus cultural competence: A critical distinction in defining physician training outcomes in multicultural education. *Journal of Health Care for the Poor and Underserved, 9*(2), 117–125. doi: 10.1353/hpu.2010.0233.

van Ryn, M., & Burke, J. (2000). The effect of patient race and socio-economic status on physician's perceptions of patients. *Social Science and Medicine, 50*, 813–828. doi: 10.1016/S0277-9536(99)00338-X.

Chapter 4

If I Die, Who Will Tell Their Stories?

Emerging Health Legacies Following the 2014–2016 Ebola Epidemic

Crystal Daugherty and Amanda Young

After losing his wife and four other members of his family in the 2014 Ebola outbreak, Akoi, a Liberian farmer, asked the question, "If I die, who will tell their stories"? Liberian culture is rich with storytelling, where narratives of suffering, loss, resilience, and survival help individuals, families, and communities make sense of both the past and present, while giving guidance for the future. We have found that included in Liberians' broad repertoire of stories are what Manoogian and her colleagues call health legacies, or intergenerational narratives that focus on how members of a family (or culture) experience and share health episodes (Manoogian, Harter, & Denham, 2010). Of interest to Manoogian and her colleagues are how the storytelling process "create[s] meaning, shape[s] identities, and provide[s] pathways to action" (p. 46). In this chapter, we argue that Akoi's story of the 2014 Ebola epidemic can be viewed as a nascent health legacy. In telling his story, he is creating a narrative legacy that he desperately wants to pass on to future generations, with the hope of avoiding the devastation of any similar epidemic.

Two years after struggling to survive so that his story could be told, Akoi and I (CD) sat inside the community center in the village of Weala. He recounted the events of 2014, when a mysterious illness, eventually identified as Ebola, overtook first a neighbor, then his wife who had cared for her, three children, and finally a grandchild. As he spoke of his sadness, his bright, youthful, amber eyes belied the deep wrinkles in his forehead and the rough calluses on his hands. He had been to the edge of death. He had suffered unbearable loss. But now, two years later, he was urgently sharing his story with me, a graduate student who had come to his village both to serve on a church-sponsored mission trip and to collect interview data for my dissertation on communication, illness, and spirituality in rural Liberia. Sitting across a small table from Akoi, I was anticipating another rich narrative from this native Liberian, where storytelling is integral to community life. Yet I realized that my privilege to engage with Akoi went beyond his culturally mandated honoring of a white visitor. Akoi was plagued with the question, "Who will tell our story?" Still grieving for his family, this heartbroken man wanted the world to know not only of their suffering but also of the quagmire of misinformation and chaos that he believed contributed to the tragedy. And so, I found myself leaning in as Akoi began his story.

THE BEGINNING OF THE 2014–2016 EBOLA EPIDEMIC

Prior to 2014, no cases of Ebola had been recorded in Western Africa (Baize, Pannetier, Oestereich, & Rieger, 2014). According to Kent Brantly, a doctor who cared for Ebola patients in Liberia and who eventually was stricken with the virus, outbreaks of Ebola in the past had been limited to small, rural communities in Central Africa (Brantly, Brantly, & Thomas, 2016). Brantly describes a "perfect storm" in the spring of 2014 that created a wave of Ebola surging through Guinea, Liberia, and Sierra Leone. The index patient, or the first person to contract the illness, is thought to have been an eighteen-month-old boy in Guinea who was bitten by a bat in December 2013 (CDC, 2017). Because of weak surveillance systems and a fragmented public health infrastructure, the virus spread to Conakry, the capital city of Guinea, and then into the neighboring countries of Liberia and Sierra Leone, where it spread through those countries' metropolitan areas. On June 17, 2014, public health officials confirmed the first case in Monrovia, the capital of Liberia (United Nations, 2014). For the first time, Ebola was striking not only isolated, rural villages but also large metropolitan areas. Regardless of the geographical context, however, misinformation, fear, unexamined cultural traditions, distrust of government, lack of experience with Ebola, poor communication, and weak infrastructure fueled the worst Ebola outbreak in history (Brantly, Brantly, & Thomas, 2015; Donovan, 2014; World Health Organization, 2015). In Weala, Akoi and his fellow villagers had never encountered Ebola; both community members and local health-care providers assumed the devastating illness and mounting deaths were a vicious form of malaria or "runny stomach" (dysentery).

Akoi's Story

Having lived most of his life in Weala, Akoi, like most of the villagers, spent his days working and providing for his family. Weala sits on the banks of the Wea River, which connects homes, neighborhoods, and villages not only with water but also with its flow of stories, relationships, and cultural norms that have guided the lives of its people for centuries. One of the strongest norms in Weala is to respond quickly and generously to neighbors in need, especially when they are sick. This tradition is not just a loving gesture. It is an integral part of a fragile health-care system. Along with most of its infrastructure, Liberia's health-care system was shattered during its two civil wars, the most recent of which ended in 2003 (Meredith, 2011). Rebuilding clinics and infrastructure in small towns like Weala has been listed as a priority in postwar reconstruction; however, the health-care system remains fragmented and sparse (Brantly, Brantly, & Thomas, 2015; Radelet, 2007; World Health Organization, 2015). Like those living along the Wea River, rural Liberians continue to rely on the cultural norms of community care to address most health-care issues. When someone becomes ill, the family's first recourse is to call for help from neighbors or to see a traditional healer, where help is often delivered both materially and in story (Manguvo & Mafuvadze, 2015). In 2014, however, the people of Weala quickly understood that for this mystery illness, the local traditional healers' efforts were fruitless. No story could explain it and no cure could stop it.

Akoi's story began with the village pastor. When a member of his family became sick in July of 2014, it was thought, as Akoi described, to be a "normal" illness, perhaps malaria or dysentery. While her illness was clearly not running a "normal" course, family and neighbors had no framework through which to understand it. Akoi lamented, "We did not know. We did not understand." Akoi explained that the sister of the pastor's wife had become ill in July after caring for a dying woman in Monrovia. When she did not recover, the pastor and his wife brought her to their home in Weala. "They didn't know. There was no awareness." Again, Akoi punctuated his story with this statement. Soon, the sister died, and the pastor's wife became ill. Now the Ebola virus had invaded Weala. But still, no one knew. No one understood. And the cultural norms of community members intimately caring for the sick continued.

Akoi explained that the sickness and death of these two women did not seem unusual. Illness and early death are part of the fabric of life in Weala. But his thinking changed on August 20 when his own wife became ill. Akoi described the scene when he and his sons came home from working on the farm that Friday. The meal was prepared, as usual. But his wife was not well. She had chills and was not able to eat. On Saturday, she was too weak to move. He continued his story:

> So the following day she started, the running stomach started. Her eyeballs became all red. We didn't know, no awareness. So we took care of her. She

wanted to use the bucket and I would help her to the bucket. My daughter would empty it. It lasted for nine days and she died on the 29th of August.

Akoi continued to reflect on the night his wife went to help the pastor's wife:

My wife went there that night to help her because she felt weak. She was very weak. We all went there but didn't enter. My wife entered the building. We didn't know. From there my wife came down with the virus.

In the months that followed, Akoi's experience was repeated in family after family in Weala. Of the 100 houses in his village, he said, "over 38 were dead," meaning that thirty-eight family units had at least one person die from Ebola. The outbreak lasted from 2014 to 2016, peaking in September 2014. By the end, there were 28,610 reported cases of Ebola across West Africa and over 11,308 deaths, resulting in a 40 percent fatality rate. Of those cases 10,675 occurred in Liberia, which reported 4,809 Ebola deaths, resulting in a 45 percent fatality rate (Center for Disease Control, 2017; World Health Organization, 2018). In the vastness of this tragedy, Akoi was desperate that his story would not be lost in the numbers.

BUILDING A FRAMEWORK OF UNDERSTANDING

Akoi's story is part of a larger qualitative data set that explores Liberian health legacies. His interview is unique, however, in that of the interviewees, only Akoi had been infected with the virus. We have chosen, therefore, to analyze Akoi's story as a single case study (Yin, 2017) using framework analysis (FA) (Ritchie & Spencer, 1994; Ritchie, Spencer, & O'Connor, 2003), which is ideally suited for single case studies (Ward, Furber, Tierney, & Swallow, 2013). Beginning with the first step of FA—thorough immersion into the data—both of us read the transcript several times, taking note of salient features that emerged and patterns that occurred. One of us (C.D.) brought firsthand experience with the data; the other (A.Y.) brought an outsider's perspective. Together we could devise a coding chart that served as a starting point to organize the data.

In step two of our FA process, we applied the basic coding scheme to the transcript by working in Dedoose (dedoose.com), a qualitative software analysis program. As we focused on each idea unit within each conversational turn, we added several subthemes to our coding scheme, as well as adding a few major themes and collapsing others. By visualizing the coding structure, we were better able to see the relationships among specific passages. Most notably, we began to see the consistency of Akoi's lament, "We didn't know," and its salience in each context where it appeared. During step 3 of FA, we created reports in Dedoose to identify all the idea units that were coded with a particular node. This process allowed us to further refine the coding scheme, ensuring that the hierarchy was accurate and that coding nodes were placed in meaningful relationships with each other. In step 4, we applied the final coding scheme to the entire manuscript and then created reports and graphics to give deeper insight into the meaning of the text. Table 4.1 illustrates our final coding scheme.

By examining the coded excerpts and our own commentary gathered in the process of step 4 of framework analysis, we were then able to create a summary of each of the identified themes. Akoi's story continues in descriptions of the texts coded by these themes.

The Impact of Ebola

While it is unlikely that one man's narrative to give us a full understanding of the impact of Ebola on Weala, we do get a picture of the multidimensional effects that the epidemic had, ranging from its ravaging symptoms for individuals to its disruption of community practices and traditions, and its ultimate death toll in the village. It devastated every household; Akoi lost the majority of his family, which included three generations. Cultural practices in Weala were disrupted, particularly their tradition of tending to the sick.

Table 4.1 Coding Scheme for Akoi's Story

1. Impact of Ebola
   a. On cultural practices
   b. On daily life
   c. On the community
   d. Symptoms
2. Resources
   a. Availability of resource
   b. Lack of resources
   c. Individual treatment
   d. Public health interventions
3. Emotional and Mental Health
   a. Fear
   b. Grief
4. Cultural
   a. Community interaction
   b. Burial practices
   c. Spirituality
5. Knowledge
   a. Awareness of not knowing
   b. Current knowledge

As the community began to understand the vicious speed with which Ebola spread, they had to stop centuries-long practices of hands-on, communal care, both for the living and the dead, regardless of where care is provided or death occurs. According to Brantly, Brantly, & Thomas (2015), it is not acceptable to leave the body of a family member at the hospital. Instead, they are taken home, where loving hands cleanse the body, and grieving family members and neighbors caress and kiss it, before wrapping it for burial. Public health officials quickly recognized that this practice increased the speed of infection exponentially. Yet, individuals who had to cease this practice suffered from the trauma of what they saw as failing their loved ones (Brantly, Brantly, & Thomas, 2015).

Resources

Most of Akoi's references to resources revealed a desperate lack of medicine, equipment, and room in the treatment centers. Akoi confirmed the limited medical resources available in Weala, prior to the epidemic (Brantly, Brantly, & Thomas, 2015; Janke, Heim, Steiner, Massaquoi, Gbanya, Frey, & Froeschi, 2017) when he described relatives caring for each other and going to the "country doctor" unless the illness seemed to be life threatening. Like many before her, Akoi's wife died at home. But when Akoi and his son became ill, they were taken to the Ebola Treatment Units (ETU) that were set up as temporary diagnostic and treatment facilities by the Liberian government and various global health organizations. In the summer of 2014, public health officials in Liberia were aware of the difficulties inherent in the ETU's, including a high mortality rate, the high incidence of patients being seen there who did not actually have Ebola but then acquired it, the difficulty of providing care for patients who had been seen at ETU's with other conditions, and the deep distrust that community members had of the facilities and their personnel (Janke et al., 2017). Despite recognizing these deficiencies, Akoi credited the government with bringing resources to his village:

> After it was getting rampant, it was getting worse, it started to be exposed. People started, the government started, the minister of health started sending the ambulance, the health team … and say that if anyone get running stomach they should be taken to the ETU.

But from a macro-level view, the lack of resources was dire. Brantly et al. (2015) describe arriving in Liberia to work in a hospital where there was not even one nasal canula available. According to Shorten and colleagues (Shorten, Brown, Jacobs, Rattenbury, Simpson, & Mepham, 2016), severe shortages of diagnostic testing materials contributed to the rapid spread of the disease in all of the affected countries. Early in the summer of 2014, the WHO Ebola Response Roadmap reported that Liberia, Sierra Leone, and Guinea were "struggling to control the escalating outbreak against a backdrop of severely compromised health systems, significant deficits in capacity, and rampant fear" (WHO, 2014, p. 4).

Emotional and Mental Health

Fear and grief were the emotions that drove Akoi's narrative as he described the events in Weala in July and August of 2014. Akoi spoke of his own fear: "Because like for me I was afraid to go to the center because when you go to the ETU they are going to spray you or you die. So I was afraid." He explained that villagers believed that patients sent to the ETU's were sprayed down with a substance that sometimes killed them. Patients and providers were gently sprayed with a bleach solution. Deceased bodies were sprayed with bleach. Equipment was sprayed. Everything was sprayed. But because so many people who were taken for treatment died, villagers formed a mistaken belief that the mysterious spray was killing them. And that fear spread as quickly as the virus itself, resulting in many people hiding from authorities, refusing to go the ETU's, and ultimately dying at home.

Akoi, his sons, and his pregnant daughter, quickly became ill after his wife's death. He described his early decision to avoid the ETU for fear of the mysterious spray. But then he decided that staying home likely meant certain death and that going to the ETU would at least give him a chance: "I make up my mind. I say, it is better to go to the hospitals, then to stay home." He called the government phone number that had been distributed in the village, asking for an ambulance to come for him and his son family. Ultimately, he had to decide which strategy was less fearful:

> But when you go to the hospital there are some people who will treat you. Maybe if you are lucky you will survive but to stay will not help you. So that is why I decided. At first I didn't want to go. I decided, I say "Let me go. If I will die, let me die at the hospital. That is the best place to die."

Grief accompanied fear throughout Akoi's story. During the interview, his posture and countenance demonstrated his resilience, but his words carried the weight of losing his family, whom he described as "all my committed people. Those who were committed to me. Very committed." As he told of his decision to seek treatment, he described one son dying in the ambulance before they got to the ETU. Another son died after Akoi and his son were taken to the ETU. His daughter, who was in labor with her first child, had to be left behind in Weala. Both she and the infant died. He had held out hope for her the entire time he was in the ETU and on his return to Weala, he enjoyed seeing the happiness of his friends and neighbors when they realized he had survived: "So when I returned they were so happy. They welcome me and very good time." But the grief he was carrying for his sons was multiplied and his hopes were dashed when he arrived at his house to find a fresh grave: "But one thing I missed my people. I was not happy when I came home and there was a fresh grave behind my house. After all of my committed people had died from me."

Cultural Factors

The theme of cultural factors fell into three subthemes: community interactions, burial practices, and spirituality. According to Akoi, one of the strongest traditions in his village is for the community to rally around a person who is sick: "Can you imagine when a female is sick, the rest of the females will go ... to draw water, to bathe the patient. Relatives, friends and other people. That is the assistance we can do in our village." It was this community tradition that led to the rapid spread of Ebola in Weala, as women in the village gathered in the pastor's home to care for his sick wife. In Weala, as throughout Western Africa, communal care for the sick extends to care for the deceased, and traditional burial practices were identified as the major factor in the spread of Ebola (WHO, 2015). Akoi described the tradition of relatives and friends washing the body of a deceased person, and at the point of the interview, he had learned that Ebola had spread rapidly through this practice. "Yes, washing the body. Sometimes you take care of the body. You will treat the body. You will have wake keeping. All of these were dangerous."

Like the rest of Liberia, spirituality in Weala is palpable but difficult to frame. The United Nation's National Population and Housing Census (2008) reports the population to be 85.6 percent Christian, 12.2 percent Muslim, 1.5 percent claiming no religion, 0.6 percent indigenous religious groups, and less than 1 percent other religious groups (e.g., Hindu or Buddhist). However, field observations from CD's three visits to Liberia suggest that in addition to a major religion (e.g., Christianity or Islam) people often adhere to indigenous religious practices in conjunction with their major religious preference. Akoi identified as Christian and he spoke often in the interview about prayer. Always, his prayers were linked to wanting to survive so that he could tell the stories of those who had already died and those who were dying around him in the ETU:

> I was strong. I was praying hard to God that I should not lose, I should go back here [Weala] to tell the stories. After all my people died, I prayed to God. Be strong because at the time, when I was admitted they had two rooms but there were dead bodies there. So I had to go to the restroom. I had to walk by the rooms and I could see people dying all over. So I prayed to God, Be strong, go by the doctor's advice, when they gave me the tablet, I make sure I take it in.

Make me strong and make sure I take it regular because I know that I lost my people. I was thinking, "If I die, who will go tell their stories?"

Akoi also spoke about a spiritual experience of being near death. While he did not elaborate on any sort of vision, he described the severity of his illness in these terms: "I went to heaven and came back. I went to heaven and I came back." When it was finally clear he would survive, he was effusive with praise to God:

As I told you I was praying! I was praying and praying. In the morning I prayed to my God. In the evening I said "Oh God help me!" and I prayed to my God. The only way. Even though the treatment helped me, over all the treatment, He had me. Here I am!

KNOWLEDGE

The most prevalent theme in Akoi's narrative was knowledge, which emerged in two subthemes: "Not knowing" and "Current knowledge." Throughout the interview, Akoi lamented the villagers' lack of knowledge about Ebola: "We did not know. No awareness." As Akoi explained his village's customs, he interspersed his story nine times with "but we didn't know." In contrast, he often acknowledged what he had learned about Ebola. He described learning that while both malaria and Ebola can cause "runny stomach," routine care will not cure Ebola. He described the change in his and the villagers' understanding of how to respond when someone became ill:

After we begin to get awareness, we started to go far from it. We started to get protections. The national government began to send ambulance in the town. You would be put in quickly and not waste time. We go far away from it. Far from it.

Though their norm had been to gather around a sick person, Akoi and the rest of the village had learned that they had to isolate themselves and the person who was ill. With that knowledge, though, came the difficult experience of countering their cultural practices of communal care for both the living and the dead.

AN EMERGING FRAMEWORK

Step 5 of framework analysis calls for a review of the indexed data by comparing themes and subthemes, checking results against original transcripts, and ensuring that the emerging framework supplies an accurate lens through which we can understand the narrative. In conducting this final analysis, we could identify three key areas that structured Akoi's emerging health legacy, both in terms of understanding his experience and in contributing to more effective communication strategies in future intercultural, crisis situations.

Lack of Knowledge: "We Didn't Know"

"We didn't know. We thought it was a normal sickness." Akoi began his story by emphasizing that in the summer of 2014, he and other villagers did not know about Ebola, and his despair in "not knowing" continued throughout his narrative. Each key point of his story was punctuated with similar words. A sick woman was brought to the village. But they didn't know. Akoi's wife helped care for the pastor's wife. But she didn't know. Akoi's wife became ill, but they didn't know. Akoi and two of his children began to take care of his wife, but they didn't know. The fever, fatigue, muscle pain, headache, diarrhea, vomiting, and sore throat the villagers saw in one another were symptoms of Ebola (CDC, 2018; WHO, 2018). But these maladies were also typical of other tropical illnesses such as malaria, typhoid, and yellow fever (CDC, 2018; WHO, 2018), which the people of Weala were familiar with. It was not until the unexplained hemorrhaging and high fatality rate of this illness emerged that Akoi and others realized that something new, something terrible, had come to their village. By September 2014, government efforts to educate people in rural areas were widespread, with high incidence areas like Weala showing impressive scores on an Ebola KAP survey (knowledge, attitudes, and practice) conducted by the CDC (Kobayashi, Beer, Bjork, Chatham-Stephens, Cherry, Arzoaquoi et al., 2015). But for Akoi, his family, and many others in Weala, that knowledge came too late. Even though they finally recognized this was a new type of sickness, they still did not understand how it was transmitted and were unaware of what treatments were available until government workers appeared in Weala, four to six weeks after the village's initial Ebola death.

Lack of Trust: "Family Could Hide You from Going to ETU"

Knowledge about this new disease and governmental health-care efforts did eventually reach Weala. Unfortunately, that knowledge was not enough to stem the crisis. Although Liberia is currently experiencing a time of political stability, it has a consistent history of unrest that includes not only governmental corruption but also war crimes that have led directly to a pervasive distrust of the Liberian health-care system (Lori & Boyle, 2011; Siekmans, Sohani, Boima, Koffa, Basil, & Laaziz, 2017; Tayler-Smith, Zachariah, Hinderaker, Manzi, De Plecker, Van Wolvelaer et al., 2012; Wagenaar, Augusto, Beste, Toomay, Wickett, Dunbar et al., 2018). That distrust was a significant barrier in stemming the spread of Ebola in the 2014–2016 epidemic (Brantly, Brantly, & Thomas, 2015; Donovan, 2014; WHO, 2015), as villagers in Weala and other rural areas hid from government health-care workers. Akoi described emergency vehicles coming to the villages to transport the sick and deceased to the ETU's. Part of the transport procedure was spraying the sick individual (or a dead body) and the interior of the ambulance with the bleach solution. For those in the village, the last time they saw their loved ones alive they were being sprayed with a chemical and loaded into an ambulance that was also being sprayed. Akoi said that many villagers believed people were being killed by the government and decided to hide themselves, those who were sick, and those who had already died. Later research confirms this practice (Coltart, Lindsey, Johnson, & Heymann, 2017) and the resulting increase in the spread of disease.

Lack of Cultural Sensitivity: "Washing the Body. You Will Treat the body."

It was not just fear that kept people away from the ETUs. While the Western biomedical model holds that hospitalization is the optimal choice for life-threatening illness, rural Liberians practice community-based, hands-on care. Their first response is often bush medicine, which can include seeking help from a traditional healer, foraging for herbs, or following protocols handed down from one generation to the next in health legacies. Their hands-on approach also includes community members gathering in the home of the ill person to offer care and comfort. While medical protocol called for isolation and a reduction in physical contact, Liberian culture called for communal care. In Akoi's narrative, the death of the pastor's wife illustrates this conflict.

Burial rites were another significant cultural barrier to stemming the spread of Ebola. During the Ebola epidemic the hands-on, intimate treatment of the dead became a point of conflict between villagers and health-care workers. Liberians were asked to not only isolate themselves but to also neglect community roles, as caregivers or grievers. Akoi could not know if knowledge of Ebola would have kept his wife from fulfilling her cultural role as a community caregiver. But in upholding her cultural and communal beliefs, Akoi and his children would also contract the Ebola virus.

AKOI'S LEGACY: IF I DIE, WHO WILL TELL THEIR STORIES?

Akoi confirmed what I (C.D.) had witnessed many times in my trips to Liberia: Liberians take their communal responsibility very seriously. Even as an outsider in Liberia, I have experienced their deep-rooted hospitality. On my first trip a team member from the United States became ill and spent the day lying on the cool floor. Later in the day I found out that one of our Liberian friends had also spent the day lying on the floor with him to provide company and comfort. Akoi highlighted that his wife provided "the assistance we can do in our village." It is that same legacy that prompted his adult children to come home and care for their mother. Akoi did not create this legacy of care. He inherited it from his family and then passed it on to his children. With the Ebola epidemic, though, that legacy had become disrupted and disjointed. Now his story, his health legacy, that he wants so earnestly to pass on to others, will include these unexpected twists and turns. But it will also include lessons learned: the difficulty of merging Western medicine with traditional health-care practices during an epidemic, the vital need for trust between villagers and government, and the challenges of making health-care decisions based on changing information during a crisis.

Akoi's health legacy is ultimately a story of faith, culture, perseverance, and survival. His extended family will grow up knowing that he survived Ebola through the integration of traditional community care and Western medical interventions. Beyond his family, Akoi's narrative teaches us about the role of knowledge and awareness in preventing and treating health problems, not just in Liberia but in other remote areas, particularly in times of crisis. His experiences with Ebola provide insight into how researchers and health-care providers across cultures should work toward reconciling cultural traditions and practices to deal with epidemics. Specifically, family health legacies in Liberia, before and after the Ebola epidemic, should be explored because they could offer insight into how multiple individuals and generations approach health not only in routine health matters but also in crisis.

A FINAL MEMORY

Akoi had moved very little during the interview. I found myself leaning closer to him, eager to cling to his story. After thanking him for the chance to listen and share his story, I asked Akoi if he wanted to add anything. He sat there for a moment and then shared a final memory:

> There was this one nurse. She was a white American lady. She was always laughing and caring. She cared for the dying people. She was really good. After I was discharged she said, "Go, take in the sights!" And, so, I have come home.

REFERENCES

Baize, S., Pannetier, D., Oestereich, L., Rieger, T., Koivogui, L., Magassouba, N., Soropogui, B., ... & Gunther, S. (2014). Emergence of Zaire Ebola virus disease in Guinea. *New England Journal of Medicine*, 371, 1218–1225.

Brantly, K., Brantly, A., & Thomas, D. (2015). *Called for life: How loving our neighbor led us into the heart of the Ebola epidemic.* Colorado Springs: Waterbrook Press.

Center for Disease Control. (2017). *History of Ebola virus disease: 2014–2016 Ebola outbreak in West Africa.* Retrieved from: https://www.cdc.gov/vhf/ebola/history/2014-2016-outbreak/index.html.

Center for Disease Control. (2018). *Ebola Virus disease: Signs and symptoms.* Retrieved from: https://www.cdc.gov/vhf/ebola/symptoms/index.html.

Coltart, C. E. M., Lindsey, G., Ghinai, I., Johnson, A. M., & Heymann, D. L. (2017). The Ebola outbreak, 2013–2016: Old lessons for new epidemics. *Philosophical Transactions, 372,* 1–24.

Donovan, G. K. (2014). Ebola, epidemics, and ethics – what we have learned. *Philosophy, Ethics, and Humanities in Medicine: PEHM, 9,* 15. http://doi.org/10.1186/1747-5341-9-15.

Janke, C., Heim, K. M., Steiner, F., Massaquoi, M., Gbanya, M. Z., Frey, C., & Froeschl, G. (2017). Beyond Ebola treatment units: Severe infection temporary treatment units as an essential element of Ebola case management during an outbreak. *BMC Infectious Diseases, 17,* 124. http://doi.org/10.1186/s12879-017-2235-x.

Kobayashi, M., Beer, K. D., Bjork, A., Chatham-Stephens, K., Cherry, C. C., Arzoaquoi, S., … Nyenswah, T. G. (2015). Community knowledge, attitudes, and practices regarding Ebola Virus Disease – Five counties, Liberia, September–October, 2014. *MMWR: Morbidity and Mortality Weekly Report, 64*(26), 714–718.

Lori, J. R., & Boyle, J. S. (2011). Cultural childbirth practices, beliefs, and traditions in post-conflict Liberia. *Health Care for Women International, 32*(6), 454–473.

Manguvo, A., & Mafuvadze, B. (2015). The impact of traditional and religious practices on the spread of Ebola in West Africa: Time for a strategic shift. *The Pan African Medical Journal, 22*(Suppl 1), 9. http://doi.org/10.11694/pamj.supp.2015.22.1.6190.

Meredith, M. (2011). *The fate of Africa: A history of the continent since independence.* New York: Public Affairs.

Manoogian, M. M., Harter, L. M., & Denham, S. A. (2010). The storied natured of health legacies in the familial experience of type 2 diabetes. *Journal of Family Communication, 10,* 40–56.

Radelet, S. (2007). Reviving economic growth in Liberia. *Center for Global Development, 133,* 1–21.

Ritchie, J., & Spencer, L. (1994). Qualitative data analysis for applied policy research by Jane Ritchie and Liz Spencer. In Bryman & R. G. Burgess (Eds.), *Analyzing qualitative data'* (pp. 173–194). London: Routledge.

Ritchie, J., Spencer, L., & O'Connor, W. (2003). Carrying out qualitative analysis. In J. Ritchie & J. Lewis (Eds.), *Qualitative research practice: A guide for social science students and researchers* (pp. 219–262). London, UK: Sage Publications.

Shorten, R. J., Brown, C. S., Jacobs, M., Rattenbury, S., Simpson, A. J., & Mepham, S. (2016). Diagnostics in Ebola virus disease in resource-rich and resource-limited settings. *PLoS Neglected Tropical Diseases, 10*(10), e0004948. http://doi.org/10.1371/journal.pntd.0004948.

Siekmans, K., Sohani, S., Boima, T., Koffa, F., Basil, L., & Laaziz, S. (2017). Community-based health care is an essential component of a resilient health system: Evidence from Ebola outbreak in Liberia. *BMC Public Health, 17*(1), 1–10.

Tayler-Smith, K., Zachariah, R., Hinderaker, S. G., Manzi, M., De Plecker, E., Van Wolvelaer, P., et al. (2012). Sexual violence in post-conflict Liberia: Survivors and their care. *Tropical Medicine & International Health, 17*(11), 1356–1360.

United Nations. (2008). *2008 National population and housing census: Preliminary results*. Retrieved from: unstats.un.org/unsd/dnss/docViewer.aspx?docID=2075.

United Nations. (2014). *Ebola response: Timeline*. Retrieved from: https://ebolaresponse.un.org/timeline.

Ward, D. J., Furber, C., Tierney, S., & Swallow, V. (2013). Using framework analysis in nursing research: A worked example. *Journal of Advanced Nursing, 69*, 2423–2431.

World Health Organization. (2014). *Ebola response roadmap*. Washington, DC: Author.

World Health Organization. (2015). *Factors that contributed to undetected spread of the Ebola virus and impeded rapid containment*. Retrieved from: http://www.who.int/csr/disease/ebola/one-year-report/factors/en/.

World Health Organization. (2018). *Ebola Virus disease: Key facts*. Retrieved from: http://www.who.int/news-room/fact-sheets/detail/ebola-virus-disease.

Yin, R. K. (2017). *Case study research: Design and methods* (4th ed.). Thousand Oaks, CA: Sage.

Part II

NARRATING PATIENTHOOD: DIFFERENCES THAT MATTER

Chapter 5

African Americans and Hospice Care

On Social Risk, Privacy Management, and Relational Health Advocacy

Patrick J. Dillon and Ambar Basu

Hospice care is a specific form of palliative care practice that is designed to provide interdisciplinary medical and support services for dying patients' (and their loved ones) physical, social, and spiritual needs. Hospice services include (1) pain and symptom management, (2) preparation for the emotional, psychosocial, and spiritual aspects, (3) lay caregiver training/support, and (4) bereavement counseling; care is most often provided in patients' homes but is also available through in-patient facilities, including hospitals and nursing homes (National Hospice and Palliative Care Organization [NHPCO], 2018). A family member or close friend typically serves as the patient's primary caregiver and—when necessary or appropriate—helps make decisions for the terminally ill person (NHPCO, 2018). In order to qualify for hospice enrollment under the Hospice Medicare Benefit, patients are required to meet two primary criteria: (1) they must have a life expectancy of six months or less; (2) they must agree to forgo curative treatment for the length of their time in hospice care (Centers for Medicare & Medicaid Services, 2008).

Approximately 1.5 million patients receive hospice care annually (NHPCO, 2018), and a number of studies indicate that hospice organizations provide "superior end-of-life care in terms of effective pain management, preservation of patient dignity, and family satisfaction when compared to alternate forms of care for terminally ill individuals" (Cagle et al., 2016, p. 27). Despite the well-documented benefits associated with hospice care, African American patients are underrepresented within the hospice population. In 2016, for example, African American patients accounted for just 8.3 percent of hospice patients (NHPCO, 2018). In recent years, there has been growing consensus that the relative underuse of hospice care by African American patients contributes to persistent disparities in the cost and quality of end-of-life care; because larger numbers of African Americans continue to die in hospitals—where they are often subject to long periods of uncontrolled pain, futile medical treatment, and increased medical expenses—they generally pay more for lower quality care at the end of life (Anderson, Green, & Payne, 2009; Hendricks Sloan et al., 2016; Hanchate, Kronman, Young-Xu, Ash, & Emanuel, 2009; Melhado & Bushy, 2011; Taylor, Ostermann, Van Houtven, Tulsky, & Steinhauser, 2007).

With the increasing recognition that disproportionate hospice enrollment may contribute to disparities in the cost and quality of end-of-life care, scholars from a variety of disciplines have sought to understand these differences by identifying population-specific barriers that may limit African Americans' participation in hospice programs. Extant research suggests that a number of factors—including reimbursement policies (particularly, the requirement that patients forgo curative care), a general mistrust of the health-care system as well as individual providers, and preferences for aggressive care—may contribute to disparate hospice enrollment (Bullock, 2011; Campbell, Williams, & Orr, 2010; Dillon, Roscoe, & Jenkins, 2012; Rhodes et al., 2017). Others have identified a reluctance to engage in formal advance care planning (e.g., Hendricks Sloan et al., 2016) and limited or inaccurate knowledge of hospice care (e.g., Cagle et al., 2016) as additional contributing factors. Studies have also noted that there is a stigma attached to hospice care among some African Americans, who equate hospice enrollment with "giving up" on one's self or a loved one, failing to trust in "God's timing," or abdicating familial caregiving responsibilities (Dillon & Basu, 2016a, 2016b; Taxis, 2006; Rhodes et al., 2017). Building from the identification of these barriers, recent studies have increasingly focused on developing educational programs and materials designed "to increase awareness and understanding of advance care planning, palliative care, and hospice among members of the African American community" (Rhodes et al., 2017, p. 510; see also Enguidanos, Kogan, Lorenz, & Taylor, 2011).

Although these existing studies provide important insights into factors that may deter and/or limit hospice enrollment among African Americans, there is a relative dearth of research focusing on the lived experiences of actual African American hospice patients and lay caregivers; as Noh and Schroepfer (2015) note, past studies have largely "focused on interviewing minority individuals who may or may not have been terminally ill and few of whom were using hospice care services" (p. 8). In essence, there is a fairly expansive body of research identifying why some African American patients and their loved ones do not (or, at least, may not) choose hospice care; there is significantly less scholarship focused on why many African Americans do choose hospice or how they make sense of their experiences with this form of care. In addressing this important gap in the literature, we have written elsewhere about the ways that some African Americans are able to navigate or avoid potential barriers to hospice enrollment (Dillon & Basu, 2016a; see also Noh & Schroepfer, 2015); we have also explored how African American patients' and lay caregivers evaluate their hospice experiences (Dillon & Roscoe, 2015) and their recommendations for increasing hospice enrollment among this population (Dillon & Basu, 2016b).

We build upon this previous work here by exploring an important "communicative dilemma" that African American hospice patients and lay caregivers face; that is, following the work of Bute and Brann (2015), we examine how patients and their loved ones "co-own and co-manage" private, potentially stigmatizing information about hospice enrollment (p. 24). We also note how some patients and lay caregivers push back against the stigma associated with hospice by becoming informal advocates for this form of care among other African Americans.

In the following section, we outline the theoretical basis for our study by describing the central tenets of Dutta's (2008) culture-centered approach to health communication (CCA) and Petronio's (2002) communication privacy management theory (CPM). We then continue by outlining our methodological approach and the findings that emerged from the data analysis process. Finally, we conclude by identifying the practical and theoretical implications of this research.

THE CULTURE-CENTERED APPROACH TO HEALTH COMMUNICATION

The culture-centered approach (CCA) argues that health meanings are situated among the interrelated constructs of culture, structure, and agency (Dutta, 2008, 2012). Within this framework, *culture* is conceptualized as dynamic, locally situated webs of meaning that are continually (re)negotiated through day-to-day interactions (Dutta, 2008). As Dutta (2012) notes, "culture is both constitutive and transformative; whereas on one hand, shared beliefs and values get passed down through generations, on the other hand, these values and beliefs are open to reinterpretations through the interactions among community members" (p. 369). *Structures* are forms of social organizing that provide or limit individuals/communities' access to resources that influence their health and well-being (Dutta, 2008). As Basu (2010) notes, examples of structures that influence health include available medical services, modes of transportation, communication channels, and health-enhancing resources (e.g., food, places to exercise, sanitary living conditions). Structures may also include avenues of civil society organizations and media platforms, as well as national and international political actors and health policies (Basu &

Dutta, 2008). These structural configurations, at all levels, often constrain the ability of marginalized populations to secure resources and engage in healthy practices (Basu, 2010; Dutta, 2008). *Agency* is defined as people's capacity to make sense of their cultural/structural realities and to work within these immediate contexts as they attempt to meet their own and their loved ones' health-related needs (Dutta, 2008).

In describing the CCA's orientation toward health disparities, Dutta (2008) argues that mainstream health communication approaches have traditionally operated within an expert-driven, top-down model to study health inequalities and to develop corresponding policies and programs to address them (see also, Airhihenbuwa, 1995, 2007; Dutta, Anaele, & Jones, 2013). Operating within this mainstream model, scholars and practitioners begin with a particular understanding of a population-specific health issue and simultaneously identify an intervention strategy to address it—typically a message-based communication program; hence, the affected populations' research participation is limited to that deemed appropriate by intervention (Dutta 2007; Dutta & Basu, 2011). This research (and the resulting intervention programs) frequently adopt a *cultural sensitivity* approach, wherein culture is understood as a static entity that acts a barrier to improved health and, therefore, must be addressed through the health communication (Dutta, 2007, 2008). Furthermore, the cultural sensitivity approach locates health issues at the individual level, and thus, offers solutions that promote individual-level behavior change rather than looking at the social and structural contexts of health experiences, as described by cultural members (Dutta & Basu, 2011).

In contrast to the mainstream, expert-driven model that defines much of health disparities scholarship in the communication discipline, the CCA is founded on "a respect for the capability of the members of marginalized communities to define their health needs and to seek out solutions that fulfill these needs" (Dutta, 2008, p. 56). Thus, scholarship grounded in the CCA privileges dialogic engagement, where those impacted by health disparities narrate their experiences in an open-ended, supportive environment (Dutta, 2008). Participants' voices are then introduced into the discursive spaces of health research and policy-making, where they have largely been absent or ignored (Dutta et al., 2013). While Dutta and Basu (2011) argue that "the very introduction of marginalized voices into the dominant [discourse]" is itself a form of social change (p. 331), studies informed by the CCA are also able to inform health-related praxis that aligns with the populations' stated needs by highlighting challenges and issues that are unlikely to emerge from research that is limited to extracting cultural characteristics to inform intervention strategies (Dutta, 2008; Dutta et al., 2013). In this chapter, for example, our analysis identifies a seemingly common dilemma among African American hospice patients and lay caregivers that has hitherto not been identified in the existing literature—that is, managing privacy concerns related to hospice enrollment. To elucidate our study's findings, in the following section we discuss the central assumptions of communication privacy management theory.

COMMUNICATION PRIVACY MANAGEMENT THEORY

Communication privacy management (CPM) theory is grounded in the assumption that people have the "right to own and regulate access to their private information" (Petronio, 2002, p. 2). CPM argues that concealing and disclosing private information is a communicative, rules-driven process; the theory employs a boundary metaphor to describe how individuals, dyads, families, and groups manage concealment and revelation practices (Petronio, 2002). It suggests that people (re)create boundaries around their private information that vary in permeability—ranging from completely permeable, wherein message about private information flow openly, to impermeable, where secrets are tightly held (Petronio, 2000).

CPM theory is organized around three primary constructs: privacy ownership, privacy control, and privacy turbulence (Petronio, 2013). *Privacy ownership* refers to the sense that people possess their private information, much like a tangible possession; thus, people can choose to provide access (in whole or in part) to the information or to keep it to themselves (Basinger, Wehrman, & McAninch, 2016; Petronio, 2002). Building from this sense of ownership, *privacy control* describes the communicative processes through which people guard their private information by implicitly or explicitly creating privacy rules pertaining to its revelation and concealment; privacy control also includes the ways people coordinate, maintain, and reconfigure privacy rules over time (Petronio, 2000, 2002). Finally, given that regulating access to private information can be challenging and unpredictable at times, people often experience *privacy turbulence*—that is, situations characterized by "breakdowns in privacy rule coordination or failures to uphold privacy expectations" (Basinger et al., 2016, p. 287; see also, Petronio, 2010). Petronio (2002) identifies several examples of privacy turbulence, ranging from intentional privacy rules violations to privacy dilemmas that occur when there are seemingly equal consequences associated with concealing and disclosing secret information.

People often develop rigid boundaries around private information that makes them vulnerable to symbolic and/or tangible consequences; this sense of vulnerability is "amplified in situations involving management of stigmatized information" (Bute & Brann, 2015, p. 26). Greene et al.'s (2012) Disclosure Decision-Making Model, for example, suggests that perceiving stigma is typically associated with decreased intentions to disclose health-related information but that this effect may be offset by other factors, such as antici-pated reactions and self-efficacy. Likewise, studies grounded in CPM have suggested that perceived stigma provides additional layers of complexity, which can influence the manner in which people develop and manage privacy boundaries (Basinger et al., 2016; Bute & Brann, 2015; Durham & Braith-waite, 2009; Steuber & Solomon, 2012). Many have argued that within the persistently death adverse culture of the United States, there is often a stigma attached to communicating about terminal illness, death, and loss (Basinger et al., 2016). Given its association with death and its palliative-focused care philosophy, hospice, too, is often stigmatized within the general US popula-tion (Connor, 2017); as noted above, studies have suggested that the stigma associated with hospice care is even more pronounced among African Ameri-cans (Campbell et al., 2010; Dillon & Basu, 2016a). However, to our knowl-edge, there are currently no published studies that have examined whether and how perceived stigma influences patients' and caregivers' conception of information about hospice care as private. Our first research question sought to address this issue:

RQ1: How do African American patients and lay caregivers describe ownership over private information pertaining to hospice care?

Although it is often associated with a single person, private information—including sensitive, potentially stigmatizing information—is frequently owned by multiple individuals. In such cases, the information is said to be *co-owned* "when multiple people claim control over a common issue, par-ticularly when the parties are highly invested in the issue" and/or in the case of shared experiences, where both parties bear responsibility for managing privacy boundaries (Bute & Brann, 2015, p. 26; see also, Durham & Braith-waite, 2009; Petronio, 2002; Steuber & Solomon, 2012). Petronio (2000, 2002) has acknowledged conditions of co-ownership since CPM's inception. Several scholars have argued, however, that privacy research has emphasized individual boundary management and disclosure decisions while largely ignoring how people collectively navigate privacy management practices—particularly as it relates to stigmatizing information (Bute & Brann, 2015; Steuber & Solomon, 2010, 2012). In response to the call for more research on how people collectively manage shared private information tied to a com-munal experience, our second and third research questions focused on how patients and lay caregivers develop and manage privacy rules pertaining to hospice enrollment:

RQ2: What rules do African American hospice patients and lay caregivers develop to manage private information pertaining to hospice enrollment?

RQ3: How do African American hospice patients and lay caregivers maintain and/or reconfigure privacy rules pertaining to hospice enrollment over time?

METHODS

Participants and Recruitment

This study involved African American patients and lay caregivers (i.e., family members and close friends) receiving hospice and/or bereavement services from a large palliative care organization located in a large city the southeast region of the United States. The Institutional Review Board approved the study and all participants provided written informed consent. We included caregivers for two important reasons: (1) hospice programs consider patients and caregivers (i.e., family members and close friends) the "unit of care" for their services, and (2) as noted above, caregivers are often the ultimate end-of-life decision makers for patients who are physically or mentally incapable of making their own care choices.

In partnership with the organization's research staff, we used an electronic medical record system to screen potential participants according to our inclusion criteria. For patients, the inclusion criteria included (1) self-identifying as African American, (2) speaking English, (3) scoring 80 percent on the Short Portable Mental Status Questionnaire, an established measure of cognitive functioning (see Pfeiffer, 1975). Caregivers were eligible to participate if they (1) served as the designated primary caregiver for a current or recently deceased (i.e., within six months of the study's start date) hospice patient, (2) were at least eighteen years of age (which was also a requirement to be a designated caregiver), and (3) spoke English. We also excluded caregivers whose loved one had died within sixty days of the study's start date as well as those who had not yet spoken to a bereavement specialist.

Twenty-six African American adults—ten patients and sixteen caregivers—volunteered to participate in the study. Six of the patients were male and four were female; they ranged in age from twenty-nine to eighty-one, with a mean age of 69.8 years. The patients' primary diagnoses were as follows: cancer ($n = 4$), heart disease ($n = 2$), lung disease ($n = 2$), kidney disease ($n = 1$), and AIDS ($n = 1$). Their time in hospice care ranged from 11 to 368 days ($M = 85$) at the time they took part in the study. All ten patients identified their religious affiliation as Christian/Protestant. By the end of time we completed the study, six of the patients were deceased, two had withdrawn from hospice, and two remained in hospice care.

The sixteen caregivers who took part in the study ranged in age from thirty-four to seventy-six years ($M = 46$). Nine were female and seven were male. They represented a range of relationships to patients, including being patients' children ($n = 7$), spouses ($n = 3$), nieces/nephews ($n = 3$), siblings ($n = 1$), friends ($n = 1$), and in-laws ($n = 1$). Three of the caregivers were connected to a patient who also participated in the study; the other thirteen caregivers were not connected to the patient sample. Fourteen of the caregivers reported their religious affiliation as Christian/Protestant; the other two caregivers stated that they were Catholics. Their loved one's time in hospice care ranged from 3 to 120 days ($M = 35$ days).

Data Collection and Analysis

The data presented here are drawn from a larger ethnographic study, which included in-depth interviews, participant-observation, and reflexive journal entries. In this chapter, we focus on the narratives that participants shared with us during the in-depth interviews. Following Riessmann (2008), we sought to "generate detailed accounts rather than brief answers or general statements" about participants' hospice experiences; hence, we followed a semi-structure interview protocol designed to focus the conversation on hospice care while also offering participants the flexibility to discuss the topic in ways that were consistent with their perspectives and priorities (see Lindlof & Taylor, 2011). As participants shared their stories, we used spontaneous probes to invite additional details and encourage further reflection. The majority of participants' chose to be interviewed at home ($n = 24$); we interviewed two participants in a private office at our partner organization's headquarters.

We conducted multiple interviews with seven participants. Among the patients, Leroy and Jane took part in three interviews each while Charles participated in four. Two primary caregivers, Carla and Richard, invited me to interview them three times, and Bridget and Robert took part in two interviews. The interviews lasted between approximately fifteen minutes and three hours, with a mean interview time of approximately thirty-seven minutes. All interviews were audio-recorded and transcribed verbatim.

We began the data analysis process concurrently with conducting the interviews. Our initial analysis was informed by constructivist grounded theory; we followed the general steps outlined by Charmaz (2006): coding data, developing inductive categories, revising the categories, writing memos to explore preliminary ideas, comparing data to existing literature, fitting data into new and existing categories, identifying where data did not fit, and revising the categories. Throughout the simultaneous processes of interviewing, transcription, and analysis, we met regularly (every two to three weeks) over a six-month period to discuss newly available data and to refine our initial thematic categories. This concurrent data collection and analysis process also allowed us to discuss emerging themes and ideas with participants during subsequent interviews and informal interactions, a process akin to "member checking" (Lincoln & Guba, 1985).

Early in the data analysis process, we recognized that participants were frequently identifying privacy concerns and privacy management practices as an important aspect of their experiences with hospice care. Hence, as the data collection process continued, we began explicitly inquiring about these issues in subsequent interviews. As we continued our analysis, we also started isolating excerpts from the interviews that pertained to privacy issues related to hospice enrollment; we then analyzed these excerpts from the standpoint of CPM theory, using its central constructs—that is, privacy ownership, privacy control, privacy turbulence—as "sensitizing concepts" (Bowen, 2006) to inform the creation of the thematic categories described in this chapter (Bute & Brann, 2015).

FINDINGS

Our findings suggest that patients and lay caregivers conceptualized information about hospice enrollment as private and established collective rules for managing the information accordingly. These privacy rules were generally effective in helping participants regulate access to information about hospice; however, as time passed and circumstances shifted, some participants described altering their concealment and disclosure practices as they increasingly became informal advocates for hospice care within their social networks.

Privacy Ownership: Hospice Enrollment and Social Risk

Participants overwhelmingly indicated that information about hospice enrollment belonged to them/their families and that their collective privacy was a major consideration in decisions to share (or not share) the information with others. Participants' sense of ownership was evident in their linguistic choices—as they frequently used terms and possessive pronouns which suggested that they possessed the information (see Basinger et al., 2016). For example, Robert (caregiver) told us, "For me, it's like, it's our story to tell. Why would we feel like we need to tell people that she's [his aunt] with hospice unless we decide they need to know?"

Consistent with Robert's description, participants frequently identified hospice enrollment as a shared experience; for instance, Mandy (patient) explained, "The hospice people keep saying this is our experience … and I feel that same way. It's not just me. We're all going through this thing."

In framing hospice enrollment as a collective experience, participants also emphasized that private information was thus co-owned by the patient and their immediate caregiver(s). They did so, as in Mandy's statement, by using a collective "we" when discussing it but also by noting the collective nature of disclosure decisions. Milton (caregiver) described it this way: "Keisha [Milton's wife] and her auntie [a hospice patient], we're like a tight circle and we have to be careful about bringing other people in … so we try to decide when to tell people together."

In addition to characterizing hospice enrollment as private, co-owned information, participants also explained why, in Milton's words, they needed to be "careful" about sharing it with other people, particularly other African Americans. Participants noted that they were protective of this information because they feared being "judged," "stigmatized," or "shunned" by others—fears that Richard (caregiver) collectively referred to as *social risks*: "I remember one of my neighbors telling me that 'hospice is like killing your parent'. You realize real quick that it's risky, like socially, to talk about it with people."

As participants discussed these risks, they generally fell into two distinct categories: (1) those who had been exposed to negative information about hospice care prior to their own experiences and (2) those who did not know about these negative associations until after they or a loved one enrolled. Mandy (patient) fell into the former category; she remembered other members of her church equating hospice care with suicide:

I remember hearing people at church saying that hospice was like some Dr. Kevorkian stuff. They said it was no better than suicide and that God wouldn't forgive you for it. It stuck with me for the longest time and made it harder to decide [hospice] was what we should … I knew that we'd have to be careful telling people.

Those in the latter category were often taken aback by others' negative reactions. For example, Milton (caregiver) recalled that a friend stopped speaking to him after saying that he and his wife were "just leaving [her aunt] to die." Similarly, Roger (caregiver) told us how his brother had become estranged from Roger's family after disagreeing with the decision to enroll their mother in hospice care:

He would only come visit Mom when nobody else was there … and he kept trying to convince her we were doing something wrong. He kept telling her, "Don't let them make you give up." When she passed, we had to beg him to even come out to the funeral.

In either case, participants frequently noted that they wished someone within the health system had prepared or reminded them to exercise caution in sharing information about hospice care. "I think somebody should say something like, 'Look some people might not react so good to this so be ready for that.' The doctor, the social worker, none of them said that," Belle said.

Privacy Rules: Developing and Enacting Disclosure Strategies

Whether the social risks and negative experiences associated with hospice were anticipated or unexpected, participants described addressing them by developing privacy rules to regulate disclosing information about it to others. Consistent with their conception of information pertaining to hospice enrollment as co-owned by patients and their immediate caregivers, participants largely described developing these privacy rules as a joint exercise. Kevin (patient) told us, for example: "We had kind of thought that, if we are going to do this hospice thing together, we needed to make some agreements about who we'd tell about it and what we were going to say to them."

Given the collective nature of the process, participants noted that developing the privacy rules around hospice was an explicit process—often developed through informal "family meetings" or created by some combination of patients and caregivers to be shared with others who co-owned the information. For instance, Keisha (caregiver) explained how, after Milton's negative interaction with his friend (described in the previous section), she and her aunt had discussed when and how they would share information about hospice with others; she said: "My auntie and me, we just talked it out. It was like, should we tell these people or these people? When do we tell them? When do we not? Stuff like that … So we talked it out and then I told [Milton] later on."

While those like Keisha and Milton developed privacy rules in reaction to specific encounters, those who anticipated negative reactions typically developed privacy rules as a precautionary measure.

Although they highlighted the collective nature of their hospice experiences, both patients and caregivers noted that such experiences were not only shared but also unique. In particular, participants were quick to emphasize that only the patients were experiencing the physical deterioration associated with terminal illness and the unique emotional/spiritual experiences of (potentially) approaching the end of life. Thus, whenever possible, participants recounted trying to privilege patients' preferences when making privacy management decisions. For example, Katherine (patient) stated:

> I didn't want them telling anybody about [hospice]. I mean it's nobody's business what I'm doing or who I got caring for me. After a while though, it got to where I knew people was wondering what was going on so I kind of told them it was okay to let certain people know … I'm glad they let me decide though; it's my life.

At the same time, however, participants also noted that the caregivers were more likely to come into contact with other people while the patient was receiving hospice care and, ultimately, after the patient's death, which led them to focus primarily on privacy strategies specific to caregivers. As Robert (caregiver) said, "We wanted to say what [my aunt] wanted us to, but we knew we were the ones who was gonna have to talk about it. I mean, she wasn't even leaving the house at that point."

In terms of the specific strategies that participants enacted, their privacy management practices generally fell into three categories: (1) avoidance, (2) testing the waters, and (3) cover stories. The first, and most popular, privacy management strategy was *avoidance*, which involved concealing all information pertaining to hospice care from other people. In many cases, it also meant actively avoiding other people so as not to have to risk discussing it; Richard (caregiver) described it this way:

> With what we'd heard about hospice, it was difficult to decide if we should tell anybody that Ma was getting services from them. I mean, you find yourself in this situation and you start worrying about her reputation, the reputation of the family. So, we kind of like closed ranks; we had this talk where it was like the hospice thing is on a need-to-know basis with everyone ... We just avoided talking about it and pretty much avoided other people. I was just going to work, taking care of Ma, and that's it.

While this was the most cited privacy management strategy, there were instances where participants described wanting and/or needing to disclose information about hospice to others.

When disclosing information about hospice care to others, participants largely relied on a strategy that Belle (caregiver) labeled *testing the waters*. She described it this way:

> I remember that we'd start bringing up hospice in conversation but not relating it to my dad. I'd mention to a neighbor that this guy I worked with mentioned his dad was in hospice. It wasn't true but I had to see how that person was going to react before I talked about Dad being in hospice ... I was testing the waters.

As Belle described in the example above, this practice involved attempts to ascertain other people's attitudes toward hospice without directly implicating themselves or their loved ones. Participants also described using this strategy as a starting point for "priming" (Bridget, caregiver) the other person for a later (or potential) disclosure; she explained: "Before we'd even made the final decision, we started telling people that the doctors had brought up hospice. And we'd like explain what it was and just try to nullify whatever misinformation they had about it."

Participants also described using *cover stories* to conceal and/or explain information that might compromise their or their loved one's hospice enroll-ment status. For example, when Julia's (caregiver) mother moved in with her and her husband Carl (caregiver) to begin hospice care, Julia told their neigh-bors that her mother "just needed a little extra help while recovering from surgery" in order to avoid mentioning hospice. Bridget (caregiver) explained that she was motivated to use a cover story when her mother started receiv-ing hospice care after hearing about a good friend's experience. She told us: "People start seeing these people coming in and out the house, wearing nurses' clothes, so her neighbors start asking. ... [She] tells them that it is her cousin, who is a nurse, just coming to visit." Bridget's family ended up using a similar tactic; however, rather than answer questions about who the hospice workers were and why they were at home, she sought to conceal their arrival. "I didn't want a bunch of people knowing my business, so I had asked the hospice people to park one street over and then come in through the back. I could [figure] they didn't like it but they went along," she told us. When one of her neighbors inquired about a person entering the home through the backdoor, Bridget explained that it was person coming to let her dog outside.

Privacy Rules: Changes over Time

In the immediate aftermath of a terminal diagnosis and the decision to enroll in hospice care, participants were (as noted above) initially motivated to protect themselves against social risks associated with hospice by develop-ing and holding to a set of privacy management strategies. However, as time passed, some participants described altering their privacy practices and being more open about discussing hospice care with others, particularly other Afri-can Americans. For patients, the increased willingness to share information about hospice care emanated from their own positive experiences and a desire for others to benefit from hospice services. Charles (patient), for example, recounted how he suggested that his neighbor ask her doctor if she would qualify for hospice care:

> I seen [Mary], that's that lady who live next door, wasn't getting on too well either. I knew she had heart disease, just like me. I thought they could probably do the same stuff they doing for me. So, I go and talk to her about [hospice], how they been helping me get by. I say, 'Next time you go, just ask your doctor about it.' She says she didn't know if she should, but I said 'What could it hurt?' So now when [the hospice workers] come see me, they go see her, too.

In addition to suggesting how others could benefit from hospice, patients also described their efforts to address misconceptions about hospice by allowing others to witness hospice care firsthand. For instance, Mandy (patient) recalled inviting others to come and visit her when she knew a hospice nurse or nurse's aide would be at her home:

> It was amazing to see how they perception shifted. I think it was because they saw how loving and caring these people was to me. People like my nurse, [Jackie], come in and say, "Hi Ms. [Mandy], how you feeling?" and then she's helping with my pills and all those things. And my friends say, "Wow. I didn't know this was what hospice did."

Others, like Betty (patient), described similar reactions to others seeing hospice providers visit their homes. She invited some friends to participate in an informal Bible-study meeting that she participated in with a Quest chaplain. "My friends were surprised, in a good way. They didn't know about the spiritual part, and I think it changed their thoughts about it," she told us. As they discussed their increased willingness to share their hospice experience, patients often described it as a form of activism. "Black people, African American people we tend to look out for others like us, and I think telling people about the good of hospice is another way to do that," Charles stated.

Several caregivers described a similar progression from initially wanting to conceal information about hospice care to attempting to "spread the word about it to members of their social network"; Milton (caregiver) stated, for example: "I think it is important to spread the word about hospice, to let others know what it can do for you, so I've taken some ownership for that." As with the patients, caregivers' willingness to share information about hospice care was linked to their positive experiences with this form of care. Geraldine (caregiver) explained:

> As we got started with [hospice] and it was just so wonderful, I knew what I needed to do to pull that curtain up, or whatever it is, so that people realize that it's something that can help you and that person who is needing that service, your loved one that you are trying to help, that this is a better way of doing it.

Other caregivers described similar experiences of advocating for hospice care by encouraging others to inquire about hospice services, providing information about hospice, and inviting others to come and witness hospice care firsthand. Taken together, participants described advocating for hospice care in these ways as a means of lessening the social risks they perceived and/or experienced for those considering hospice care in the future. For example, Keisha (caregiver) said: "People sometimes assume the worst about things, especially something like hospice, where they have no knowledge of it ... I take it as an opportunity to make sure more people know what hospice has to offer. Not everybody is going to accept [it], but there is people who will if they know more."

DISCUSSION

The goal of this study was to examine the lived experiences of African American hospice patients and lay caregivers through the dual lens of the Culture-Centered Approach (CCA) and Communication Privacy Management (CPM) theory. More specifically, our analysis focuses on identifying (1) how patients and caregivers conceptualized private information about hospice enrollment, (2) what rules they developed to manage this private information, and (3) whether these privacy management practices shifted over time.

Our findings indicate that patients and caregivers largely conceptualize hospice enrollment as private information that is co-owned by patients and their immediate caregivers; they further note that keeping the information private is necessitated by the "social risks" associated with hospice care in their interactions with other African Americans. As noted in the introduction, existing studies highlight the ways insufficient knowledge and perceived cultural incongruencies contribute to the stigma attached to hospice care among African Americans (see, for example, Bullock, 2011; Cagle et al., 2016; Dillon & Basu, 2016a). However, to our knowledge, this is the first study to document how African American patients and caregivers who choose hospice care experience and respond to the relational consequences that emanate from this stigma through the use of privacy management practices. In doing so, this study lends additional empirical support to the assertion that perceived stigma is a key factor in concealment/disclosure practices pertaining to health-related information (Greene et al., 2012; Petronio, 2000) and extends it to a new care context.

This study also addresses the need for additional research regarding how people manage the co-ownership of private information (Bute & Brann, 2015; Steuber & Solomon, 2010, 2012). Our analysis suggests that patients and caregivers work together to develop shared privacy management strategies; despite the collective nature of this process, however, participants frequently describe designating patients as the primary owners of the private information and thus privileging their preferences in developing/enacting privacy rules. Bute and Brann (2015) identified a similar trend in their study of how romantic couples manage private information about pregnancy loss; they label this practice *embodied ownership*, which they define as "the ways that co-owners of private information defer to the owner who embodied the experience central to the private information at hand" (p. 37). Ultimately, this finding provides additional support to Petronio's (2002) claim that co-ownership of private information does not necessarily imply equal ownership of that information; hence, certain people may have greater control of when and how co-owned information is shared (see also Bute & Brann, 2015).

Our findings also provide insights into the range of privacy management practices that patients and caregivers develop around information pertaining to hospice enrollment. From the standpoint of the CCA, these privacy practices exemplify participants' agentive capacity to develop sophisticated communicative strategies that are responsive to and allow them to function within their cultural and structural environments (Dutta, 2008, 2012; Dutta et al., 2013). At the same time, participants' descriptions of their privacy management practices also allude to some of the practical implications of this work. For one, the commonality of the experiences that necessitated such practices suggests that the social risks associated with hospice care, as well as how to manage such risks, should be a point of discussion as health-care providers help patients/caregivers make decisions about hospice enrollment. Extant research suggests that health-care providers often struggle to provide patients and their loved ones with a holistic sense of their end-of-life care options and/or to adequately prepare them for the varied experiences that might accompany specific options (Roscoe, Tullis, Reich, McCaffrey, 2013). In recent years, provider training programs focusing specifically on improving communication about palliative and end-of-life care have demonstrated promising results (Rucker & Browning, 2015; Smith, O'Sullivan, Lo, & Chen, 2013); however, to this point, these training programs have focused on issues such as available care services, advance directives, prognosis, brain death, and withdrawal of life support (Rucker & Browning, 2015). The narratives presented in this chapter suggest that these training programs—and the subsequent conversations—should also address the larger social context where end-of-life care decisions are made.

Another noteworthy finding from this analysis was participants' progression from protecting information about hospice care to actively promoting it within their social network—a practice we describe elsewhere as a form "relational health advocacy" (Dillon & Basu, 2016b). A similar trend was identified by Webel and Higgins (2012) among a sample of African American women living with HIV; the authors discovered that—as the women came to accept their diagnosis over time—they increasingly inhabited (and identified with) the social role of "advocate," as they engaged in formal and informal efforts to promote awareness of HIV risk behaviors and available health services. Like the women in Webel and Higgins (2012) study, patients and caregivers' narratives demonstrate their agency—in enacting local, practical solutions to respond their health-related circumstances and simultaneously address a marker of health disparity (Dutta et al., 2013). Participants' first-hand understanding of the challenges associated with hospice enrollment and their willingness to share their experiences support the use of role model stories to promote hospice enrollment (see Enguidanos et al., 2011). However, rather than focusing exclusively on message-based approaches (Rhodes et al., 2017), participants' stories also suggest that hospice organizations should identify ways to formalize relational forms of hospice advocacy—perhaps through a peer health worker program (see Dillon & Basu, 2016b; Rosenthal et al., 2010).

Beyond the need to explore alternative mechanisms for disseminating information about hospice care to those who may qualify for it (and their loved ones), the social risks identified in this study indicate a need for broader outreach efforts aimed at promoting increased knowledge and wider acceptance of hospice care—within the African American population and beyond. A recent cross-sectional study by Cagle et al. (2016) identified a number of misconceptions about hospice care among the study participants. The authors also noted that participants' knowledge of hospice—which was highest among those who were more educated, worked in the medical field, were non-Hispanic—was associated with their attitudes toward it. Patients and caregivers do not make end-of-life care decisions in isolation; they make them within sociocultural environments that influence their initial choices and their subsequent experiences with hospice care. By ensuring that the wider populations that inhabit these same sociocultural environments are more educated about hospice care, scholars and practitioners can potentially lessen the misconceptions and stigma that make these experiences more difficult than they need to be (Cagle et al., 2016; Dillon & Basu, 2016b).

CONCLUSION

This study was limited by our use of a convenience sample in two specific ways. First, in the majority of cases, we were only able to interview one of the people who co-owned and managed private information about hospice care. Future studies should follow Bute and Brann (2015) by including all participants who are considered to be co-owners of private information. Second, the patients and caregivers who volunteered to participate in this study were overwhelmingly satisfied with their hospice experiences. Future studies should attempt to include a broader sample of hospice patients and caregivers, including those who were dissatisfied with their care in order to ascertain how it impacts how they manage information about hospice care.

Participants in this study also indicated that they were able to reach a consensus on how to manage shared information about hospice care and described largely adhering to their established privacy rules. Future studies should examine what happens when patients and caregivers do not agree on privacy rules and/or when one or more people violate the privacy rules—that is, experience what Petronio (2002) describes as boundary turbulence. Future research should also focus on developing programs and intervention materials to address the practical issues identified here (i.e., training providers to discuss social risks associated with hospice, promoting greater awareness about hospice). There is a vast body of research focusing on hospice enrollment among African Americans, but—to our knowledge—there are currently no interventions that have demonstrated the ability to increase hospice enrollment or improve hospice experiences among this population.

Despite its limitations, this study provides novel insights regarding how African American patients and lay caregivers manage the "communicative dilemma" of concealing and revealing information about hospice care. Our findings suggest that these patients and caregivers experience and/or anticipate social risks associated with hospice enrollment and develop shared privacy rules to regulate the disclosure of information pertaining to hospice. Over time, however, many patients and caregivers shift from concealing information about hospice care to explicitly advocating for this form of care within their social network. We look forward to seeing how other scholars and practitioners build upon this research in the future.

REFERENCES

Airhihenbuwa, C. O. (1995). *Health and culture: Beyond the Western paradigm.* Thousand Oaks, CA: Sage.

Airhihenbuwa, C. O. (2007). *Healing our differences: The crisis of global health and the politics of identity.* Lanham, MD: Rowman & Littlefield.

Anderson, K. O., Green, C. R., & Payne, R. (2009). Racial and ethnic disparities in pain: Causes and consequences of unequal care. *The Journal of Pain, 10*(12), 1187–1204. doi: 10.1016/j.jpain.2009.10.002.

Basinger, E. D., Wehrman, E. C., & McAninch, K. G. (2016). Grief communication and privacy rules: Examining the communication of individuals bereaved by the death of a family member. *Journal of Family Communication, 16*(4), 285–302. doi: 10.1080/15267431.2016.1182534.

Basu, A. (2010). Communicating health as an impossibility: Sex work, HIV/AIDS, and the dance of hope and hopelessness. *Southern Communication Journal, 75,* 413–432. doi: 10.1080/1041794x.2010.504452.

Basu, A., & Dutta, M. J. (2008). Participatory change in a campaign led by sex workers: Connecting resistance to action-oriented agency. *Qualitative Health Research, 18,* 106–119. doi: 10.1177/1049732307309373.

Bowen, G. A. (2006). Grounded theory and sensitizing concepts. *International Journal of Qualitative Methods, 5*(3), 1–9.

Bullock, K. (2011). The influence of culture on end-of-life decision making. *Journal of Social Work in End-Of-Life & Palliative Care, 7*(1), 83–98. doi: 10.1080/15524256.2011.548048.

Bute, J. J., & Brann, M. (2015). Co-ownership of private information in the miscarriage context. *Journal of Applied Communication Research, 43*, 23–43. doi: 10.1080/00909882.2014.982686.

Cagle, J. G., Van Dussen, D. J., Culler, K. L., Carrion, I., Hong, S., Guralnik, J., & Zimmerman, S. (2016). Knowledge about hospice: Exploring misconceptions, attitudes, and preferences for care. *American Journal of Hospice and Palliative Medicine, 33*(1), 27–33. doi: 10.1177/1049909114546885.

Campbell, C. L., Williams, I. C., & Orr, T. (2010). Factors that impact end-of-life decisions making in African Americans with advanced cancer. *Journal of Hospice & Palliative Nursing, 12*, 214–224. doi: 10.1016/j.jpainsymman.2010.10.189.

Centers for Medicare & Medicaid Services. (2008). Hospice conditions of participation final rule. Retrieved from: http://edocket.access.gpo.gov/2008/pdf/08-1305.pdf.

Charmaz, K. (2006). *Constructing grounded theory: A practical guide through qualitative analysis*. London: Sage.

Connor, S. R. (2017). *Hospice and palliative care: The essential guide* (3rd ed.). New York: Routledge.

Dillon, P. J., & Basu, A. (2016a). African Americans and hospice care: A culture-centered exploration of enrollment disparities. *Health Communication, 31*(11), 1385–1394. doi: 10.1080/10410236.2015.1072886.

Dillon, P. J., & Basu, A. (2016b). Toward eliminating hospice enrollment disparities among African Americans: A qualitative study. *Journal of Health Care for the Poor and Underserved, 27*, 219–237. doi: 10.1353/hpu.2016.0014.

Dillon, P. J., & Roscoe, L. A. (2015). African Americans and hospice care: A narrative analysis. *Narrative Inquiry in Bioethics, 5*, 151–165. doi: 10.1353/nib.2015.0049.

Dillon, P. J., Roscoe, L. A., & Jenkins, J. J. (2012). African Americans and decisions about hospice care: Implications for health message design. *Howard Journal of Communications, 23*, 175–193. doi: 10.1080/10646175.2012.667724.

Durham, W., & Braithwaite, D. O. (2009). Communication privacy management within the family planning trajectories of voluntarily child-free couples. *Journal of Family Communication, 9*, 43–65. doi: 10.1080/15267430802561600.

Dutta, M. (2008). *Communicating health: A culture-centered approach*. Cambridge, UK: Polity Press.

Dutta, M. J. (2012). Hunger as health: Culture-centered interrogations of alternative rationalities of health. *Communication Monographs, 79*, 366–384. doi: 10.1080/03637751.2012.697632.

Dutta, M. J., Anaele, A., & Jones, C. (2013). Voices of hunger: Addressing health disparities through the culture-centered approach. *Journal of Communication, 63*, 159–180. doi: 10.1111/jcom.12009.

Dutta, M. J., & Basu, A. (2011). Culture, communication, and health: A guiding framework. In T. L. Thompson, R. Parrott, & J. F. Nussbaum (Eds.), *The Routledge handbook of health communication* (2nd ed., pp. 320–334). New York: Routledge.

Enguidanos, S., Kogan, A. C., Lorenz, K., & Taylor, G. (2011). Use of role model stories to overcome barriers to hospice among African Americans. *Journal of Palliative Medicine, 14*(2), 161–168. doi: 10.1089/jpm.2010.0380.

Greene, K., Magsamen-Conrad, K., Venetis, M. K., Checton, M. G., Bagdasarov, Z., & Banerjee, S. C. (2012). Assessing health diagnosis disclose decisions in relationships: Testing the disclosure decision-making model. *Health Communication, 27*, 356–368. doi: 10.1080/ 10410236.2011.586988.

Hanchate, A., Kronman, A. C., Young-Xu, Y., Ash, A. S., & Emanuel E. (2009). Racial and ethnic differences in end-of-life costs: Why do minorities cost more than whites? *Archives of Internal Medicine, 169*, 493–501. doi: 10.1001/ archinternmed.2008.616.

Hendricks Sloan, D., Peters, T., Johnson, K. S., Bowie, J. V., Ting, Y., & Aslakson, R. (2016). Church-based health promotion focused on advance care planning and end-of-life care at Black Baptist churches: A cross-sectional survey. *Journal of Palliative Medicine, 19*(2), 190–194. doi: 10.1089/jpm.2015.0319.

Lincoln, Y. S, & Guba, E. A. (1985). *Naturalistic inquiry.* Beverly Hills, CA: Sage.

Lindlof, T. R., & Taylor, B. C. (2011). *Qualitative communication research methods* (3rd ed.). Thousand Oaks, CA: Sage.

Melhado, L., & Bushy, A. (2011). Exploring uncertainty in advance care planning in African Americans: Does low health literacy influence decision making preference at end of life. *American Journal of Hospice & Palliative Medicine, 28,* 495–500. doi: 10.1177/1049909110398005.

National Hospice and Palliative Care Organization. (2018). *NHPCO facts and figures: Hospice care in America.* Retrieved from: www.nhpco.org/sites/default/files/ public/Statistics_Research/2017_Facts_Figures.pdf.

Noh, H., & Schroepfer, T. (2015). Terminally ill African American elders' access to and use of hospice care. *American Journal of Hospice & Palliative Care, 32,* 286–297. doi: 10.1177/1049909113518092.

Petronio, S. (2000). The boundaries of privacy: Praxis of everyday life. In S. Petronio (Ed.), *Balancing the secrets of private disclosures* (pp. 37–50). Mahwah, NJ: Lawrence Erlbaum.

Petronio, S. (2002). *Boundaries of privacy: Dialectics of disclosure.* Albany, NY: State University of New York Press.

Petronio, S. (2013). Brief status report on communication privacy management theory. *Journal of Family Communication, 13,* 6–14. doi: 10.1080/15267431.2013.743426.

Pfeiffer, E. (1975). A short portable mental status questionnaire for the assessment of organic brain deficit in elderly patients. *Journal of American Geriatrics Society, 23,* 433–441. doi: 10.1111/j.1532-5415.1975.tb00927.

Rhodes, R. L., Elwood, B., Lee, S. C., Tiro, J. A., Halm, E. A., & Skinner, C. S. (2017). The desires of their hearts: The multidisciplinary perspectives of African Americans on end-of-life care in the African American community. *American Journal of Hospice and Palliative Medicine, 34*(6), 510–517. doi: 10.1177/ 1049909116631776.

Riessman, C. K. (2008). *Narrative methods for the human sciences.* Thousand Oaks, CA: Sage.

Roscoe, L. A., Tullis, J. A., Reich, R. R., & McCaffrey, J. C. (2013). Beyond good intentions and patient perceptions: Competing definitions of effective communication in head and neck cancer care at the end of life. *Health Communication, 28,* 183–192. doi: 10.1080/10410236.2012.666957.

Rosenthal, E. L., Brownstein, J. N., Rush, C. H, ... Fox, D. J. (2010). Community health workers: Part of the solution. *Health Affairs, 29,* 1338–1342. doi: 10.1377/hlthaff.2010.0081.

Rucker, B., & Browning, D. M. (2015). Practicing end-of-life conversations: Physician communication training program in palliative care. *Journal of Social Work in End-of-Life & Palliative Care, 11*(2), 132–146. doi: 10.1080/15524256.2015.1074140.

Smith, L., O'Sullivan, P., Lo, B., & Chen, H. (2013). An educational intervention to improve resident comfort with communication at the end of life. *Journal of Palliative Medicine, 16*(1), 54–59. doi: 10.1089/jpm.2012.0173.

Steuber, K. R., & Solomon, D. H. (2010). "So, when are you two having a baby?" Managing information about infertility within social networks. In M. Miller-Day (Ed.), *Family communication, connections, and health transitions: Going through this together* (pp. 297–322). New York, NY: Peter Lang.

Steuber, K. R., & Solomon, D. H. (2012). Relational uncertainty, partner interference, and privacy boundary turbulence: Explaining spousal discrepancies in infertility disclosures. *Journal of Social and Personal Relationships, 29,* 3–27. doi: 10.1177/0265407511406896.

Taylor Jr., D. H., Ostermann, J., Van Houtven, C. H., Tulsky, J. A., & Steinhauser, K. (2007). What length of hospice use maximizes reduction in medical expenditures near death in the US Medicare program? *Social Science & Medicine, 65*(7), 1466–1478. doi: 10.1377/hlthaff.2012.0851.

Taxis, J. C. (2006). Attitudes, values, and questions of African Americans regarding participation in hospice programs. *Journal of Hospice & Palliative Nursing, 8,* 77–85. doi: 10.1097/00129191-200603000-00011.

Webel, A. R., & Higgins, P. A. (2012). The relationship between social roles and self-management behavior in women living with HIV/AIDS. *Women's Health Issues, 22*(1), e27–e33. doi: 10.1016/j.whi.2011.05.010.

Chapter 6

"Can You Please Direct Me to a Doctor That Has a Heart?"

A Stage IV Breast Cancer Patient Narrative

Andrea L. Meluch

It was a sunny morning in June, the first time I met Riley Jackson.[1] I was working with a nonprofit organization that provided cancer wellness services to adults diagnosed with cancer, and I was recruiting participants for my research. I was interested in the experiences of people diagnosed with cancer who used the services and resources offered at this center (see Meluch, 2016). Clients who chose to participate in my study were interviewed to better understand their experiences at the cancer wellness organization, with their family members, and with their health-care providers following their diagnoses.

I had come to the center that morning to give a short presentation about my study and recruit potential participants from one of the center's weekly yoga classes. The yoga class was held in a large multipurpose room. About twenty women had spread out their yoga mats around the room and were busy chatting when I was introduced by the yoga instructor. I explained to the class the purpose of my study, how the interviews would take place, that participants would receive a $20 gift card to a local grocery store for their time, and that my study had been approved by my university's institutional review board. After I finished speaking, several of the participants decided to give me their phone numbers and email addresses to be interviewed. I first noticed Riley when she gave me her contact information. She did not say much to me when she signed up and I left immediately afterwards so that their yoga class could start. Later I met Riley on several occasions and interviewed her about her experiences being diagnosed with, and treated for, breast cancer.

Riley Jackson is a thirty-four-year-old wife and mother diagnosed with stage IV breast cancer. Riley's breast cancer was repeatedly misdiagnosed by physicians after she found a lump in her breast and had it examined. Riley's husband was unemployed at the time of her diagnosis, and she and her family were living with her aunt and uncle because they could not afford to pay for rent on their own. This chapter tells Riley's life narrative, using her own words, leading up to and through her cancer journey. First, relevant literature will be summarized to help situate Riley's story within a wider understanding of the ways that health-care providers interact with individuals of low socioeconomic status. Second, Riley's upbringing and young adulthood will be discussed. Last, the chapter will describe Riley's various medical upheavals, including repeatedly being misdiagnosed, and her perceptions of the health-care system. Riley's narrative is one that recounts perceptions of being failed by health-care providers and her search for a correct diagnosis and proper care, despite limited financial resources.

SOCIOECONOMIC DISPARITIES AND CANCER

In the United States, many individuals experience health disparities due to gender, race, age, geographical region, ability, and socioeconomic status (Adler & Rehkopf, 2008). These health disparities can manifest in reduced access to preventive medicine (e.g., mammograms, pap smears), higher rates of chronic conditions (e.g., cancer, diabetes), and poorer health outcomes (e.g., quality of life, survival rate). Those who experience health disparities often do so because of their intersectionality (e.g., combinations of identity factors, such as race, socioeconomic status, and gender) and, thus, multiple social categorizations are often considered when examining health disparities (Adler & Rehkopf, 2008; van Ryn & Burke, 2000). Socioeconomic status is determined by one's income, educational background, and occupation (American Psychological Association, 2018). Individuals who have limited financial resources lack educational credentials, and/or are unemployed or are employed as unskilled laborers, may be considered to have low socioeconomic status.

Health communication scholars have found marked differences in provider-patient communication between patients from disadvantaged socioeconomic classes when compared to wealthier segments of the patient population (Ndiaye, Krieger, Warren, & Hecht, 2011; Willems, De Maesschalck, Deveugele, Derese, & Maexeneer, 2005). For example, in their systematic review of original research articles and meta-analyses examining patient socioeconomic status and doctor-patient communication, Willems et al. (2005) found that patients from more disadvantaged socioeconomic classes receive a more direct consulting style when interacting with their physicians. Further, Willems et al.'s analysis also found that patients of lower socioeconomic status receive less information regarding their medical conditions from their physicians when compared to patients with a higher socioeconomic status.

Physician-patient communication is interactive and, as such, patient communication style influences physician communication. However, patients of lower socioeconomic status are often less likely to actively participate in the medical encounter, which in turn influences how physicians communicate with them. Willems et al. (2005) note:

> Patients from a lower social class and doctors often find themselves in a vicious circle. These patients' communication and actions (e.g. less question asking, less opinion giving, less affective expressiveness, less preference for decision making) elicit a less involving behaviour [*sic*] from the doctor, with less partnership building utterances, which discourages the patient to adopt a more active communication style. (p. 143)

Thus, patients from lower social classes often do not experience the same interactions with physicians that patients with a higher median income do because physicians often misperceive the meaning of patients' passive behaviors. However, such physician perceptions are not accurate because patients from lower social classes are concerned about their health and health-care and often want to participate in the conversation. Physicians beliefs about patients' perceived lack of engagement in medical encounters are especially problematic when the patient is diagnosed with cancer or another serious illness.

Cancer diagnoses and mortality rates vary by age, race, sex, and class (DeSantis, Ma, Sauer, Newman, & Jemal, 2017). Breast cancer diagnoses continue to be the most common cancer diagnosis among women and are the second leading cause of cancer deaths in women, following lung cancer (American Cancer Society, 2018). Breast cancer diagnoses are more common among African American women when compared to other races and have increased slightly in recent years (American Cancer Society, 2018). Socioeconomics are a key factor influencing differences in cancer diagnoses (i.e., stage of cancer at diagnosis) and aggressiveness in treatment decisions among people diagnosed with cancer (Siegel, Ma, Zou, & Jemal, 2014; Wells & Horm, 1992). Researchers have found that lower median income and education are key indicators of diagnosis at later cancer stages (Wells & Horm, 1992) and are also associated with lower survival rates (Bradley, Given, & Roberts, 2002).

Socioeconomic status can influence physician-patient communication and medical treatment for women diagnosed with breast cancer (Maly, Liu, Leake, Thind, & Diamant, 2010; Mills et al., 2006; Royak-Schaler et al., 2008). For example, Maly et al. (2010) found that cancer patients of color from lower socioeconomic statuses were less likely to discuss their symptoms (e.g., pain, depression) with physicians and, thus, did not receive the same symptom resolution as white women from higher socioeconomic statuses. Similarly, in their systematic review, Mills et al. (2006) found that socioeconomic status is a barrier for cancer patients to be included in clinical trials and, thus, these patients were less likely to experience health benefits due to participation in clinical trials. Health disparities affecting people diagnosed with cancer continue to be a pressing concern for researchers and health-care practitioners.

RILEY'S NARRATIVE

The following sections show Riley's narration of her upbringing, early adulthood, challenges related to receiving a correct diagnosis, and concerns following her diagnosis and cancer treatment. Riley's experience highlights the health disparities that many women in the United States face because of their socioeconomic status and lack of structural support. Further, Riley's interactions within the health-care system reflect the issues that people from a lower socioeconomic status face when interacting with physicians (e.g., direct consulting style). Struggles to receive adequate care for individuals from lower socioeconomic classes are well documented and often lead to delayed and more aggressive cancer diagnoses, as Riley's narrative demonstrates.

Riley's Adolescence and Early Adulthood

When Riley sat down for her first interview session she was very open when telling her story to me. The first question I asked her was, "So tell me a little bit about you, just some background information." Riley responded to this question by telling me about her upbringing and early adulthood. Her story ended up taking the better part of the initial interview time and so we decided to schedule additional meetings. Riley started our conversation by talking about her childhood:

> My parents gave me away when I was four years old. My dad was a meth cook. My mom was a drug addict and a drunk. I lived with my aunt from four 'til I was seven, then my mom dropped my sister off, who was six months old, with my grandmother, my mom's mom. Never came back. I ended up going to live with my grandmother from seven to thirteen ... My aunt is a wonderful woman. Her and my uncle took me in. When I lived with grandma, I lived with [aunt and uncle].

When she was thirteen Riley decided to try to live with her mother. Riley did not live with her mother very long. She then went to live with her paternal grandparents:

My [paternal] grandpa hated women. He constantly would tell me, if I was going to eat something, he would tell me I was going to get fat, so I'd throw the food in the trash. I was ninety-seven pounds in ninth grade. If he saw a razor from me shaving my legs he'd break it. I wasn't allowed to go out with my friends, but I was allowed to go out with my [paternal] uncle and my aunt who allowed me to smoke [marijuana] at fourteen years old ... I was offered coke, meth [from uncle].

Just before tenth grade, Riley returned to live with her maternal aunt and uncle who had raised her for most of her life. She stayed with them until her senior year of high school. During her senior year of high school, her uncle received an out-of-state job that required her aunt and uncle to move. Riley decided to stay and graduate from the high school she had been attending. She attempted to rent her own apartment, however, legally at her age she was not able to and when her landlord found out her age she lost her apartment and was homeless.

Since Riley could not legally rent an apartment and felt she had nowhere else to turn, she decided to join the military. However, her time in the military was short-lived:

The second week [of boot camp] I started noticing that my legs were hurting. My shins were hurting. I went to the petty officer and I told her that I thought I needed to go to medical ... I continued to walk, run, jump, do everything and ended up with stress fractures all the way from my feet all the way up to my tibia, my fibula, up to my knees, up into my hip all the way up there.

Riley left the military due to her medical issues and moved with a friend she made in the military to another state. She jumped from job to job for a while and then started dating her boyfriend. After they had been dating for a short period of time, she found out that she was pregnant.

Found out on Monday that I was pregnant. Found out on that Friday that I was four months pregnant and I was having a little boy. My now husband wanted me to have an abortion. I told him, "Well, you can leave." We weren't married at that point. I said, "You have a choice. You can leave, just sign over all the parental rights. I won't come after you for anything. I can do this perfectly on my own." He changed his tune and said, "Well, I want to be with you."

Riley went on to have her son and then marry her husband. About a year later her husband lost his job and they decided to move to be with her aunt and uncle because they could not afford their rent on their own.

Riley's Struggle to Receive the Correct Diagnosis

Riley found a small lump in her breast roughly two years after she gave birth to her son. At the time, Riley, her husband, and her son had just moved to live with her aunt and uncle. Riley had started working full-time and was very busy. Riley's aunt gave her the name of her family doctor to go have the lump checked out. Riley said:

> I found the lump two months after I moved. I went into my aunt's general doctor and [the doctor] was like, "Yeah. You need to get this checked out by a breast surgeon immediately." I felt like, "Oh my God, there's something really wrong with me." My aunt decided that she would go with me to the doctor because she was really concerned. We sat there for two and a half hours with no explanation [from the health-care staff] ... Finally, after two and a half hours, this nurse comes out, gets me and she takes me back [to the exam room]. She's asking me my height and my weight. I told her my height and she goes, "No you're not. You're much taller than that." I'm like, "I have heels on." I get in the room. She tells me to take my shirt off. She asks me like two or three questions, then she leaves. I wait another 15 minutes for this doctor to come in.
>
> [The doctor] walks in, asks me like two or three questions. She feels the lump in my boob. She tells me it's fibrocystic breast tissue and she'll order an ultrasound just to confirm her findings. [The doctor said] that I can try primrose oil and vitamin E to help relieve the discomfort because it was painful. It was a little tiny lump ... [The doctor] was in the room no more than five minutes. Five to seven minutes at max. She told me that I could take the primrose oil and vitamin E but she thought it was just a placebo ... She's like, "If I were you, I wouldn't even waste my money on it." I was like, "Okay."

Riley left that appointment and decided to not try the primrose oil and vitamin E suggestions since her physician did not seem to believe that using those treatments would be effective. Riley was frustrated by the long wait to see the physician and the lack of time the physician spent with her but felt that, moving forward, she at least had a correct diagnosis. Riley scheduled the ultrasound, but felt confident that ultrasound would confirm the physician's original diagnosis.

Riley made the appointment to get an ultrasound and the ultrasound came back with inconclusive findings. Riley explained:

> Okay, now, there's a lump in my breast. The first doctor could feel it. I could feel it. They didn't do another ultrasound. [The doctor] goes, "Unless something

extreme changes, like, catastrophic changes don't worry about it. You've got fibrocystic breast tissue. You're going to get more lumps and bumps. It's going to be painful." She tells me again about the primrose oil and vitamin E.

Riley continued to believe the physician's advice following her ultrasound and began finding additional lumps in the coming months. At her annual gynecologist check-up Riley asked her gynecologist about the lumps she was finding.

I said, "You know, at this point, it's red. The whole area is red." It's a larger area. Quite a bit larger and I'm like, "You know, there's something wrong." He sends me back to the same hospital. He sends me back to the same place where I had the first ultrasound. I get an ultrasound. I get a mammogram. He sends me to go see the same doctors. I did everything I could. Finagled everything. I go there, I'm sitting there for thirty minutes before they tell me that they've known for an hour that they weren't going to see me. They didn't call me. They waited 'til I sat there for thirty minutes. Apparently, they had a surgery, an emergency surgery or something. I'm really so upset. They're like, "Well, maybe we can get you in in a few weeks." I'm like, "No, there's something wrong and you guys need to freaking see me." At that point I was just mad. I didn't believe them. I thought they were stupid to begin with. I called down to where they had done the scans and things. I said, "Can you please direct me to a doctor that has a heart?"

Riley was in pain and was getting very frustrated with her health-care providers and options. Riley felt that it was obvious that something was wrong with her health because she could feel lumps in her breast tissue and was experiencing tenderness and pain in these areas. However, Riley also felt that she was consistently getting dismissed by her physicians despite evidence to suggest that something was very wrong. Upon a nurse's referral Riley went to a different physician to get another opinion.

I went to [another physician]. I told him everything. Talked with him. I'm like, "I need a biopsy. I would like you to biopsy my breast." He's like, "Why would you disfigure your breast like that? That's absolutely absurd." I'm like, "Okay?" He goes, "You have fibrocystic breast tissue. We can just drain the cysts." I'm like, "Okay? Nobody ever told me that I can do that." [I have a] mammogram to have the cysts drained. They do all that. The radiologist comes in [and says], "I can't drain something that's not there. You have an infection."

The radiologist told Riley that the infection in her breast was the result of breastfeeding her son, but she stated that she was skeptical of that diagnosis because she had "only breastfed for a day and half" and her son was now two years old. Riley then went back to the doctor to discuss her options. Riley's

physician similarly did not believe that she had an infection and told her
that the diagnosis was still fibrocystic breast tissue. However, the physician
decided to write her a prescription for antibiotics since the radiologist told her
that she had an infection. Riley explained:

> I said, "Then why are you writing me a prescription for antibiotics?" He goes,
> "Some people would think it was negligent of me not to." I said, "I consider that
> over prescribing. If you know I don't have something, why are you giving me
> medicine for something I don't have?" I got the prescription. I took the prescrip-
> tion. This is two rounds of antibiotics.
>
> While I was sitting there [at a follow-up appointment] and he's writing out
> that script I look at him and I'm like, "This is ridiculous. You guys have no idea
> what the hell is going on." He goes, "Maybe you should get a second opinion."
> I said, "I've talked to two other doctors and two radiologists. None of you can
> seem to figure out what the hell is going on." He's frustrated and mad at me.
> Throws the prescription at me. I walked out to the front. I [went to] the lady at
> the front desk I'm like, "You get me the number to another fucking hospital."
> I sat in front of their door sobbing while I called [another hospital] to see if I
> could get an appointment.

Riley was determined to get the correct diagnosis. She explained how she
felt that her situation was only getting worse:

> At this point I have a ten-centimeter mass in my breast. It is oozing puss out the
> nipple that is brownish in color. My lymph nodes are hanging down and pulling
> on my skin so hard that I can barely write. I'm having trouble driving with my
> arm because it's just so full. I would call it my fat armpit because it hung down.

Riley's health concerns were further complicated by the fact that her
husband had lost his job and they were going to lose their COBRA[2] health
coverage in a matter of weeks.

> Now, my husband has been without a job for almost two years. His COBRA
> insurance is about to end. I'm working for [a company] and you can get [low
> quality health] insurance ... It's basically go get your own damn insurance,
> we're not going to help you in any darn way. This is back in 2010 [before the
> Affordable Care and Patient Protection Act].

Riley decided to go ahead with the appointment at the new hospital even
though she was going to be losing her health insurance soon.

> I got an appointment. I went down and got all my films, everything. I took
> them with me to my first appointment [at a new hospital]. They asked that I
> bring in all of my ultrasounds, mammograms and so on and so forth ... [At the

appointment] they get me in the gown and I'm sitting there … they take me to ultrasound room, let me undress and a doctor walks in. Right there I know something's off. She sits down. She starts the ultrasound and within a minute she looks at me and she goes, "We need to biopsy this immediately." While she starts trying to get a biopsy room, she sends me for a MRI [and] a CAT scan.

Riley explained that she was very concerned about the reaction she was receiving from the physician at this new hospital. After Riley came out of the CAT scan she said she saw "twelve doctors who were not there when [she] went in" and this made her feel like "something's really wrong." Her physician quickly came back and sat Riley down to explain her situation to her.

I go to the doctor I was supposed to see and she's like, "Well, there's three possibilities." She goes, "One, can be an infection. But why you would only have it on one side and not the other? Doesn't make sense." She's like, "That doesn't really make sense. It could be an infection but you went through two rounds of antibiotics so that seems a little silly that it wouldn't of went away. Or it's cancer." I was like, "Okay." She goes, "There's a very slim possibility that it's anything else. We're going to hope for that [that it is something else], but I'm pretty sure it's cancer." I'm thinking, "Okay, they got it wrong the first time so [maybe they are wrong]."

Riley explained that she was not sure that she trusted this new physician's diagnosis because she had been let down so many times before. Her experience searching for a diagnosis at this point had been going on for more than a year and she had received multiple and conflicting diagnoses.

When Riley went in for her biopsy the physician again told her that she believed that Riley had breast cancer. However, Riley was concerned about what she was going to do since she was about to lose her COBRA health insurance:

I'm like sitting there when she tells me this and I just burst out in tears because this is October. On January 1, I lose my insurance. I looked at her and I just burst into tears. I'm like, "How am I going to do this? I can't afford this." She looked at me and she goes, "I've already got you set up to start chemo November 1st." This is October 13th and this is before she's even sent [the biopsy] out. She's already got me set up to start chemo in 15 days or 17 days. She really was 100%. She had me set up to see a doctor for my mastectomy. She had everything set up as quickly as she could.

I told her I was losing my insurance and she looked at me, she goes, "You show up. I don't care. You show up. We will find a way to take care of this. I don't care. You show up to every appointment that is booked for you. You show up." She goes, "We will figure it out. [Name of hospital] will help you. They will pay for it if need be. You are not going to die because you can't pay."

I'm like, I have no understanding as to what she's talking about at that point.
I'm still freaking out that I am going to have no insurance. I can't pay all these
huge medical bills. I'm 29 and I've got breast cancer. I left that day and I'm
like, "Oh my god."

Riley went home and waited to get the results of her biopsy even though
she knew that her physician felt certain that she was going to receive a cancer
diagnosis. Two days later Riley's physician called her:

She goes, "I am so sorry to tell you this. You have breast cancer." She goes, "It's
stage IIIC, maybe Stage IV but we don't know and we won't be able to tell you
because we have to do the surgery.

Finally, after more than a year of conflicting diagnoses, multiple physicians
and tests, and incorrect treatments, Riley had the correct diagnosis. Unfortunately, Riley's diagnosis also came when she was about to lose her health
insurance and her husband was without work.

Riley later found out that when she initially went in to her have lump
examined that the breast cancer was likely at an early stage. However, Riley
always felt that those first physicians that she went to "rushed" through her
appointments. She explained that she believes that her health-care providers
rushed her "because they're paid per patient or what-not." Riley compared
her current health-care providers to her previous providers. She said, "That's
what's different with [the new hospital], in my opinion, is they're not just
rushing you through." As I was interviewing Riley, to confirm my understanding of her statements I asked her, "[This new hospital] gives you the
time that you need?" She replied, "They do! If you need to sit there and talk
to your doctor for a little bit, you're allowed to. The next person will be seen.
They will be taken care of in the exact same manner." Thus, Riley did not
believe that she was treated the same as other patients at the first hospital that
she went to and that was the reason why her cancer was not diagnosed early.

Riley explained that she believed that had her cancer been caught at that
early stage that she would have had a much different prognosis:

If they [the physicians I first went to] would have taken it out, I probably would
have lived a long, long, long, long life and never had a recurrence. But, since
they ignored it, it sat there and it festered and it festered and it festered and it
festered and it broke out of that capsule and it continue to grow. It became an
extremely aggressive cancer.

Riley also believed that part of the reason that she received a delayed
cancer diagnosis was because she did not have superior quality health insurance at the time that she was seeking treatment. She said, "I think [health]

insurance needs to go away. I think [health] insurance should be a non-profit. Just plain and simple."

Lacking private health insurance and having a low income have both been found to be significant predictors of being diagnosed with late-stage cancer (Lannin et al., 1998). Riley was using a COBRA plan for health insurance, and her husband was unemployed at the time that she found the lump on her breast. Riley stated that she believes both of those factors contributed to her delayed cancer diagnosis. Further, Riley's experience feeling rushed by her health-care providers similarly matches other research on patient-physician communication and socioeconomic status. Mainly, physicians are more direct in their consultation style with individuals from lower socioeconomic classes (Willems et al., 2005), which can lead patients to lack trust in their physicians (Becker & Newsom, 2003).

Working with Health-care Providers Post-Cancer Diagnosis

Riley's physician informed her that she had a ten-centimeter mass in her breast and cancer in her lymph nodes as well. Riley had been biopsied in five different places and each of those biopsies were positive for cancer. After several months and two rounds of chemotherapy, Riley had a double mastectomy to remove both of her breasts. She then went through a round of radiation therapy. However, with her new team of health-care providers Riley felt like she was in good hands.

> After I changed hospitals ... they were a lot more caring in many different ways. They would explain things and continue on until I understood ... The nurses really reach out to you. They wanted to know ... They had so many helpful people pointing me in directions that I needed to go ... There was [a social worker] who came up and offered to help me with [the] financial [aspects].

Riley found many of the resources and services that her hospital connected her with to be very helpful in managing the financial and emotional burdens associated with her cancer treatment:

> I've really felt that [Hospital] was great with just helping explain, teach me, help me financially to navigate things. They are also the people that told me about [Cancer Wellness Organization] ... They gave me other options of support outside of the realm of the hospital ... [They referred me to an organization that] helps you like with your house payment while you're sick. Taught me how to get my prescriptions at a lower cost by just paying cash. A lot of places will cut it in half. Also, gave me a little card to help with prescriptions. They helped me a lot financially. Their financial aid program [at hospital provided] over three million dollars for me because I did not have any insurance and was

unable to get any insurance. Without the health care law [the Patient Protection and Affordable Care Act], if they ever get rid of it, I will never be able to get insurance again.

Riley holds very positive opinions of her current health-care organization and the overall care she received since she began her treatment there. Her positive perceptions of the care she is receiving indicate that her interactions with these providers are different than those she experienced previously. Specifically, she felt "rushed" by her previous physicians, whereas she perceives that her new health-care providers (e.g., nurses, oncologist) spend more time with her to help her "understand" her health care and ensure that she has access to important cancer care resources (e.g., financial assistance, wellness support).

CONCLUDING THOUGHTS

Riley's experience finding the correct diagnosis and interacting with her initial health-care providers was laden with complications and tension. Riley's descriptions of her experiences at different health-care organizations illustrate and highlight the struggle that some individuals face when interacting with health-care providers. That is, some individuals may not perceive that their health-care providers are acting appropriately (e.g., spending adequate time with the patient, providing clear information) or providing satisfactory care (Mulley, Trimble, & Elwyn, 2012).

Riley's experiences were outliers when compared to the other participants that were included in my initial research. Her upbringing, misdiagnosis, and young age at the time of diagnosis contrasted with the stories that other men and women diagnosed with cancer shared with me (see Meluch, 2016). However, the differences in Riley's experience from other stories shared by many women diagnosed with breast cancer are critical to examine. Today breast cancer is generally caught in its early stages and women diagnosed in the early stages often have a high survival rate (DeSantis et al., 2017). Thus, Riley's experience of being misdiagnosed and later being diagnosed with an advanced stage cancer is markedly different from the experiences of many of her peers (i.e., young women diagnosed with breast cancer). In addition, Riley also expressed how she believed her financial struggles were a barrier in allowing her to effectively meet her health-care needs.

Riley's experience demonstrates how some women diagnosed with breast cancer may experience health disparities in the U,nited States. In addition, Riley's interactions and relationships with her early health-care providers indicate that there are often structural barriers faced by individuals from lower socioeconomic statuses when attempting to receive health care. The challenges that Riley faced are not unique to her because many other women, especially women of color, from low socioeconomic statuses are experiencing similar issues (e.g., delayed and more advanced diagnosis) when being diagnosed with cancer (DeSantis et al., 2017). However, Riley's story provides an important narrative describing the lived experience of such struggles, which is useful when attempting to understand how women from low socioeconomic statuses navigate their health-care needs.

NOTES

1. A pseudonym is used throughout the chapter to protect the confidentiality of the subject.

2. COBRA (Consolidated Omnibus Budget Reconciliation Act) provides individuals who no longer qualify for health insurance through employer (e.g., due to loss of job) to continue on their group health insurance plan for a limited period of time (U.S. Centers for Medicare & Medicaid Services, 2018).

REFERENCES

Adler, N. E., & Rehkopf, D. H. (2008). U.S. disparities in health: Descriptions, causes, and mechanisms. *Annual Review of Public Health, 29*, 235–252.

American Cancer Society. (2018). How common is breast cancer? Retrieved from: https://www.cancer.org/cancer/breast-cancer/about/how-common-is-breast-canc er.html.

American Psychological Association. (2018). SES intersecting. Retrieved from: http://www.apa.org/pi/ses/resources/publications/index.aspx.

Becker, G., & Newsom, E. (2003). Socioeconomic status and dissatisfaction with health care among chronically ill African Americans. *American Journal of Public Health, 93*, 742–748.

Bradley, C. J., Given, C. W., & Roberts, C. (2002). Race, socioeconomic status, and breast cancer treatment and survival. *Journal of the National Cancer Institute, 94*, 490–496.

DeSantis, C. E., Ma, J., Sauer, A. G., Newman, L. A., & Jemal, A. (2017). Breast cancer statistics, 2017, racial disparity in mortality by state. *CA: A Cancer Journal for Clinicians, 67*, 439–448.

Lannin, D. R., Matthews, H. F., Mitchell, J., Swanson, M. S., Swanson, F. H., & Edwards, M. S. (1998). Influence of socioeconomic and cultural factors on racial differences in late-stage presentation of breast cancer. *JAMA, 279*, 1801–1807.

Maly, R. C., Liu, Y., Leake, B., Thinkd, A., & Diamant, A. L. (2010). Treatment-related symptoms among underserved women with breast cancer: The impact of physician-patient communication. *Breast Cancer Research Treatment, 119*, 707–716.

Meluch, A. L. (2016). *Understanding the organizational and institutional origins of social support in a cancer support center* (Doctoral dissertation). Retrieved from: https://etd.ohiolink.edu/pg_10?0::NO:10:P10_ACCESSION_NUM:kent146 6944822.

Mills, E. J., Seely, D., Rachlis, B., Griffith, L., Wu, P., ..., & Wright, J. R. (2006). Barriers to participation in clinical trials of cancer: A meta-analysis and systematic review of patient-reported factors. *Lancet Oncology, 7,* 141–148.

Mulley, A. G., Trimble, C., & Elwyn, G. (2012). Stop the silent misdiagnosis: Patients' preferences matter. *BMJ, 345,* e6572–e6578.

Ndiaye, K., Krieger, J. L., Warren, J. R., & Hecht, M. L. (2011). Communication and health disparities. In T. L. Thompson, R. Parrott, & J. F. Nussbaum (Eds.), *The Routledge handbook of health communication* (2nd ed.). New York: Routledge.

Royak-Schaler, R., Passmore, S. R., Gadalla, S., Hoy, M. K., Zhan, M., ..., & Hutchison, A. P. (2008). Exploring patient-physician communication in breast cancer care for African American women following primary treatment. *Oncology Nursing Forum, 35,* 836–843.

Siegel, R., Ma, J., Zou, Z., & Jemal, A. (2014). Cancer statistics 2014. *A Cancer Journal for Clinicians, 64,* 9–29.

U.S. Centers for Medicare and Medicaid Services. (2018). COBRA coverage and the marketplace. Retrieved from: https://www.healthcare.gov/unemployed/cobra-c overage/.

van Ryn, M., & Burke, J. (2000). The effect of patient race and socio-economic status on physicians' perceptions of patients. *Social Science & Medicine, 50,* 813–828.

Willems, S., De Maesschalck, S., Deveugele, M., Derese, A., & De Maeseneer, J. (2005). Socio-economic status of the patient and doctor-patient communication: Does it make a difference? *Patient Education and Counseling, 56,* 139–146.

Wells, B. L., & Horm, J. W. (1992). Stage at diagnosis in breast cancer: Race and socioeconomic factors. *American Journal of Public Health, 82,* 1383–1385.

Chapter 7

Exploring the Effects of Patient-Provider Communication on the Lives of Women with Vulvodynia

Elizabeth A. Hintz and Maria K. Venetis

Vulvodynia, defined as "vulvar pain of at least three months' duration, without clear identifiable cause" is experienced by one in four women in the United States during their lives (Bornstein et al., 2016; Reed et al., 2012). With no single identifiable cause or cure, vulvodynia is poorly understood and often ineffectively treated. Women, on average, visit three or more providers before receiving a diagnosis, and one study found that only 1.4 percent of women fitting the diagnostic criteria for vulvodynia received an accurate diagnosis at all (Harlow & Stewart, 2003; Reed et al., 2012). Consequently, medical interactions for patients seeking treatment are often unhelpful. For this study, twenty-six women with vulvodynia completed in-depth interviews that included their experiences of patienthood. This chapter explores vulvodynia as an interpersonal phenomenon, highlighting the provider and health-care system-related factors that delay help seeking and diagnosis and outlining the physical, relational, and psychological effects of the illness. First, vulvodynia will be defined, and its effects explored. Then, standards of patient-centered communication (PCC), the diagnostic protocol for treating vulvodynia, barriers for physicians treating patients, barriers for patients seeking treatment, and participant accounts of medical interactions and their implications will be described. Finally, practical advice for improving the medical experience and upholding standards of PCC will be offered.

NARRATING THE EXPERIENCE OF VULVODYNIA

Willow was in her late twenties when the symptoms of vulvodynia began. She was in a long-term relationship and had plans for marriage and children.

Not knowing what vulvodynia was, she assumed that the burning she suddenly began experiencing was indicative of a yeast infection. She went to her doctor, who prescribed her antifungal medication. Yet, her symptoms did not improve. After a month of self-treatments for this nonexistent yeast infection, her partner began expressing frustration about the absence of sex in their relationship. Willow returned to her doctor, determined to figure out what was wrong. After tests for multiple bacterial infections and STDs returned negative results, her doctor dismissed her pain as being "all in her head" and encouraged her to seek psychiatric care. Disheartened, and fearing a similar interaction with another doctor, Willow forsook seeking treatment altogether. She tried to ignore the pain, and continued to engage in painful intercourse to satisfy her partner's needs. Eventually, the pain worsened, and all sexual intercourse with her partner halted. The relationship began to turn toxic. After Willow's doctor had failed to find a problem and told her that her pain was "all in her head," her partner began to treat her poorly. Frustrated by the provider's inability to diagnose her symptoms, her partner began telling her that she was lying to avoid having sex with him and that she was faking the pain. Eventually, Willow's partner ended their relationship, citing her unwillingness to engage in intercourse as the primary reason for dissolving the relationship. After her relationship ended, it would take another three years for Willow to receive an accurate diagnosis of vulvodynia. This experience changed the way that Willow viewed herself. She felt "defective," being unable to perform a task that she felt was necessary to maintain a relationship. She felt helpless and blamed herself for having the pain. To return to seeking medical care, she had to overcome feeling that her pain was a psychological issue, as had been suggested by a previous provider. In 2017, Willow became connected with a clinic specializing in the treatment of vulvodynia. She received a correct diagnosis and crafted a treatment plan that would help her to better manage her symptoms. Willow's story is not unique.

Vulvodynia Explained

Definition

Vulvodynia is defined as "vulvar pain of at least three months' duration, without clear identifiable cause, which may have potential associated factors" (Bornstein et al., 2016, p. 747). Most commonly triggered during penetrative intercourse with a partner, a burning or stinging pain around the opening of the vagina is the chief complaint of those suffering from vulvodynia (Rosen et al., 2014). Although vulvodynia often presents as pain with intercourse, it is a complex pain disorder. For example, vulvodynia is associated with risk factors linked to genetics, inflammation, musculoskeletal disorders, and neurological mechanisms. Furthermore, the effects of vulvodynia are physical, interpersonal, and psychological in nature.

Physical Effects

Despite being characterized by its connection to painful intercourse, the physical effects of vulvodynia often affect a woman's entire life. The nature of pain that accompanies vulvodynia can be severe. For some women, pain is so intense that full-time employment is not possible, making them eligible for disability benefits (NVA, 2010). Furthermore, the location of the physical pain, independent of severity, disrupts daily functioning, and may limit activities such as sitting, bike riding, and tampon use (Bois et al., 2016). Sexual functioning also suffers, as women with vulvodynia commonly report a low sex drive and orgasm difficulties (Donaldson & Meana, 2011). For these reasons, receiving an accurate diagnosis and beginning treatment are urgent matters for women with vulvodynia.

Psychological Effects

Women with vulvodynia experience heightened anxiety and depression. Other pertinent psychological factors related to vulvodynia include pain catastrophizing (Sullivan et al., 2001), fear of pain, hypervigilance to pain, lower pain self-efficacy, negative attributions about the pain, avoidance of sex, emotional dysregulation, negative affect, and negative self-assessment (Bornstein et al., 2016; Donaldson & Meana, 2011). Together, these effects allow us to understand how the world outside of the provider's office may affect the medical interaction. The psychological effects can have a cumulative and negative effect on how a woman views herself and her relationship. Thus, as the search for a diagnosis and effective treatment continues across time, interactions with providers can become emotionally charged (Goldstein, Pukall, & Goldstein, 2009; NVA, 2016).

Interpersonal Effects

The physical and psychological challenges of living with vulvodynia also threaten the feminine identity as women with vulvodynia relate to their partners (Kaler, 2006), particularly as vulvodynia challenges notions of what it means to be female, sexual, and in a relationship with a man (Hintz, 2018; Kaler, 2006). Over time, vulvodynia begins to take a toll on interpersonal relationships (Hintz, 2018). Women who are in relationships often experience emotional distance, increased conflict, partner dissatisfaction, and infidelity or abandonment fears because of vulvodynia (Donaldson & Meana, 2011; Smith & Pukall, 2011). Conversations about vulvodynia call into question notions about the roles of sex and intimacy within the relationship. These conversations are often difficult, addressing shifts within the relationship, changes in the way a woman views herself, and vulvodynia as it obstructs daily activity (Hintz, 2018). Furthermore, 77 percent of women reported fearing that pain would end their relationships (Gordon et al., 2003). Unhelpful interactions with medical providers, then, come not only at the expense of patient health, but also the relationships that deteriorate as symptoms persist.

Vulvodynia and the Medical Interaction

Patient-centered Communication

The quality of a medical interaction is often measured in terms of its ability to adhere to the tenets of patient-centered communication (PCC), one component of patient-centered care. An interaction following PCC principles is one that (a) elicits the patient perspective, (b) understands the patient within the psychosocial context, (c) produces a value-concordant mutual understanding of the problem and its treatment, and (d) shares decision-making power and responsibility to a degree comfortable for the patient (Epstein et al., 2005). Women with vulvodynia, however, often have many medical interactions before their condition is diagnosed, suggesting the inability to achieve a mutual understanding of the medical issue (Harlow & Stewart, 2003). Multiple interactions with various providers could result from provider referrals to specialists, but are also likely to result from unhelpful visits in which the legitimacy of pain is questioned by the provider. These visits prompt women with vulvodynia to seek additional medical care (Pukall et al., 2016). Such efforts to prevent undermining patients' experience of pain align with tenets of PCC, and result in providers soliciting, understanding, and affirming patient expressions of pain, and acknowledging their isolation and frustration at being disbelieved. In fact, when providers fail to recognize patient pain and, instead, suggest a psychological explanation for pain, patients may perceive this diagnosis as demeaning and a denial of the patient's pain and experiences. When recognizing pain, providers should also empower the patient with health-care options to counter feelings of helplessness associated with pain (Newton, Southall, Raphael, Ashford, & LeMarchand, 2013). Similarly, acknowledging the emotional component of vulvodynia, recommended by both Epstein et al. (2005) and Newton et al. (2013), is also recognized by leading physicians in the treatment of vulvodynia as essential for promoting treatment adherence (Goldstein et al., 2009). Together, these articles provide standards by which communication in medical interactions for patients with vulvodynia can be judged. Next, the diagnostic protocol for treating vulvodynia will be overviewed.

Diagnostic Protocol

To understand what women with vulvodynia experience in medical interactions with providers, it is necessary to begin by overviewing the protocol for diagnosing and evaluating a patient presenting with symptoms of vulvodynia. The International Society for the Study of Vulvovaginal Disease (ISSVD), a leading authority in the classification, treatment, and clinical management of vulvodynia, explicate a "vulvodynia algorithm," a flowchart of sorts, for the proper treatment of vulvodynia as an exclusionary illness (Haefner et al., 2005). When a patient presenting with symptoms enters a medical provider's office, the medical provider should first begin by soliciting a comprehensive medical and sexual history. In the absence of infection, inflammation, neoplasia (i.e., abnormal tissue growth), or a neurological disorder, the specific location and subtype of vulvodynia (i.e., generalized or localized) should be determined. To do so, a cotton swab test should be performed, whereby the provider lightly touches a cotton swab to the vestibule in several locations and records patient reports of discomfort and severity. If a patient reports tenderness or burning during the cotton swab test, a yeast culture should be taken. If the results of the yeast culture are negative (i.e., the patient does not have a yeast infection), a variety of possible treatments can be explored with the patient, including topical medications, injections, biofeedback, physical therapy, and cognitive behavioral therapy. Should those treatments provide adequate relief, treatment is halted. If adequate relief is not provided, and the patient desires additional treatment, a vestibulectomy, where a portion of the vulva is surgically removed, becomes an option (Haefner et al., 2005).

Barriers for Providers

Although this "algorithm" exists to successfully diagnose and treat women with vulvodynia, providers face many issues that make diagnoses difficult. In 2012, the National Institute of Health (NIH) compiled and released a Research Plan on vulvodynia that detailed many of these issues encountered by providers. First, providers are often reluctant to probe for information about sexual wellness, which may contribute to delays in diagnoses. Many studies have underscored the need for increasing the quantity and duration of sexual conversations in medical environments (e.g., Fuzzell, Fedesco, Alexander, Fortenberry, & Shields, 2016). In fact, one study found that 80 percent of all conversations in medical environments about vulvodynia were initiated by the patient (Donaldson & Meana, 2011). This lack of inquiry (by the provider) and reluctance to seek help (on the part of the patient) contribute greatly to problems identifying and labeling the disorder and prolong the cognitive search for causal attributions (Donaldson & Meana, 2011; NVA, 2016). Providers also report low levels of efficacy and express a lack of confidence in their ability to treat women with genital pain (Abdolrasulnia et al., 2010). As one physician explained, "women with genital pain often make us feel that we do not know what we are doing" (Binik, Bergeron, & Khalife, 2007, p. 141).

Second, a fundamental lack of standardized definitions and terminology to describe vulvodynia complicate communication in medical interactions. Patients struggle to find information about vulvodynia, as providers often use multiple terms for the same condition (such as vulvar vestibulitis, vestibulo-dynia, vestibulitis, provoked vestibulitis). Since 2012, the ISSVD, International Society for the Study of Women's Sexual Health (ISSWSH), and the International Pelvic Pain Society (IPPS) have jointly crafted new terminology for vulvar pain to "acknowledge the complexity of clinical presentation and pathophysiology ... and [incorporate] new information ... since the last terminology published in 2003" (Bornstein et al., 2016).

Third, the inclusion of dyspareunia (i.e., painful intercourse) in the Diagnostic and Statistical Manual of Mental Disorders (DSM) as a "sexual dysfunction due to a general medical condition" in the DSM-IV and as a "genito-pelvic pain/penetration disorder" in the DSM-V has remained controversial (Binik, 2005; Vieira-Baptista & Lima-Silva, 2016). The inclusion of vulvodynia in the DSM often results in a purely psychiatric approach to its treatment, which has detrimental effects, as Willow described earlier. A psychological ascription for physical pain may prolong the diagnostic process or turn women away from seeking further treatment altogether. Thus, "all suspected cases of dyspareunia or vaginismus should be evaluated by a medical professional with differentiation in this area before a pure psychological cause for the complaints can be assumed" (Vieira-Baptista & Lima-Silva, 2016, p. 354). However, as physicians who specialize in the treatment of vulvodynia are few, and general practitioners of gynecology are often not trained in its diagnosis or treatment, the experiences of women seeking treatment are often unhelpful (NIH, 2012; Reed, 2006).

Barriers for Patients

Women with vulvodynia often encounter barriers with providers and healthcare systems from the onset of symptoms to diagnosis. These barriers may help us to understand why the average woman will see numerous providers before receiving a diagnosis (Harlow & Stewart, 2003). When symptoms first begin, women encounter difficulty identifying the problem and labeling the disorder (Donaldson & Meana, 2011). This issue is exacerbated by a lack of standardized terminology and a complicated set of symptoms and comorbid symptoms (NIH, 2012). Lacking the terminology to describe the condition and the language to effectively convey the feeling of pain, women with vulvodynia often report low levels of efficacy for engaging in talk about the condition with close others (Donaldson & Meana, 2011; Hintz, 2018). However, for women with vulvodynia, the success of interactions, both medical and interpersonal, depends on one's ability to communicate her pain. The social validation of pain, like other nonvisible illnesses, relies upon the sufferer's ability to communicate the experience of pain in a way that is accessible to the listener.

Furthermore, the stigma associated with sexual disorders, a fear of the severity of the diagnosis, faith in spontaneous remission, and a lack of confidence in the medical system act as barriers to seeking and receiving treatment (Donaldson & Meana, 2011). It has been suggested that, for those facing illness, "stigma processes are a leading barrier to health promotion, treatment, and support" (Smith, 2011, p. 455). A lack of confidence in a medical cure can be present from the onset of symptoms and may be caused by many factors. These factors include doubting the possibility of a cure, considering the condition a component of a larger physical (e.g., he is too big for me), relational (e.g., maybe I don't like him as much as I thought I did) or psychological issue (e.g., perhaps some repressed trauma is making having sex difficult?), or not viewing the condition as a medical problem (e.g., we need to use more lubricant). For these reasons, one study of 208 women meeting the diagnostic criteria for vulvodynia found that over 51.4 percent ($n = 107$) did not seek traditional medical treatment, often turning to complementary (i.e., alternative) health treatments and products instead (Haefner et al., 2005; Reed et al., 2012). Of the remaining 48.6 percent ($n = 101$) of women who did seek treatment, only 1.4 percent ($n = 3$) were correctly diagnosed with vulvodynia (Reed et al., 2012).

Participant Interviews

To better understand how PCC principles are both upheld and violated in medical interactions, interview data gathered by the first author will be included below. Twenty-six women with vulvodynia, who were recruited via condition-specific forums and the first author's social media sites, participated in semi-structured interviews where they described the experience of living with vulvodynia. The interview opened with a generic prompt, "tell me about your experience with vulvodynia," subsequent questions exploring the experiences of seeking treatment and receiving a diagnosis. To participate in the study, all participants were required to be biologically female, over the age of eighteen, reside within the United States, and have been diagnosed with vulvodynia by a medical professional. Participants ranged in age from twenty to fifty-two years ($M = 28$, $SD = 6.7$), and 77 percent ($n = 20$) had localized vulvodynia (i.e., vulvar pain only with touch or pressure). Interviews took place via phone call and were recorded for later transcription. All interviews were transcribed verbatim by the first author.

PATIENT EXPERIENCES AND THE ROLE OF COMMUNICATION

Clear criteria have been outlined above for the diagnosis and treatment of vulvodynia, yet barriers for providers and patients, as explored above, can complicate this process. We know that patients entering these medical interactions face many physical, relational, and psychological issues that degrade over time as diagnosis and treatment are sought. Barriers faced by providers and patients prolong the search for causal attributions, consequently sexual and relational health continues to decline until a diagnosis is made and treatment begins (Donaldson & Meana, 2011). Thus, the lived experience of seeking treatment differs from the prescribed process outlined by the ISSVD, and medical interactions are often emotionally charged. Participants described both positive and negative interactions with medical providers and detailed the problems they faced when interacting with physicians. These narratives are useful for understanding the lived experience of seeking treatment for vulvodynia and may offer practical advice for the medical community in terms of how PCC principles are best upheld. The following exemplars are taken from qualitative interview data with women who suffer from vulvodynia.

Negative Medical Interactions

Many participants detailed negative or unhelpful interactions with medical providers. Most often, these interactions took place early in the patient's treatment seeking process and occurred with a provider who did not specialize in the treatment of vulvodynia. What happens when a provider does not know how to treat a patient? As vulvodynia is a diagnosis by omission, common illnesses must first be ruled out before a diagnosis of vulvodynia can be made. A woman at her first medical appointment presenting with burning pain should likely be tested for STDs and a yeast infection, but when negative results are returned, other treatment options should be pursued (NIH, 2012). Yet, women reported being retested for STDs, infections, urinary tract infections (UTIs) at each appointment, even having the condition or infection in question was impossible and the women themselves knew and expressed that they did not have that infection or illness. Two participants described interactions during which this took place.

> Yeah, over the course of like those two years, uhm, and I mean people were-some doctors were genuinely stumped. … Uhm, but then others were kind

of blatantly rude, like, I was asked-they were like, "Are you sure there's no, like, possibility of your husband cheating on you? Like, you could like, be getting like, herpes." And I was like, haha! Like, the audacity. (Participant #1)

So when you go to the doctor and say, "Oh, it hurts when I have sex" they say "Do you have an STD?" and "You need more lube." And when you try to explain, "No, I promise I don't need more lube," everyone's response is "Well, have you tried this one obscure lubricant that I heard of one time that is not sold anywhere?" (Laughing) (Participant #10)

These accounts demonstrate several violations of PCC principles. Although these providers may not understand protocol for treating vulvodynia, respecting patient legitimacy and dignity remain essential components of a successful medical interaction. PCC advocates for an elicitation of the patient perspective and a share of decision-making power and responsibility (Epstein et al., 2005). In the context of unexplained pain, shared decision-making cannot take place without an understanding and affirmation of the patient's story of pain (i.e., expressing belief in the patient's account of her symptoms) (Newton et al., 2013). In these instances, the provider indirectly expresses disbelief about the symptoms of pain. In the first example, a provider resorts to making negative inferences about the patient's life, suggesting that her husband may have given her a sexually transmitted infection (STI). The second example similarly illustrates how the patient's assertion that lubrication is not the issue is discounted by the provider. After these interactions, patients not only felt frustrated, but were tasked with seeking out other providers who would legitimize their concerns and diagnose them. Other participants described instances of how providers failed to uphold principles of PCC when facing symptoms that stumped them.

I remember [my doctor] going in after the second antibiotic didn't work and she said something like, "Well nothing seems to be working, I don't know, do you have any ideas?" Like as in, did I know what was wrong with me, which is not what I want to hear from a doctor. (Participant #9)

...when I did try to bring it up with my gynecologist and my doctors, they could never find anything wrong. So obviously in their limited knowledge of it, they couldn't figure out what it was. So they were like, "Oh, it's just in your head. You should drink a bottle of wine before having sex." Or, "You should just try to be more confident." Stupid things like that. (Participant #32)

Then I became depressed because I started realizing that doctors didn't know what I had. ... Doctors thought that I was abused or raped. They told me to read these books like "The Art of Marriage," and I just didn't understand what was wrong. (Participant #35)

While it is often not possible for women and their providers to come to a mutual understanding of the problem and its treatment, the principles of PCC must be upheld in interactions where symptoms remain unexplained. Yet, our first example demonstrates a violation of shared decision-making whereby the provider admits to the patient that her ideas for treating the symptoms have proven unsuccessful. Her solicitation of the patient's perspective is perceived as being insensitive and dismissive, and the provider fails to empower the patient with other health-care options. Consequently, this participant then sought out another provider. The second example not only delegitimizes the patient's pain, but also makes negative attributions about her personality and sexual prowess. The third example makes similar negative personal attributions that relegate symptoms of pain to inexperience or abuse, shifting the burden of healing the illness from the provider to the patient. It is important to be cautious when delivering psychologic explanations for pain, as described in the second example above, as these may be interpreted as a denial of the existence of pain altogether. Psychological ascriptions for pain appear frequently when providers feel unequipped to treat an illness, rely on gendered stereotypes to evaluate the complaints of female patients, or are threatened by their own inability to treat a patient (Netwon et al., 2013).

These interactions offer insight into the experiences of women seeking treatment for vulvodynia. While not all medical interactions for women are negative, these situations do occur, often with devastating consequences for the patients. Fearing judgment, some women delay help seeking. As one participant explained, "I knew I should've sought treatment right away, but … I had major anxiety about going into the doctor and telling the doctor that I thought that there was something wrong. Because I thought that they were just going to discount me." (Participant #15). After a negative medical interaction occurs, women may feel discouraged from seeking treatment. Another participant felt that her negative interaction discouraged her from pursuing treatment.

> Once I figured out what it was that I was dealing with I tried to approach my current gynecologist about it and she was not very receptive to what it was that I was dealing with. I think that she had never really heard of it or wasn't able to provide me with any sort of pathway to treatment, and that ended really poorly. So that experience to me was a little bit traumatic … that kind of put me off of seeking treatment for it. It really discouraged me from going in and trying to find other doctors that were willing to do it. (Participant #8)

Furthermore, their relationships may suffer if partners interpret the lack of a diagnosis as personal rejection (Hintz, 2018). The providers included in the above examples were not specialists trained to diagnose and treat vulvodynia. However, the maltreatment of vulvodynia outlined above, a condition that affects an estimated 25 percent of the female population during their lives, points to a gap in gynecological training that must be addressed (Pukall et al., 2016; Reed et al., 2012). In the short term, by upholding principles of PCC in these interactions, even when a diagnosis is not made, such interactions can be positive rather than invalidating experiences.

Positive Medical Interactions

Participants described positive interactions most often with current providers, the specialists who have diagnosed them and provided treatment. These providers often upheld tenets of PCC, acknowledging the emotional component of managing vulvodynia and validating feelings of frustration and the long process that precedes an appointment where a positive diagnosis can be made. For example, three participants described meeting their specialists for the first time.

> I sat there for like an hour and told this doctor everything and she was like "Yeah, I've heard all of this before." Are you kidding me!? Like, no way. Everybody said I was crazy. She's like, "You're not crazy." And so, since January I've been getting treatment and relief finally, it's been amazing. Instead of telling me I'm out of my mind. (Participant #13)

At the start of her interaction with a patient, this provider had upheld several principles of PCC. First, by saying "Yeah, I've heard this all before," the provider expressed that she understood and affirmed the patient's story of her pain. When she said, "You're not crazy," the provider reinforced this affirmation. Another participant shared a similar story about meeting her provider.

> And the first appointment I had with her, she was like going through this little questionnaire that they had me fill out for the first meeting or appointment. And she was like, "This is an absurd question, but what do you use for lubricant?" And I was like, "Well uh, I don't need any of them, but I have a lot of them." And she says, "Yeah, by the time you make it to me you probably have at least a dozen of them." Like yeah, I'm just hoarding a drawer full of various lubricants because I apparently need to be able to outwit lubricants for a doctor to take me seriously (laughing). (Participant #10)

The provider in this example used their first meeting to acknowledge the isolation and frustration of being disbelieved. She prefaces a question understood to be a sore spot for her patients with "This is an absurd question," signaling to the patient that she understands what the patient has likely endured prior to their appointment. She accomplishes this again in the next statement, where she uses humor to address the large collection of unnecessary lubricant amassed by the patient. Another patient detailed a positive interaction with her specialist.

> This doctor took a look and he was almost crying because he understood how much pain I was in. He was the one who helped me and told me what I needed to know in terms of lifestyle. He gave me some steroid cream to control it and he helped me manage it. Now it just comes and goes once a month, maybe. Used to be constantly. (Participant #30)

These accounts of positive interactions underscore the importance of validating the experience of pain and feelings of frustration in the medical interaction. In this example, the patient's provider expressed empathy to acknowledge the patient's pain, and empowered her with information and treatment options to reduce her feelings of helplessness (Newton et al., 2013). Expertise also played a role in determining the valence of the medical interaction. By validating the emotional experience of living with the condition, being trained in its diagnosis and treatment, and working with others in other areas of medicine, providers can begin to improve the patient experience of seeking treatment for vulvodynia.

IMPROVING THE PATIENT EXPERIENCE

To help medical providers better understand how women with unexplained health problems have been viewed historically in medical interactions, it may be useful to draw parallels between vulvodynia and hysteria, the first mental illness imputed specifically to women. Women with nonvisible health issues have a long history of being mistreated, disbelieved, and degraded in medical interactions. Until 1980 (when it was removed from the DSM-III), hysteria, characterized by a wide array of symptoms, afflicted urban, upper, and middle-class women between the ages of fifteen and forty (Smith-Rosenberg, 1972, p. 660). Medicine today still stumbles to provide adequate care for illnesses like chronic pain, where women often report negative experiences with physicians who are unequipped to help them or rely on the "histrionic" female stereotype, where women are viewed as melodramatic and theatrical (Newton et al., 2013; Smith-Rosenberg, 1972; Werner, Isaksen, & Malterud, 2004; Werner & Malterud, 2003). Negative stereotypes manifest in the ascription of purely psychological solutions for physical problems and provide a lens through which a practitioner views their female patient. As one physician treating women with chronic pelvic pain reported, "I think that if women are fat and tearful then there's likely to be a psychological component" (McGowan, Pitts, & Carter, 1999, p. 312).

While hysteria was a disease of yesteryear, the historical context of hysteria shares some striking similarities with the issues faced by women with vulvodynia today. For example, participants often reported experiencing the questioning of their legitimacy and being disbelieved at the hands of medical providers. Many participants reported being told that the pain was purely psychological after traditional tests for common infections and conditions were negative. The unwillingness of providers to credit the health complaints of women has negative implications for the patient and their relationship. Therefore, keeping the experiences and historical context outlined above in mind, several broad recommendations can be made for improving the experiences of women seeking treatment for vulvodynia by upholding the tenets of PCC.

Participants emphasized the importance of being believed when reporting vulvar pain to a practitioner (Newton et al., 2013). This skepticism is often expressed when a physician suggests that the pain is "all in the mind" of a female patient (Werner & Malterud, 2003). A patient may seek purely psychological treatment for a physical problem and not receive any subsequent medical care. Or, a woman may then feel discouraged from seeking help, fearing that a similar interaction may take place a second time. Furthermore, when a provider expresses skepticism about the validity of a woman's pain, de facto permission is given to a woman's partner to express similar disbelief. If a doctor does not believe a woman's pain, her partner may feel personally rejected when she refuses to engage in painful intercourse.

This skepticism also shifts the burden of responsibility for resolving pain from the physician and medical system to the individual. Yet, a patient does not have the access to the information and resources necessary to resolve pain on her own. When a physician expresses skepticism about a woman's pain, women in turn often report feeling skeptical about the medical system in general. Many women with vulvodynia who see multiple physicians to no avail seek alternative or holistic practitioners for cures outside of the realm of traditional medical care (Haefner et al., 2005). These women, who have often rejected traditional medicine as a source of information or treatment for vulvodynia, are susceptible to the influence of those who have claimed to "cure" vulvodynia naturally. Women who are distrusting of or dissatisfied with traditional treatments may also seek alternative treatments.

Supporting the principles of PCC for those with unexplained pain means providing health-care options to empower patients and reduce feelings of hopelessness (Netwon et al., 2013). One strategy for upholding this principle in the face of an uncertain diagnosis might include a referral to a specialist if a provider has ruled out all possible alternatives within their own realm of expertise and thus cannot adequately treat vulvodynia. When treated incorrectly, participants were often given steroids, which thin vulvar tissue, unnecessary antibiotics, creams or ointments for yeast infections that they did not have, and sometimes reported having unnecessary surgery or biopsies, all of which served to worsen the discomfort they were feeling (Goldstein et al., 2009). Skepticism also manifests in advice given by physicians that implies that a woman is not having sex correctly. Advising women to find new boyfriends, use more lubricant, or try more foreplay are often forms of unhelpful advice given to sufferers.

Another important and often overlooked component of treating vulvodynia involves addressing the emotional component of living with the condition (Netwon et al., 2013). Goldstein et al. (2009) described the importance of addressing this emotional component. Women may travel across the country, pay thousands of dollars for treatments, or wait extended periods of time to see specialists who treat vulvodynia. During these waiting periods, physical and relational health tend to decline. Women are likely to feel guilt and shame when they experience illness, and vulvodynia is threatening to feminine identities and problematic for the heterosexual relationships that reinforce them (Haug, 1992; Shallcross, Dickson, Nunns, Mackenzie, & Kiemle, 2018). Women often enter appointments prepared to defend their legitimacy, and these appointments tend to be emotionally charged. When patients are emotionally charged, and these feelings of, for example, urgently and anxiously wanting the pain to stop, are not addressed, compliance with treatments that do not produce immediate results is poor (Goldstein et al., 2009). Thus, addressing the emotional component of living with vulvodynia, perhaps by setting realistic expectations about what to expect, can facilitate compliance with treatments that produce long-term (rather than short-term) relief.

In summary, medical providers interacting with women who have vulvodynia should strive to uphold the tenets of PCC by affirming patient stories of pain and addressing the emotional toll of living with vulvodynia. In doing so, patients are treated correctly sooner and hold realistic expectations about disease course and treatment.

CONCLUSION

Ample opportunity exists for future research in this area. First, while examples were utilized to exemplify the upholding and violation of PCC principles, a larger sample size would provide additional insight concerning what an average experience looks like for women seeking treatment. Furthermore, a larger data set would allow for an understanding of how provider characteristics (e.g., personality) that affect the interaction. Second, it is important to reiterate that many providers treating women with vulvodynia are simply doing their best given the barriers they face. However, this study makes several recommendations to ensure that all medical interactions are steps in the right direction, not invalidating and delegitimizing. Third, all of the women interviewed for this study had received a diagnosis. Thus, the inclusion of women with symptoms of vulvodynia who have seen multiple providers but have not received a diagnosis may offer additional insight.

This chapter explored vulvodynia as an interpersonal phenomenon, highlighted the interpersonal and structural factors that delay help seeking and diagnosis, and outlined the physical, interpersonal, and psychological effects of the illness. First, vulvodynia was defined and its effects explored. Then, the diagnostic protocol for treatment, barriers for physicians treating patients, barriers for patients seeking treatment, and participant accounts of medical interactions were described. Finally, practical advice for improving the medical experience was offered. This chapter extends our understanding of the experiences of women with chronic, unexplained illness in medical interactions. By narrating these experiences of patienthood, we gain an understanding of the role of patient-provider communication as it benefits and harms the lives of vulvodynia patients in this unique context.

REFERENCES

Abdolrasulnia, M., Shewchuk, R. M., Roepke, N., Granstaff, U. S., Dean, J., Foster, J. A., Goldstein, A. T., & Casebeer, L. (2010). Management of female sexual problems: Perceived barriers, practice patterns, and confidence among primary care physicians and gynecologists. *The Journal of Sexual Medicine, 7*, 2499–2508. doi: 10.1111/j.1743-6109.2010.01857.x.

Binik, Y. M. (2005). Should dyspareunia be retained as a sexual dysfunction in DSM-V? A painful classification decision. *Archives of Sexual Behavior, 34*, 11–21. doi: 10.1007/s10508-005-0998-4.

Binik, Y. M., Bergeron S., & Khalife, S. (2007). Dyspareunia and vaginismus: So-called sexual pain. In S. R. Leiblum (Ed.), *Principles and practice of sex therapy* (pp. 124–156). New York: Guilford Press.

Bois, K., Bergeron, S., Rosen, N., Mayrand, M. H., Brassard, A., & Sadikaj, G. (2016). Intimacy, sexual satisfaction, and sexual distress in vulvodynia couples: An observational study. *Health Psychology, 35*, 531. Retrieved from: https://papyrus.bib.umontreal.ca/xmlui/bitstream/handle/1866/13936/Health%20Psychology_Bois%20et%20al%20Final.pdf?sequence=2.

Bornstein, J., Goldstein, A. T., Stockdale, C. K., Bergeron, S., Pukall, C., Zolnoun, D., ... & Starke, N. B. (2016). 2015 ISSVD, ISSWSH, and IPPS consensus terminology and classification of persistent vulvar pain and vulvodynia. *The Journal of Sexual Medicine, 13*, 607–612. doi: 10.1016/j.jsxm.2016.02.167.

Donaldson, R. L., & Meana, M. (2011). Early dyspareunia experience in young women: Confusion, consequences, and help-seeking barriers. *The Journal of Sexual Medicine, 8*, 814–823. doi: 10.1111/j.1743-6109.2010.02150.x.

Epstein, R. M., Franks, P., Fiscella, K., Shields, C. G., Meldrum, S. C., Kravitz, R. L., & Duberstein, P. R. (2005). Measuring patient-centered communication in Patient-Physician consultations: Theoretical and practical issues. *Social Science and Medicine*, *61*, 1516–1528. doi: 10.1016/j.socscimed.2005.02.001.

Fuzzell, L., Fedesco, H. N., Alexander, S. C., Fortenberry, J. D., & Shields, C. G. (2016). "I just think that doctors need to ask more questions": Sexual minority and majority adolescents' experiences talking about sexuality with healthcare providers. *Patient Education and Counseling*, *99*, 1467–1472. doi: 10.1016/j.pec.2016.06.004.

Goldstein, A., Pukall, C., & Goldstein, I. (Eds.). (2009). *Female sexual pain disorders: Evaluation and management*. John Wiley & Sons.

Gordon, A. S., Panahian-Jand, M., McComb, F., Melegari, C., & Sharp, S. (2003). Characteristics of women with vulvar pain disorders: Responses to a Web-based survey. *Journal of Sex & Marital Therapy*, *29*, 45–58. doi: 10.1080/713847126.

Haefner, H. K., Collins, M. E., Davis, G. D., Edwards, L., Foster, D. C., Hartmann, E. D. H., ... & Piper, C. K. (2005). The vulvodynia guideline. *Journal of Lower Genital Tract Disease*, *9*, 40–51.

Harlow, B. L., & Stewart, E. G. (2003). A population-based assessment of chronic unexplained vulvar pain: Have we underestimated the prevalence of vulvodynia? *Journal of the American Medical Women's Association (1972)*, *58*, 82–88.

Haug, F. (1992). Morals also have two genders. In F. Haug (Ed.), *Beyond female masochism. Memory-work and politics* (pp. 31–52). London, New York: Verso.

Hintz, E. A. (2018). Purdue University. The vulvar vernacular: Communicative dilemmas experienced by women with chronic genital pain (Master's thesis).

Kaler, A. (2006). Unreal women: Sex, gender, identity and the lived experience of vulvar pain. *Feminist Review*, *82*, 50–75.

McGowan, L., Pitts, M., & Carter, D. C. (1999). Chronic pelvic pain: The general practitioner's perspective. *Psychology, Health & Medicine*, *4*, 303–317. doi: 10.1080/135485099106234.

National Institute of Health. (2012). *Research plan on Vulvodynia* (Rep.). Retrieved from: https://www1.nichd.nih.gov/publications/pubs/documents/NIH_Vulvod ynia_Plan_April2012.pdf.

National Vulvodynia Association. (2010). How to apply for disability benefits: A self-help guide for women with vulvodynia. [Brochure]. N.P.

National Vulvodynia Association. (2016). Vulvodynia: A common and under-recognized pain disorder in women and female adolescents–integrating current knowledge into clinical practice [PowerPoint slides]. Retrieved from: https://cm e.dannemiller.com/articles/activity?id=570.

Newton, B. J., Southall, J. L., Raphael, J. H., Ashford, R. L., & LeMarchand, K. (2013). A narrative review of the impact of disbelief in chronic pain. *Pain Management Nursing*, *14*, 161–171. doi: 10.1016/j.pmn.2010.09.001.

Pukall, C. F., Goldstein, A. T., Bergeron, S., Foster, D., Stein, A., Kellogg-Spadt, S., & Bachmann, G. (2016). Vulvodynia: Definition, prevalence, impact, and pathophysiological factors. *The Journal of Sexual Medicine*, *13*, 291–304. doi: 10.1016/j.jsxm.2015.12.021.

Reed, B. D. (2006). Vulvodynia: Diagnosis and management. *American Family Physician, 73*(7), 1231–1238.

Reed, B. D., Harlow, S. D., Sen, A., Legocki, L. J., Edwards, R. M., Arato, N., & Haefner, H. K. (2012). Prevalence and demographic characteristics of vulvodynia in a population-based sample. *American Journal of Obstetrics and Gynecology, 206*, 170–e1. doi: 10.1016/j.ajog.2011.08.012.

Rosen, N. O., Bergeron, S., Sadikaj, G., Glowacka, M., Baxter, M. L., & Delisle, I. (2014). Relationship satisfaction moderates the associations between male partner responses and depression in women with vulvodynia: A dyadic daily experience study. *PAIN, 155*, 1374–1383. doi: 10.1016/j.pain.2014.04.017.

Shallcross, R., Dickson, J. M., Nunns, D., Mackenzie, C., & Kiemle, G. (2018). Women's subjective experiences of living with vulvodynia: A systematic review and meta-ethnography. *Archives of Sexual Behavior, 47*, 577–595. doi: 10.1007/s10508-017-1026-1.

Smith, R. A. (2011). Stigma communication and health. *Handbook of Health Communication, 2*, 455–372.

Smith, K. B., & Pukall, C. F. (2011). A systematic review of relationship adjustment and sexual satisfaction among women with provoked vestibulodynia. *Journal of Sex Research, 48*, 166–191. doi: 10.1080/00224499.2011.555016.

Smith-Rosenberg, C. (1972). The hysterical woman: Sex roles and role conflict in 19th-century America. *Social Research*, 652–678. Retrieved from: http://www.jstor.org/stable/40970115.

Sullivan, M., Thorn, B., Haythornthwaite, J., Keefe, K., Martine, M., Bradley, L., & Lefebvre, J. (2001). Theoretical perspectives on the relation between catastrophising and pain. *Clinical Journal of Pain, 17*, 52–64.

Werner, A., & Malterud, K. (2003). It is hard work behaving as a credible patient: Encounters between women with chronic pain and their doctors. *Social Science & Medicine, 57*, 1409–1419. doi: 10.1016/S0277-9536(02)00520-8.

Werner, A., Isaksen, L. W., & Malterud, K. (2004). 'I am not the kind of woman who complains of everything': Illness stories on self and shame in women with chronic pain. *Social Science & Medicine, 59*, 1035–1045. doi: 10.1016/j.socscimed.2003.12.001.

Vieira-Baptista, P., & Lima-Silva, J. (2016). Is the DSM-V leading to the non-diagnosis of vulvodynia? *Journal of Lower Genital Tract Disease, 20*, 354–355. doi: 10.1097/LGT.0000000000000250.

Chapter 8

Queer Patienthood

Laura E. Brown

Communication between patients, providers, and patients' close others can influence a range of health predictors, health experiences, and health outcomes. Duggan and Thompson (2011) outline a number of these areas of influence, including patient satisfaction, quality of life for the patient and their relational partners, medical adherence to a treatment plan, instances of malpractice lawsuits against care providers, and the relative success or failure of health interventions. Interpersonal communication in health contexts is an important predictor and mediator of health-related outcomes like managing uncertainty (Brashers, 2001; Mishel, 1988) and adherence to a medication regimen. Queerness influences a wide range of health-related processes and outcomes: health-care utilization and access to care, stigma, discrimination, violence, trauma, substance use, mental health, sexual health, cancer, and chronic disease (Sharman, 2016).

Communication influences the successful or unsuccessful navigation of structural inequalities (e.g., policy, economic) and barriers to health and wellness that exist in the United States. Although lesbian, gay, bisexual, transgender, queer, and additional gender and sexual minorities (LGBTQ+; GSM) people face many of the same health issues as cisgender, heterosexual people, gender and sexual minorities have additional concerns with which they must deal.

Experiences of health, illness, wellness, and the health-care system for queer people and patients are unique in meaningful ways. This chapter describes better and worse queer patienthood experiences, provides an overview of key terms and concepts, offers a snapshot of health disparities and how stigmatizing communication influences health outcomes, and concludes with a vision of queer patienthood for the future.

TERMS AND ACRONYMS

Throughout this chapter, the terms and acronyms LGBTQ+, queer, and GSM will be used. These terms and acronyms have some overlap in meaning, however, identity is dynamic and personal to individuals. In Table 8.1, key definitions are provided (LGBTQIA Resource Center Glossary, 2014). In communication studies, queer can be used as a noun, an adjective, or a verb (West, 2018). In this chapter, queer will be used as an adjective to describe a patient population.

Having common language, and specific definitions, can be helpful in conceptualizing all of the small moments that contribute to a greater sense of understanding when considering an interaction holistically. Of course, language is shifting rapidly to be more specific, more inclusive, or more accurate all the time. Thanks in part to millennials on Tumblr, artists, writers, and queer theorists, we have an ever-expanding and ever more vibrant vocabulary with which to express the dynamism of identities and proclivities and experiences

Table 8.1   Key Definitions

Sex assigned at birth	A medically constructed categorization assigned by health-care providers, usually based on the appearance of genitalia. Although many sexes exist, newborns are often labeled "M" for male or "F" for female.
Gender	A social construct used to classify a person as a woman, a man, or another identity. Gender does not necessarily match sex assigned at birth.
Gender expression	How a person expresses themselves to others by dress, appearance, and behavior
Gender identity	An internal sense of one's self as a woman, man, or another identity.
Cisgender	A person is cisgender when their gender aligns with their sex assigned at birth
Transgender	An umbrella term for anyone whose gender does not align with their sex assigned at birth. Medical transition (e.g., hormone replacement therapy, surgeries) is not necessary for a person to be transgender.
Gender pronouns	Words used to refer to a person in the third person include: they/them/theirs, ze/hir/hirs, she/her/hers, and he/him/his.
LGBTQ+	An umbrella term and abbreviation for lesbian, gay, bisexual, transgender, and queer. The addition sign makes space for people who are questioning, intersex, asexual, and multiple additional identity categories.
Queer	Historically, this word has been used as a slur. Some people have reclaimed this word, and often use it to signal an anti-assimilationist position. Queer can encompass multiple aspects of identity.

and each other. Although this can be a point of consternation for those who are just beginning to consider gender and sexuality and health, it is well worth learning the basics of the language of LGBTQ+ identity and experience.

One communication issue that GSM confront in health settings is a double bind. That is, a contradictory desire to self-disclose GSM status to further develop an interpersonal relationship while simultaneously fearing social rejection (Wells & Kline, 1987). Gershman (1983) describes the twin anxieties of revealing or concealing one's GSM status as a "Catch 22." Dindia (1998) states, "Social systems involve contradictory and opposing forces (e.g., openness-closedness) ... Individuals continually face the contradictory impulses to be open and disclosive versus closed and protective of the self or of other" (p. 84). The question of disclosure occurs in a larger context of health disparities and stigma. Listening to the narratives of LGBTQ+ patients is one of the best tools scholars and practitioners have in fostering inclusivity and health equity.

MEMORABLE MESSAGES ABOUT LGBTQ+ HEALTH CARE

In a study of patients' memorable messages about sexual orientation and receiving health care, participants ($n = 119$) described their memories of when someone told them about going to the doctor and its relation to sexual orientation (Brown, 2015). Participants could be cisgender or transgender, so long as they did not identify as heterosexual. Four themes emerged from an exploratory thematic analysis of these data: (1) stigma, heterosexism, and discrimination (65%); (2) safer sex practices (35%); (3) "coming out" and disclosure of sexual orientation (20%); and (4) finding a health-care provider (11%). These themes resulted from the descriptive codes (i.e., topical codes) and process codes (i.e., action codes) initially assigned to each memorable message description. In some instances, messages contained more than one topic.

Occasionally, messages that contained stigma, heterosexism, or discrimination also included messages about safer sex practices and coming out disclosures. For example, one participant explained,

> Multiple lesbian friends of mine tell me how that even though they disclose their orientation they are treated as if they still have sex with men. Often asked to start birth control in case they start sleeping with men.

Messages like this one may make participants feel socially supported and in solidarity with one another, or messages like this may make participants feel pessimistic about their chances of receiving tailored care from competent providers. In summary, memorable messages contained some material that may have been interpreted negatively and other information that may have been positively received.

Participants received conflicting advice about whether or not to disclose their sexual orientation to a health-care provider. Notably, 20 percent of descriptions of memorable messages illustrated themes about "coming out" and disclosure of sexual orientation. One individual wrote that someone said to them, "Remember to inform them when they don't ask." Alternatively, another individual reported, "I remember a friend telling me that it would be embarrassing if I went to a doctor and identified as bisexual, and that I should just say I'm straight instead."

Some participants reported receiving messages containing factually incorrect information. For example, one woman explained, "My parent assumed that because I had only same-sex relationships, I would not need to be tested for STIs." Another individual wrote that he was told, "All gay people will need a doctor because they will get AIDS." Although these conflicting, and sometimes factually incorrect, messages were reported as influential for the way people interacted with health-care providers since the time of reception, other experiences over time may have had a larger predictive influence over coming out disclosure decision-making processes.

Care as Process

For many LGBTQ+ patients, encountering the health-care system occurs long before stepping into a clinic or office setting. Individuals both access routine care (e.g., receiving the annual flu vaccination) as an LGBTQ+ person, and access LGBTQ+ specific care (e.g., a transgender man receiving a prescription for testosterone).

Queer patients often engage in information seeking before making an appointment with a new health-care provider. Although many non-LGBTQ+ individuals also engage in pre-visit information seeking, this is a unique process for queer patients because of the stigma, prejudice, and discrimination that exist. Even if an individual has not personally been discriminated against by a health-care provider (e.g., refused treatment after making a coming out disclosure), stories of discrimination get circulated among queer communities, thereby reifying individual patient expectations and fears. Many times, the veracity of the story is less important than the fact of the story's existence; the underlying narrative of prejudicial health-care providers creates anxiety, uncertainty, and a need for additional information, even and especially when one needs care. Word of mouth, asking friends and acquaintances for recommendations, and searching online for reviews and professional biographical blurbs are common ways that queer individuals go about finding LGBTQ+ affirming, or at least tolerant, providers. Some queer individuals learn to scour these brief blurbs for any clue that a provider will be a safe choice.

Receiving a recommendation for a LGBTQ+ affirming health-care provider is only the beginning. Practical questions related to access remain. For example, is transportation available, affordable, safe, and reliable? Is the provider accepting new patients? Does the queer individual have health insurance?

For a brief period, the Affordable Care Act made it so that the vast majority of LGBTQ+ individuals had health insurance, either through an employer or the system commonly referred to as Obamacare. The Out2Enroll campaign specifically targeted uninsured queer individuals. Although these are issues that all individuals face (e.g., transportation), queer patients are disproportionately affected. Many LGBTQ+ people report not having a primary care provider, and going to the doctor much less frequently than cisgender, heterosexual people. This is both a problem of access and of utilization. Even if a queer patient has had positive past experiences with health-care providers, it is usually the negative experiences that are remembered the most. Having just a few negative experiences interacting with the health-care system discourages individuals from seeking care in the future.

Receiving Care

The waiting room experience, from the décor to interpersonal interactions with front desk staff can contribute to the overall stress or lack thereof of a doctor's visit. Visual cues like what kinds of people are featured in framed wall art can offer clues as to whether or not a patient feels like the clinic is "right" for them. Non-discrimination policies can be displayed in waiting areas, or posted on a clinic's website. Non-discrimination policies might protect patients, employees, or both. Without this information available, and without a federal mandate ensuring equitable access and care, LGBTQ+ patients are often left wondering how they can expect to be treated.

It is common for pre-visit questionnaires to be completed by patients either online or in person in the waiting area. While best practices for intake forms do exist, they have not been widely adopted. Patients tell stories about the harmful idiosyncrasies on intake forms, and these narratives need to inform best practices. This is important for two reasons: first, to make patients feel welcome, and second, to ensure the accuracy of the information providers are collecting on the forms. Typical necessary revisions include deleting binary language that does not reflect the vibrant and varied realities of many individuals' genders, romantic or sexual behaviors, and sexual and sexual orientation identities. Gender diverse, genderqueer, and gender nonconforming are labels that individuals who do not experience gender as a binary might use to describe themselves (Donatone & Rachlin, 2013).

Binary forms make it difficult, if not impossible, for queer individuals to make themselves visible in health-care settings. Transgender patients may have more than one legal name, and it may be different from the name they use in their daily lives. Distinguishing which names and pronouns individuals use from the names and pronouns their insurance might need to be able to process their visit is necessary. If a practice must ask for one's legal name, then an additional note should be included to explain why this question is necessary. Binary questions about gender that include only the options "male" and "female" do not reflect the lived experiences and identities of LGBTQ+ people, not to mention the few marital status response options that are typically available. Since the Defense of Marriage Act was overturned, many more LGBTQ+ individuals have become married, however, many queer relationships are more complicated than simply "single, married, divorced, or widowed." This question becomes practically important when visitation rights and the roles of support people are considered.

In most cases, a nurse opens the door into the waiting area and calls out a patient's name. This can be problematic when gendered prefixes are used (e.g., Mr. or Mrs.), especially if a patient's name and gender marker ("F" or "M") on the insurance card is inaccurate, but still being used for identification purposes. Words that people sometimes use because they have been taught that they signal politeness (e.g., "ma'am" or "sir") often accomplish the opposite goal if not used mindfully with queer patients. If verifying patients' identities is a concern for staff, one procedural change can be to call patients by last name only, at least until the provider establishes an ongoing trusting relationship with the patient. If information beyond last name needs to be verified, phone numbers or addresses can be more inclusive and affirming than the use of first names.

Now imagine an alternate scenario in which a queer patient has a positive experience interacting with the health-care system. What could this look like? Pre-appointment, it might be the case that the patient knows exactly where and how to search for LGBTQ+ affirming providers. After making an appointment with an affirming provider, someone who is taking on new patients and who accepts insurance, the patient can feel more confident upon arrival to the physical setting of the clinic.

Many other seemingly small, yet meaningful, factors can influence the patient experience. For example, imagine in this scenario that the patient enters the waiting room and immediately sees a rainbow-colored sticker accompanied by a simple, easy-to-read non-discrimination policy. Ideally, non-discrimination policies cover race, ethnicity, religion, age, sexual orientation, gender identity and expression, and disability status. Something as minor as a rainbow sticker signals to the patient that there is at least one person in the clinic who is likely to be a LGBTQ+ ally. Waiting room wall art that is inclusive of different types of relationships or magazines or brochures positively featuring elements of LGBTQ+ life can also signal allyship.

Imagine that the front office staff have small stickers on their nametags that indicate which pronouns they use. This aligns with recommendations that health-care professionals first disclose which pronouns they use before asking a patient which pronouns they use. Seeing a pronoun sticker on the nametag of whomever greets patients at the clinic signals to queer patients that they can safely share their own pronouns. For patients who are not in the know about gender pronouns, the sticker gives them an opportunity to ask. In this way, front office staff can serve as front-line educators for queer patient inclusivity.

Practice makes perfect when it comes to correctly using peoples' gender pronouns. If a mistake is made, individuals should immediately correct the language, offer a simple and sincere apology, and move on. This approach avoids burdening the patient with the responsibility of providing social support or consolation. Practicing using the correct pronouns makes it easier to avoid making mistakes in the future.

Expert recommendations and best practices for collecting gender data outline a two-step process (Cahill & Makadon, 2013; Fenway Guide to LGBT Health, 2015). Patients should be asked two separate questions: First, what is your gender? According to the Fenway Guide to LGBT Health (2015), answer choices should include male, female, transgender male/trans man/FTM, transgender female/trans woman/MTF, genderqueer, an additional category with an option to write in a response, and decline to answer. Patients should be instructed to check or circle all that apply. Second, what is your sex assigned at birth? Recommended answer choices include male, female, or decline to answer. Patients should be instructed to check just one box.

This eliminates common issues that crop up because of the binary, and overly simplistic, nature of many patient intake forms. For example, some women identify both as "transgender woman" and as "woman." Which single box should this woman check? From the health-care professional perspective, imagine that you are a nurse who sees that a patient has checked the "transgender" box on a patient intake form. What knowledge is gained by this checked box? It is impossible to know which of the many, and varied, genders encompassed by the term "transgender" a patient is communicating here. Transgender and genderqueer patient narratives are a way that cisgender men and cisgender women can understand the problem of binary systems (e.g., Harbin, Beagan, & Goldberg, 2012). Although expert recommendations have not been widely implemented, in part because they have not been mandated, the recommendations do exist. Organ inventories can be another way to assess patient needs; however, it should be clear to the patient why an organ inventory is necessary.

Sexual orientation as a blend of attraction, behavior, and in some cases, political identity, is another powerful binary structure. That is, the binary system of sexual orientation allows for only one kind of pairing—that of a heterosexual cisgender woman with a heterosexual cisgender man. Expert recommendations and best practices also exist for asking about sexual orientation. The Fenway Guide to LGBT Health (2015) recommends asking: Do you think of yourself as? With answer choices including lesbian, gay, or homosexual, straight or heterosexual, bisexual, something else, and don't know. Changing the phrasing of medical history questions on forms and in conversation to be inclusive of a range of sexualities would "alleviate the burden of repeated disclosure" for the patient (Boehmer & Case, 2004, p. 1888). Sexual behaviors should be asked separately from sexual orientation or sexual identity.

Relationship questions can include answer choices like "in a committed relationship" and should make space for patients to describe other meaningful relationships they have. Being a new patient and completing a form that captures the complexity of identity and behaviors from the start of the visit, and being correctly named when called to the exam room, sets the tone for a positive patient-provider interaction. Patient narratives are space-making, and a tool to dismantle binary structures. Taking patient narratives seriously is one way that health-care experiences can be reimagined and evolve to better reflect the care-related needs of LGBTQ+ people.

There are many opportunities for the exam itself to go well or poorly. Intake interviews are common parts of all doctor's visits. A negative intake interview can be characterized by communication behaviors such as asking inappropriate or irrelevant questions, making assumptions about sexual orientation identities or behaviors based on perceived gender, failing to use accurate gender pronouns, hyper-focusing on GSM components of identity, hyper-sexualizing patients, or engaging in stigmatizing nonverbal communication like avoiding eye contact or touch. These are examples of ways that prejudice can be communicatively enacted. Negative experiences ensure that LGBTQ+ patients do not feel welcome in the health-care space. Additionally, stigmatizing and prejudicial communication has measureable consequences for negative health outcomes.

What does a positive intake interview look like? Imagine that providers ask open-ended questions rather than making assumptions. It is acceptable, and often a required part of the process, to confirm what patients have written down, and it can be helpful for patients if providers explain why they are asking questions that may seem overly personal or invasive, especially questions about sensitive topics like sexual practices or genitals. Communication, including provider-patient interactions, visual cues, and word choices, influences the experiences and outcomes of LGBTQ+ health.

Health Outcomes and Disparities

According to Ndiaye and colleagues (2011), there is a lack of research attention to LGBTQ+ health disparities, and this lack of attention is "a form of disparity [itself] because it impedes the development of treatments" (p. 472). The authors suggest that scholars first acknowledge that LGBTQ+ people experience health differently than cisgender, heterosexual people experience health. Next, the authors suggested that researchers study LGBTQ+ people beyond the domain of sexual behaviors so as not to neglect other important health issues.

Illnesses do not distinguish their host on the basis of sexual identity, however, sexual identity translates to health and communication differences between groups. Relieving health disparities is a "complex communication task" (Ndiaye, Krieger, Warren, & Hecht, 2011, p. 470). Certain populations are likely to contract specific diseases or face various challenges when obtaining treatment or even routine, preventive care.

Despite relatively recent policy changes like the overturning of the Defense of Marriage Act, there is still much work to be done at the policy level to ensure equitable care for all. Notably, there is no national-level protection against sexual minority status-related discrimination (Human Rights Campaign, 2013). States that do not allow same-sex marriage, and states in which individuals can be fired for being LGBTQ+ complicate employment, economic, and health insurance issues for LGBTQ+ people.

Stigma, discrimination, prejudice, and the denial of civil and human rights are separate, yet highly interconnected, processes. If stigma is defined as an attribute that is discrediting to the individual who exhibits it (Goffman, 1963), then discrimination can be thought of as systematized stigma. According to Healthy People 2020, stigma happens on an individual, or micro, level. Discrimination happens at a group, or mezzo, level. The denial of civil and human rights happens on a policy, or macro, level. Prejudice can be communicated through stigmatizing behavior, discrimination, or the denial of civil and human rights for a group. Discrimination and prejudice have health consequences for LGBTQ+ people and patients.

Some researchers have conceptualized the experience of discrimination and prejudice as minority stress. Antonovsky (1979) defined stress as "the strain that remains when tension is not successfully overcome" (p. 3). Stress can be a precursor or a consequence of becoming ill, and stress affects the physical, emotional, cognitive, behavioral, physiological, and social aspects of life (Bendelow, 2009). Minority stress is chronic and socially or communicatively based. Minority stress is additive (Meyer, 2007). In other words, queer individuals must deal with the stress that a cisgender, heterosexual patient would not ordinarily deal with in encountering health-care providers. This additive stress puts more pressure on the LGBTQ+ individual to adapt to a potentially unpleasant and stigmatizing communication event.

Existing programs of research have identified some trends in terms of LGBTQ+ physical and mental health (e.g., Ryan, Wortley, Easton, Pederson, & Greenwood, 2001). Biologically speaking, queer people are qualitatively no different from anyone else (Byne, 2007), so it is important to investigate reasons beyond the body that help explain why these differences in health outcomes exist. It is not enough to know that LGBTQ+ individuals are at greater risk for a host of health issues and illnesses; further investigation is necessary and can move the United States toward a more equitable system of care, which would help meet the stated goals of the national Healthy People 2020 program. Conceptualizing bodies as "acting mind-body units" (Freund, 1990, p. 457) means that social experiences and cultural factors produce physical reactions in the body. Feeling powerless, blameworthy or having thoughts and emotions invalidated from those with more social power (e.g., physicians, cisgender people, heterosexuals) can affect physical functioning. If minority stress is chronic, it can affect neurohormonal regulation (Bendelow, 2009), which is necessary for good cardiovascular health.

Substance abuse is a sizable issue in queer communities. For instance, LGB individuals are up to 40 percent more likely to smoke cigarettes than heterosexual individuals (Ryan et al., 2001). Smoking leads to a variety of health issues including lung cancer, heart disease, bone thinning, and emphysema. Cigarette use accounts for approximately 30 percent of all deaths from cancer (American Cancer Society, 2013). Lesbians and gay men have higher rates of alcohol consumption, which is linked to increased rates of physical violence, sexually transmitted infections (STIs), and chronic diseases (Woodial & Brindle, 2008).

Cisgender lesbian and bisexual women have an increased risk of breast and gynecological cancers, some STIs, obesity, and heart disease. In one study of the women who had sex with women in the past three years, 92 percent reported in engaging in unprotected oral sex, 25 percent engaged in vaginal fisting without using a latex barrier, and 29 percent reported sharing dildos without using a latex barrier (Lemp et al., 1995). The increased risk of breast and gynecological cancers can be at least partially attributed to this group being less likely to receive preventive medicine including annual check-ups, pap smears, and breast exams (Matthews, Brandenburgh, Johnson, & Hughes, 2004). There is no simple biological reason why queer cisgender women are more affected than heterosexual cisgender women, which suggests that more research is needed to understand the health behaviors (e.g., accessing care) and interpersonal communication (e.g., disclosure) of SGMs.

Queer men have a greater risk of methamphetamine use, disordered eating, and HIV contraction than their cisgender, heterosexual counterparts (Diaz, 2007). Disordered eating includes anorexia and bulimia. Internalized homophobia is related to body shame, which mediates the relationship between body surveillance and disordered eating (Wiseman & Moradi, 2010). Cultural standards of masculinity and attractiveness and media messages can also contribute to body shame and body surveillance. Disordered eating has harmful physical effects like kidney, cardiovascular, and dental damage.

Differences exist between the mental health of SGMs and cisgender heterosexuals in the United States. Depression and anxiety, like the physical health issues explicated above, are more likely to affect LGBTQ+ people. Some of the mental health challenges that LGBTQ+ people face can be linked explicitly to SGM identification, such as navigating anti-queer violence and decisions about coming out (Woodial & Brindle, 2008). Domestic partner violence in same-gender relationships can involve threats of "outing" someone against their will as a means of control. Bullying is an important mental health issue for adolescent and young adult LGBTQ+ students. Over 85 percent of queer adolescents reported being verbally harassed because of their SGM status, and about half of those adolescents reported physical harassment (Russell, Ryan, Toomey, Diaz, & Sanchez, 2011). There is a strong positive correlation between experiencing verbal or physical harassment and lower self-esteem and poor social adjustment. Additionally, victimization is linked to higher suicide rates among LGBTQ+ individuals (e.g., Haas et al., 2010).

COMMUNICATION APPROACHES TO ADDRESSING LGBTQ+ HEALTH DISPARITIES

Historically, perhaps the most common recommendation to providers who interact with LGBTQ+ individuals is to de-medicalize GSM statuses. In other words, providers should avoid suggesting that being LGBTQ+ is an illness or medical abnormality. Since the 1970s, medical textbooks and research monographs have made more specific recommendations to providers (for a more complete history, see Martos, Wilson, & Meyer, 2017). These recommendations include using gender non-specific pronouns when referring to sexual partners, explaining why detailed questions about sexual activity must be asked before soliciting that information, interacting with colleagues non-discriminatorily (i.e., modeling good behavior), asking if it is okay to ask about sexual history before doing so, and using direct, normalizing language (e.g., "many women experience difficulty with" or "it is not uncommon to experience"; Washer, 2009). Some researchers have recommended that physicians and other care providers use behaviorally focused language rather than identity-focused language (Bonvicini & Perlin, 2003). Just as with heterosexual patients, it is preferable for providers to use clear and simple language.

Other researchers have argued for a model of cultural competency. In general, cultural competency involves perceiving LGBTQ+ people as being part of a community and facing community-wide challenges like increased risk for alcohol and cigarette use and abuse, increased risk of methamphetamine use, among cisgender gay men, and so on (Woodial & Brindle, 2008). Other recommendations based in a cultural competency model include being aware of perceived or enacted stigma rooted in heterosexism, cissexism, transphobia, and homophobia, creating a welcoming environment by using inclusive language, and recognizing one's own potential for discriminatory thoughts and behavior. In their focus groups of LGBTQ+ patients and in their focus groups of providers who treat LGBTQ+ patients, Wilkerson and colleagues (2011) identified structural components (e.g., decor), systemic components (e.g., policies and forms), and interpersonal components (e.g., a trusting provider-patient relationship) that contribute to an overall culturally competent clinic. They reported, "Trust appeared to be inextricably linked to feeling safe in the clinical space and influenced decisions by health care providers and patients to come out as LGBT" (p. 383). Although the authors offered many recommendations for modifying structural components (e.g., place a rainbow sticker on the door) and systemic components (e.g., ask about pronouns on medical intake forms), they offered almost no recommendations about the interpersonal components. Rather, they noted that just one negative provider-patient interaction can damage a clinic's reputation within a local LGBTQ+ community.

Dismantling Binaries and Barriers

Many of the communication challenges that present themselves in clinical settings and patient-provider contexts stem from binary structures of identity and behavior relating to gender and sexuality. The problematic nature of the binary system of gender and sexuality is often invisible (Ahmed, 2006) to those who are cisgender and heterosexual. Patient narratives render systems of privilege visible. However, it is not enough to collect narratives, or listen to stories, or express sorrow or regret at the ways in which health-care systems are not constructed to care for the bodies, minds, and lives of LGBTQ+ people. Good intentions including the intention to "treat all patients equally" are often not enough. It is not enough to promote LGBTQ+ affirming policies that can take months, or years, to be implemented and can just as quickly be overturned.

The best tools we have are our bodies and our abilities as communicators. Action and engagement can take many different forms for communication scholars, educators, and advocates. Action and engagement can look like providing clinic trainings for the two-step process of data collection for gender, it can look like designing and distributing informative half-sheets on what gender pronouns are and how to use them, it can look like scribbling out sections on patient intake forms and revising them so they mirror lived realities, and it can look like creating the infrastructure necessary so that more LGBTQ+ people become providers.

CONCLUSION

As a final note, I would like to acknowledge my intersecting identities and note how all peoples' identities influence perception and narrative. As a queer, white, educated, able-bodied (for now) woman, I need to leave space for that which I do not perceive because of my various privileges and oppressions. Queer patienthood is continually spooling out from time, it is always in development, it is a dynamic process in and of itself—and this dynamism is something that must be honored, even within an idealized vision of what queer patienthood can look like in the future.

REFERENCES

Ahmed, S. (2006). *Queer phenomenology*. Durham, NC: Duke University Press.

American Cancer Society. (2013). Cancer facts for lesbian and bisexual women. Retrieved from: http://www.cancer.org/healthy/findcancerearly/womenshealth/cancer-facts-for-lesbians-and-bisexual women.

Antonovsky, A. (1979). *Health, stress and coping*. San Francisco, CA: Jossey-Bass.

Bendelow, G. (2009). *Health, emotion, and the body*. Cambridge, UK: Polity Press.

Boehmer, U., & Case, P. (2004). Physicians don't ask, sometimes patients tell: Disclosure of sexual orientation among women with breast carcinoma. *Cancer, 101*(8), 1882–1889.

Bonvicini, K. A., & Perlin, M. J. (2003). The same but different: Clinician-patient communication with gay and lesbian patients. *Patient Education and Counseling, 51*(2), 115–122. doi: 10.1016/S0738-3991(02)00189-1.

Brashers, D. E. (2001). Communication and uncertainty management. *Journal of Communication, 51*(3), 477–497. doi: 10.1111/j.1460-2466.2001.tb02892.x.

Brown, L. E. (2015). Modeling lesbian, gay, and bisexual patient disclosures: An exploration of the role of memorable messages, past experiences, perceived visibility, screening behaviors, and efficacy (Doctoral dissertation). Retrieved from: the University of Texas Library.

Byne, W. (2007). Biology and sexual minority status. In I. H. Meyer & M. E. Northridge (Eds.), *The health of sexual minorities: Public health perspectives on lesbian, gay, bisexual, and transgender populations* (pp. 65–90). New York: Springer.

Cahill, S. R., & Makadon, H. (2013). Sexual orientation and gender identity data collection in clinical settings and in electronic health records: A key to ending LGBT health disparities. *LGBT Health, 1*(1), 4–41.

Diaz, R. M. (2007). Methamphetamine use and its relation to HIV risk: Data from Latino gay men in San Francisco. In I. H. Meyer & M. E. Northridge (Eds.), *The health of sexual minorities: Public health perspectives on lesbian, gay, bisexual and transgender populations* (pp. 584–603). New York: Springer.

Dindia, K. (1998). "Going into and coming out of the closet": The dialectics of stigma disclosure. In B. M. Montgomery & L. A. Baxter (Eds.), *Dialectical approaches to studying personal relationships* (pp. 83–108). Mahwah, NJ: Erlbaum Associates.

Donatone, B., & Rachlin, K. (2013). An intake template for transgender, transsexual, genderqueer, gender nonconforming, and gender variant college students seeking mental health services. *Journal of College Student Psychotherapy, 27*, 200–211. doi: 10.1080/87568225.2013.798221.

Duggan, A. P., & Thompson, T. L. (2011). Provider-patient interaction and related outcomes. In T. L. Thompson, R. Parrott, & J. F. Nussbaum (Eds.), *The Routledge handbook of health communication* (2nd ed., pp. 414–427). New York: Routledge.

Freund, P. (1990). The expressive body: A common ground for the sociology of emotions and health and illness. *Sociology of Health and Illness, 12*(4), 452–477.

Gershman, H. (1983). The stress of coming out. *American Journal of Psychoanalysis, 43*, 129–138.

Goffman, E. (1963). *Stigma: Notes on the management of spoiled identity*. Englewood Cliffs, NJ: Prentice Hall.

Haas, A. P., Ellason, M., Mays, V. M., Mathy, R. M., Cochran, S. D., D'Augelli, A. R., ... Clayton, P. J. (2010). Suicide and suicide risk in lesbian, gay, bisexual, and transgender populations: Review and recommendations. *Journal of Homosexuality, 58*(1), 10–51. doi: 10.1080/00918369.2011.534038.

Harbin, A., Beagan, B., & Goldberg, L. (2012). Discomfort, judgment, and health care for queers. *Bioethical Inquiry, 9*, 149–160.

Healthy People 2020. (2013). Lesbian, gay, bisexual, and transgender health. Retrieved from: http://www.healthypeople.gov/2020/topicsobjectives2020/overv iew.aspx?topicid=25.

Human Rights Campaign. (2013). Employment non-discrimination act. Retrieved from: http://www.hrc.org/campaigns/employment-non-discrimination-act.

Lemp, G. F., Jones, M., Kellogg, T. A., Nieri, G. N., Anderson, L., Withum, D., & Katz, M. (1995). HIV seroprevalence and risk behaviors among lesbians and bisexual women in San Francisco and Berkeley, California. *American Journal of Public Health, 85*, 1549–1552. doi: 10.2105/AJPH.85.11.1549.

LGBTQIA Resource Center Glossary. (2014). In UC Davis lesbian gay bisexual transgender queer intersex asexual resource center. Retrieved from: http://lgbtrc.u cdavis.edu/lgbt-education/lgbtqia-glossary.

Makadon, H. J., Mayer, K. H., Potter, J., & Goldhammer, H. (2015). *Fenway guide to lesbian, gay, bisexual, and transgender health* (2nd ed.). Philadelphia, PA: American College of Physicians.

Martos, A. J., Wilson, P. A., & Meyer, I. H. (2017). Lesbian, gay, bisexual, and transgender (LGBT) health services in the United States: Origins, evolution, and contemporary landscape. *PLoS ONE, 12*(7), 1–18.

Matthews, A. K., Brandenburg, D. L., Johnson, T. P., & Hughes, T. L. (2004). Correlates of underutilization of gynecological cancer screening among lesbian and heterosexual women. *Preventive Medicine, 38*(1), 105–113.

Meyer, I. (2007). Prejudice and discrimination as social stressors. In I. H. Meyer & M. E. Northridge (Eds.), *The health of sexual minorities: Public health perspectives on lesbian, gay, bisexual and transgender populations* (pp. 242–267). New York: Springer.

Mishel, M. H. (1988). Uncertainty in illness. *Journal of Nursing Scholarship, 20*(4), 225–232. doi: 10.1111/j.1547-5069.1988.tb00082.x.

Ndiaye, K., Krieger, J. L., Warren, J. R., & Hecht, M. L. (2011). Communication and health disparities. In T. L. Thompson, R. Parrott, & J. F. Nussbaum (Eds.), *The Routledge handbook of health communication* (2nd ed., pp. 469–481). New York: Routledge.

Russell, S. T., Ryan, C., Toomey, R. B., Diaz, R. M., & Sanchez, J. (2011). Lesbian, gay, bisexual, and transgender adolescent school victimization: Implications for young adult health and adjustment. *Journal of School Health, 81*(5), 223–230. doi: 10.1111/j.1746-1561. 2011.00583.x.

Ryan, H., Wortley, P. M., Easton, A., Pederson, L., & Greenwood, G. (2001). Smoking among lesbians, gays, and bisexuals: A review of the literature. *American Journal of Preventive Medicine, 21*(2), 142–149.

Sharman, Z. (2016). *The remedy: Queer and trans voices on health and health care.* Vancouver, BC: Arsenal Pulp Press.

Washer, P. (2009). *Clinical communication skills.* New York: Oxford University Press.

Wells, J. W., & Kline, W. B. (1987). Self-disclosure of homosexual orientation. *Journal of Social Psychology, 127*, 191–197. doi: 10.1080/00224545.1987.9713679.

West, I. N. (2018). *Queer perspectives in communication studies.* Oxford Research Encyclopedia of Communication.

Wilkerson, J. M., Rybicki, S., Barber, C. A., & Smolenski, D. J. (2011). Creating a culturally competent clinical environment for LGBT patients. *Journal of Gay & Lesbian Social Services, 23*(3), 376–394. doi: 10.1080/10538720.2011.589254.

Wiseman, M. C., & Moradi, B. (2010). Body image and eating disorder symptoms in sexual minority men: A test and extension of objectification theory. *Journal of Counseling Psychology, 57*(2), 154–166. doi: 10.1037/a0018937.

Woodial, K., & Brindle, K. (2008). Culture and sexual orientation. In M. A. Perez & R. R. Luquis (Eds.), *Cultural competence in health education and health promotion* (pp. 213–230). San Francisco, CA: Jossey-Bass.

Chapter 9

An Autoethnographic Account of Navigating Patienthood as a Person with Hearing Impairment

Alexis Z. Johnson

According to the National Institute on Deafness and Other Communication Disorders (NIDCD) (2017) approximately 37.5 million American adults aged eighteen and over report some trouble hearing. Despite the number of people affected by hearing impairment, the hard of hearing and deaf population are underrepresented. In addition, there remains a lack of resources in the medical field presenting a unique subset of challenges for the hearing impaired. This autoethnography focuses on my experience of coping with and navigating the health-care system as a person with hearing impairment. The autoethnographic account explores face-to-face encounters with doctors and other medical practitioners, and the communication barriers that come with hearing loss that effect my decision-making, health, and quality of life as a patient. My stories illustrate more generally how those with hearing impairments are disempowered in the medical world, and often struggle to make informed decisions because of the lack of resources for them in hospital settings. I offer reflections on life changing experiences as a patient struggling to communicate effectively with medical practitioners because of my hearing loss.

THE HEARING LOSS

"Alexis," my mother called from the other room.

It was a typical childhood Saturday morning for me. I was watching my favorite Spider-Man cartoon and eating cereal.

"Alexis!" My mother continued to shout. She had something important she needed to discuss with me and was growing concerned I was not answering her.

I continued to stare at the screen in awe of the complexity I was witnessing on television.

"What is wrong with you? Why are you ignoring me? Alexis!" My mother continued.

She finally had grown tired of waiting for me to respond. My mother came storming into the room with a look of fury on her face.

"Didn't you hear me?" She screamed.

"What?" I responded. I was genuinely confused as to why she was so angry with me. All I had been doing was watching some good old comic cartoons.

"Alexis!" She screamed, continuing to raise her voice. "Didn't you hear me?"

"Oh, Mom. I didn't hear anything." I said looking confused.

These types of conversations became commonplace over the next couple of years. Finally, a school counselor reached out to my parents and asked if I had ever been tested for hearing loss. They informed my parents that I was not responsive at school. At first, I would get in trouble in the classroom. It was the same routine of me being yelled at by my teacher. I had a cold once that was so severe it obstructed my ears, making hearing almost impossible. The teacher had been so aggravated by my behavior that she threw my books out of the window in an effort to get my attention. I cried, feeling completely lost. I didn't understand why I couldn't hear anything and everybody around me attributed this to a behavioral issue. My school grew concerned about how consistently I was unable to respond, and my look of surprise when they said they had tried to talk to me.

At seven years old I was diagnosed with a moderate to severe 60-70 decibel sensorineural hearing loss in both ears. My hearing loss was unique because I had difficulty hearing both high and low frequencies; I was described as "tone deaf." Being hearing impaired presented numerous challenges in the bio-medical field. For me, these issues were fairly significant being diagnosed at a young age. This was—in part—because I needed to learn how to navigate these challenges as a child. Much like invisible illness, it is not always obvious that somebody lives with a hearing impairment. However, it is common for people to suffer from some degree of hearing loss, whether it be moderate or severe.

***

Hearing losses affect approximately 37.5 million people in the United States (National Institute on Deafness and Other Communication Disorders, 2017). One in six U.S. adults have some trouble hearing and one in three older adults (70+) will have a hearing loss (NIDCD, 2017). Unfortunately, many adults go without treatment for their hearing loss. The National Institute on Deafness and Other Communication Disorders (NIDCD) (2017) found that 28.8

million adults could benefit from using hearing aids. However, only one in four U.S. adults, ages twenty or over, who may benefit from hearing aids have used them. In fact, on average, people live ten years or more with hearing loss before seeking hearing aids (Davis et al., 2007). This is problematic because people rely on their senses to build their world, conceptualize things, and to reason (Verma et al., 2017). While some may benefit from hearing aids, others may not. There are several different types as well as reasons why someone develops hearing loss, which can be permanent or temporary.

Specifically, the Hearing Loss Association of America (2018) describes three main types of hearing loss. Conductive hearing loss is due to problems with the ear drum, ear canal, or middle ear bones. Conductive loses can result from malformation in the ear, fluid in the ear, allergies, ear infections, benign tumors, impacted earwax, and more. The second type is a sensorineural hearing loss. A sensorineural hearing loss is different from a conductive loss—in that—it is caused with problems of the inner ear and is nerve related. There are many ways that a person can develop or have a sensorineural hearing loss. These include exposure to loud noise, aging, trauma, virus/disease, autoimmune diseases, Meniere's disease, and others. Finally, individuals have potential to have a mixed hearing loss that is a combination of conductive damage as well auditory nerve damage (sensorineural) (Hearing Loss Association of America, 2018).

My loss was characterized as being irreversible sensorineural hearing loss that could be managed with hearing aids. Research suggests that hearing aids can improve health-related quality of life in adults who have a permanent sensorineural hearing loss (Chisolm et al., 2007). Unfortunately, however, I fell into the atypical statistic, not seeking the use of hearing aids for over twenty years. I was also informed that my hearing loss would progress as I aged (Davis et al., 2007), and I was advised to consider cochlear implants in the future. The audiologist and doctors struggled to understand how I had such a severe loss. One doctor suggested it could have potentially been present at birth, others thought that it was because of a tonsil and adenoid surgery I had a few months prior to my hearing loss diagnosis. Regardless of how the loss developed I now needed to face the realities and struggles that come with a hearing impairment. My identity and my narratives of patienthood as a hearing-impaired person became forever interwoven. They transformed into a story ripe with uncertainty and challenges.

AUTOETHNOGRAPHY OF PATIENTHOOD

I turned to autoethnography to capture my experiences as a moderate-severe hearing -impaired individual navigating the health-care system. In particular,

I focused on the many challenges that may result from working with an audiologist, but also in other facets of the biomedical world. I used Carol Rambo's layered accounts (Ronai, 2002) as a means to reflexively interrogate the multiplicity of my experiences, emotions, and identities that constituted my narratives in the medical world as a hearing-impaired individual. Consistent with Rambo's work on layered accounts, I move forward and back through time writing from a variety of perspectives from my childhood, young adulthood, with hearing aids and without, and also as an autoethnographer in the communication discipline. My hope is that by layering my experiences from different vantage points I will be able to move beyond my own experiences in the deaf/hard of hearing community and provide insight into larger cultural issues that others may face in the biomedical world (Ellis, 2004; Ronai, 1992).

In particular, I am drawn to the method of autoethnography because of its focus on "reflexively writing the self into and through ethnographic text, isolating that space where memory, history, performance, and meaning intersect" (Denzin, 2014, p. 22). My narratives are more than a collection of stories: they focus on current issues surrounding an underrepresented population, in this case the hearing-impaired community. Autoethnography also allows me to shed light on some of the larger sociocultural implications that exist between hearing loss and communication in the biomedical world. The method offers invaluable perspectives on a multitude of issues surrounding race, gender, and other hybrid and/or stigmatized identities in society (Adams, Jones, & Ellis, 2015, Denzin, 2014). As aforementioned, the hearing-impaired community often does not seek help in the medical world. Thus, my goal is to use my own lived experiences to understand why those in this community may not get the assistance they need in medicine, and how this might influence decisions made pertaining to their loss and health. I hope that by sharing my own challenging narratives within this context that I may shed light on the stigma that surrounds this community. Additionally, my goal is to bring voice to a population that may otherwise be unheard.

The "You Will Never" Approach in Medicine

I will never forget the words that were written on my charts pertaining to my hearing loss. They wrote "a hearing loss of this degree is considered communicatively handicapping." Something I learned early on with a hearing loss diagnosis is that in the medical world you are often faced with the conversations of "you will never" with your doctors. In my case many audiologist told me what I would never be capable of. I was an aspiring actress and singer. The lack of background noise in my daily life drew me to music. Music provided a means to add noise to my otherwise silent life, and more importantly it allowed me to get out of my head. I enjoyed listening, but I also enjoyed singing and joined choir at a young age. I walked into my usual six month hearing test and check-up when my doctor asked me what was going on at school. I told her about my newfound excitement for this year's song line up for choir. She was silent as pressure filled my ears and the machine measured the reactivity of the nerves. After the test, she delivered news that shattered my heart into a million little pieces making it beyond repair.

"You know," she said. "You will never be able to really sing. Your type of hearing loss makes it nearly impossible for you to hear pitch and tone. We are surprised you don't have a speech impediment.

My mother was there with me and could see the look of anguish on my face. She tried to encourage me after the appointment, but I was unable to have a coherent conversation. I was just delivered news that the one thing that brought some joy to my life, I would never excel at because of my disability. That year I was told by my choir director that I often fell flat while singing, but I couldn't tell. I couldn't hear if I was flat or on pitch. I didn't even really know what "normal" sounded like. His critiques, coupled with the audiologist definitive statement, made me feel like I was left with no other choice but to discontinue my pursuit of music. I stuck with acting, always longing to be in the school musicals, but never having the courage to audition.

In addition to being told I couldn't sing, there were countless other moments where I was told I would never be able to lead a normal life because of my hearing impairment. I had to tolerate sitting at the front of the class because I did not have hearing aids to support my loss. This resulted in bullying by my peers. I was told I was a teacher's pet and a nerd. I shrugged off the bullying and tried to ignore something that was not in my control. However, I felt too ashamed to tell anyone that I was hearing impaired. I made the informed decision that being bullied because I was considered a nerd was a far greater alternative then being bullied for a disability.

In addition to being bullied, my doctors expressed concern that I would struggle in school. It was after this revelation, while in middle school, that I noticed my grades deteriorating. That was not all the doctors had to report. They also emphasized how my interpersonal relationships had potential to be strained as a result of my loss and so I began to isolate myself. I had few friends growing up because I was concerned I would be judged when I requested clarification of what was said in numerous conversations. I lost friends, had trouble talking to my parents, my education was negatively influenced, I was bullied, and most importantly, lost passion for a dream I long held onto from my childhood, I would never be a singer. I lost all sense of self-confidence, fell into a deep depression, and felt that I was now defined by my hearing loss. It took control over almost every facet of my daily life.

***

The "you will never" approach to my hearing loss presented newfound challenges and emotions that I never imagined were possible. I had self-doubt about my ability to communicate because I was labeled as "communicatively handicapped." Research suggests that the impact of a hearing loss not only effects the individual, but also the families and friends of the individual with hearing impairment on a daily basis. Hearing loss can potentially reduce an individual's ability to communicate effectively with others (Verma et al., 2017; Arlinger, 2003). From my own experience, I established that it was difficult to reach out to others. Indeed, the cloud of oppression, coercion, and bad news seemed to follow closely. My joy for extracurricular activities was easily broken by friends, family members, and/or medical practitioners who insisted I would not have the capacity to partake in the activity. Thus, I silenced myself and concealed my hearing loss to the best of my ability. Unfortunately, this type of silencing can lead to difficulties maintaining relationships and may alienate the individual with the hearing loss (Verma et al., 2017).

One explanation for isolation with hearing loss could be that hearing loss has potential to decrease an individual's self-esteem, or feelings of self-worth (Stephanie et al., 2014). Lower self-esteem is often associated with greater feelings of loneliness and complications coping with stressful life events. A study by Stephanie and colleagues (2014) found that hearing-impaired children experience lower levels of self-esteem in a variety of social domains. These findings are compelling, because they are consistent with my own narrative and discovery of self-esteem issues. Nonetheless, self-esteem does not always affect a singular aspect of an individual's life. Issues with self-esteem may also have emotional and behavioral repercussions as well (Harter, 2006; Stephanie et al., 2014; Cole et al., 2001).

Specifically, emotional shifts may lead to the development of depression, anxiety, and other mental health issues (Wayner and Abrahamson, 2001; Kramer et al., 2002; Gopinath et al., 2009). Jones & White (1990) profess that people with hearing impairment are more vulnerable to depression and symptoms of anxiety (Monzani et al., 2008) than the general population. Other studies corroborated these findings for individuals with profound and mild to moderate hearing impairments (Hallam et al., 2006; Monzani et al., 2008). Despite these findings, there is limited attention on the psychosocial needs of people with hearing loss (Hallam et al., 2006). Therefore, it is plausible that these residual effects have potential to have negative repercussions on one's quality of life. I found myself not only plagued by the fear of communicating with others, questioning my abilities, but also experiencing a superabundance of depression and anxiety. I scarcely sought help from others thinking I was exaggerating my disability. In spite of that, there are other complex issues that may need to be addressed in general medical care.

In my experience, my hearing loss went beyond the scope of dealing with depression and judgment from my peers. I found that I was handled and regarded divergently by medical practitioners. This differentiation of treatment led to difficulty making informed decisions and sensing that my doctor's didn't care. Ultimately, I felt a decline in my overall well-being as a result of issues that presented themselves in the most mundane appointments regarding other aspects of my health. In fact, individuals with hearing loss often report poorer quality of life and a decline in overall health (McCormack & Fortnum, 2013), which may result from other incidents regarding their health (McShea, 2015).

The Assumption of Hearing

My experience afforded me the opportunity to make observations of how I was treated before and after having hearing aids during doctor's appointments. Fundamentally, this granted me insight into how decision-making, assumptions about abilities, and medicine treats a disability like hearing loss. I have dealt with hearing loss most of my life, but I found that many are stunned to hear I have such a profound hearing loss at my age. It seems that the cultural assumption lies in the notion that older adults face hearing loss and younger adults are immune to its affliction. In fact, my audiologist said "I'm not used to having someone so young with such a severe loss in my office." Additionally, there are stereotypes that exist regarding speech impairment for those who have a hearing loss. I am often told that I don't "sound" hearing impaired which causes people to question the authenticity of my disability. Thus, my age coupled with my seemingly normal speaking serves as a means of masking my disability. Hence, I am treated as a typical patient by medical practitioners. Many doctors, outside of audiologists, presume that I am able to hear well. As a result, I often have doctors check my ears bluntly push the light into my ear. I promptly hear "oh" from the doctor. I scarcely receive an apology for potentially damaging my expensive hearing aids.

"Could you remove those so I can examine you," doctors often say.

"Yes, I am sorry," I reply.

While my ears are being examined, doctors often continue to carry on a normal conversation. Unfortunately, I exert myself to hear what they are saying. Not only do I have a medical device obstructing my ear, but I generally am not able to hear most people without my ability to lip read.

"Okay you can put them back in," doctors say.

"Huh?" I find myself replying.

The doctor usually doesn't repeat what they said. They continue to speak as I catch on to context clues that it is safe to put my hearing aids back in. I have never been asked if I would like an American Sign Language (ASL) interpreter. I don't speak fluent ASL as I was not in any way formally taught, but I still find it precarious that these services are not offered once doctors discover that I have a hearing impairment.

Adversity exists in what seems like a disregard for my hearing impairment, but also in the approach medical practitioners take to communicate with me. I attempt to hear different accents and am incapable to comprehend speech that is quiet or spoken at a fast pace. I have had copious encounters with doctors who parallel the described speech patterns. If I don't have somebody with me to explain what the doctor said, I often make a strong effort to interpret what was spoken on my own. This diminishes my confidence that I am executing the correct decisions about other aspects of my health. Additionally, when I request information to be repeated medical practitioners often appear mildly annoyed. While this behavior shouldn't cause me to feel like a burden, it often does. During appointments I observe that I seek to conceal my hearing loss. Occasionally I also agree with my doctors without asking appropriate questions or understanding the medical condition or tests.

While face-to-face doctor appointments can be intimidating, I do have the gift of lip reading to help me trudge through them. Worse than doctors' appointments are receiving information over the phone regarding my health. Likewise, setting up appointments with staff can be burdensome. My hearing aids are troublesome to use over the phone, unless I have it on speaker. They shrill and scream in their high pitched resistance to being covered, they are amplifiers after all. Thus, I am often not able to answer the phone in a public setting if I am awaiting news regarding my health. Not unless I want everyone in the vicinity to know that my white blood cell count and kidney counts are off due to my autoimmune disease. Once I do have time to be in a more private setting I am on the other side of the phone hoping that the nurse calling speaks slowly and pronounces words with a bit more exaggeration so it is easier for me to know what was said. There have been numerous times I have misheard a medical practitioner over the phone, sought information on what I thought I heard, and was horrified to learn I was dying from a rare disease. For appointments, I often second guess if I've written down the correct date and time because there are times I mishear staff. I typically call several times before my appointment confirming the date and time and I am not always greeted in a friendly manner.

***

Regrettably, while hearing impairment is common, medical practitioners are often unaware of patients hearing abilities and their skills with this demographic can be limited (Heron & Wharrad, 2000). Studies demonstrate communicative issues have potential to arise between patients with a hearing loss and practitioners (Hines, 2000; Mick et al., 2014). In particular, patients may make an effort to conceal their disability from their medical practitioners because of how they are treated (Hines, 2000). I frequently consider whether I should wear my hearing aids to my doctor's office. If I elect to wear them the doctor may be forceful and disregard my disability, handling the situation poorly. Yet, if I don't wear them I endure breaches in my capacity to understand and maintain a productive conversation. Hearing aids also do not produce a complete natural listening experience; they are hearing their world through a microphone that amplifies sound. Therefore, a noisy hospital setting can be laborious for the patient to pick up what the doctor has said (Slaven, 2003).

In a study by Hines (2000), participants were asked whether their doctors were accommodating in their communication. In total, 64% of hearing-impaired individuals in the study reported that while doctors made an effort, they used inappropriate methods and lacked effective communication skills in this context; 36% of participants felt that their doctors made little or no effort. Individuals who were deaf have also criticized medical practitioners for their lack of understanding and empathy during appointments (Mackenzie & Smith, 2009). Sadly, many medical practitioners and staff members do not have adequate training on how to work with the hearing-impaired and deaf community. Consequently, they may lack the communication skills needed to answer patient's questions and address their concerns. The lapse in communication between medical practitioners and patients may also result in patient's not receiving additional resources that could benefit them (Hines, 2000). The participant's experiences in these studies resonated with my own encounters in the biomedical world. I often formed perceptions that my doctors lacked consideration and sensitivity to my hearing loss. Indeed, once they discovered I had loss, I was not offered additional services and communication was not adapted to fit my needs.

In addition to having the resources to make decisions about healthcare, individuals with hearing impairment have another choice that can impact their quality of life and health. This outcome lays in the ability to afford and maintain hearing aids. Hearing aids remain an expensive investment. It is an investment that does not last a lifetime either. Hearing aids degrade and malfunction over the years. They may also not be utilized because of the stigma connected to them and the amount of time it takes to adjust to them.

As your Hearing Abilities Decrease your Debt Increases

Despite pressures from several audiologists, my parents elected not to purchase me hearing aids. An audiologist informed my parents that I would have tremendous strain in school because of the magnitude of my hearing impairment. The doctors discussed my options and because I was only seven years old I was not able to partake in that decision-making process. It was either that I got hearing aids to help amplify sound or the doctors would write a note for my teachers that said I had to sit in the front of the class. That note would also come with a detailed explanation of my disability and the complications I may have in the course. Though my parents wanted to provide me with the best opportunities they could, hearing aids were and remain incredibly expensive. They told my parents that the cost of hearing aids would range from 5,000 to 10,000 dollars for an acceptable pair of hearing aids. At the time, my parents made too much money for government support, but too little money to be able to afford to buy them for me. Additionally, my mother also worried about the stigma that comes with a hearing disability. She was reluctant to subject me to potential bullying because of my hearing aids (Hetu, 1996). They opted for the note option and so began my life as someone who needed to adapt the way that they communicated to function in society.

I became a master lip reader. When I was unable to see somebody's lips moving I felt slightly panicked. If somebody tried to call me from another room I still was not able to hear them. I spent years adapting the best that I could; however, I still struggled in school, had hindrances maintaining relationships, and I felt lost. My world was silent and I found myself drawn to music to break the silence that encompassed my life. I wanted more than anything to understand why someone tapping their pencil was annoying. A strange, but telling example of how hearing impairment has potential to influence our lives.

It wasn't until I was eighteen years old that I finally got my first pair of hearing aids. I had learned some basic American Sign Language (ASL) and relied heavily on lip reading until that day. My dad was informed that his insurance was now covering hearing aids for those considered to have a moderate to severe hearing loss. I was deemed more than qualified to get fitted for my own pair of hearing aids. My dad was still unsure if he wanted to have to pay part of his deductible on the hearing aids.

"You really think she needs these?" he asked the doctor.

"Do you not see her looking at you and then looking at me when we speak? She is staring at our lips. She clearly relies on lip reading." He responded to my father.

"Everybody looks at someone who is speaking, that's not uncommon." My dad replied.

"Here, let me get the point across to you." He covered his mouth slightly as to not distort the sound significantly. I heard a slight noise, but it was unintelligible. I could not understand any of it.

"What did I say," he asked.

I shrugged my shoulders as I looked at my dad to see if he heard the doctor. My dad glanced back at me, his eyes grew wide with anticipation.

"I have no idea," I replied feeling defeated. That familiar feeling plagued me for my entire life. It impeded in my friendships, family, and education.

"Are you serious, you are lying to the doctor," my dad looked at me. "Didn't you hear him? He clearly said "Hi Alexis, would you like to get fitted for hearing aids?""

I shook my head no.

"I told you. She relies on lip reading to make sense of the language."

That day I got measured for my hearing aids and my audiologist went through some important information about the process. He explained that it would take some time for my mind to adjust to sounds. He shared how many sounds were foreign to my brain and that I would likely get headaches the first few months of wearing hearing aids. When the doctor got the hearing aids in I was overwhelmed with the amount of sounds. The air-conditioning unit in the office kicked on and I felt my heart skip a beat.

"What was that?" I inquired.

"What was what?" He responded. "Oh the air? Yeah that makes noise."

I looked in awe as I tried to discover where this loud, almost grumbling noise was coming from. I left the office, opened my car, and prepared to drive home with the gift of sound. On the way home, I went to turn left and turned on my signal. I heard a clicking noise I had never heard before in my car. I was convinced something was wrong and called my father. After a long winded explanation from me and some troubleshooting he determined I did not know that the signal makes noise. Other noises soon bombarded me and it became too much. I got headaches daily from these noises. I felt overwhelmed trying to figure out "what that sound was" and being looked at like I was some sort of cavewoman who had never left her cave. I discontinued wearing the hearing aids after two weeks of trying. I decided that lip reading and not hearing people was easier then dealing with the burden of sound.

Flash forward a decade and the topic of getting hearing aids resurfaced. My husband expressed concern regarding my inability to hear. I think he grew tired of having the TV on excessively loud, trying to have normal conversations with me, and not surprisingly not being able to talk to me if I left the room. He encouraged me that there was nothing wrong with my hearing impairment, convinced me that it was actually a problem, and shared how he felt it could improve our relationship and my quality of life. I had expressed my discomfort in the classroom, being unable to hear students. I shared with my audiologist that my hearing loss was negatively impacting my job as a professor, and that I had tried to deal with it for nearly five years to no avail. I finally came to the conclusion that it was time to try to fix my ears again. I sought out a new audiologist, enrolled in a program to try to get me affordable hearing aids, and got another test only confirming my need to get hearing aids. My doctor said that the technology had gotten much more advanced since the last time I got hearing aids, told me I was likely fitted with the wrong type of hearing aids for my loss, and shared news that there were hearing aids that were made specifically for my type of loss. She made the process feel like I was picking out a brand new outfit. We discussed the size of the hearing aids I'd like and I was able to pick from what felt like fifty different colors. Some were normal hair colors, others were fun colors, I opted for the white hearing aids. I wanted something that would stand out. I wanted to finally embrace my identity that I had worked so hard over the years to minimize out of lack of confidence and stigma.

The next two months consisted of endless migraines. I felt regret, uncertainty, and questioned whether I should be wearing this $6,000 pair of hearing aids. I decided to continue to power through the difficult adjustment and eventually the pain went away. Looking back two years later and I am in disbelief that I could function in society without my hearing aids. My audiologist and I call them "my ears" and when I'm not wearing my ears I can tell. I struggle to hear someone, even in a quiet setting having a one on one conversation. I feel naked without my hearing aids. I was fortunate to have qualified for a program to obtain my hearing aids. However, many are not able to get benefits from the government or health insurance. As a result, so many are having to live in the same silent world that I had to live in for so many years. There are also many that may be able to afford hearing aids, but are concerned by the stigma deterring them from getting the assistance they need.

***

Getting used to hearing aids is demanding (Mueller & Powers, 2001) and requires consistent use to result in greater benefits (Munro, 2008). In addition, clinical observations made by an audiologist suggest that new hearing aid users must allow for a period of time to adjust to amplification (Munro, 2008; Brooks, 1989; Dillion, 2012). Use of hearing aids has been found to be low (Popelka et al., 1998) and in general people who own hearing aids may not wear them frequently enough for the adjustment (Housgaard & Ruf, 2011; Harley et al., 2010). In my experience, my most recent audiologist explained that wearing hearing aids is virtually retraining your brain to understand new sounds. My hearing loss is also particular and very few hearing aids are able to work with my type of loss. Specifically, users who have loss in the high frequency region may have more aversive and negative experiences when first using hearing aids (Palmer et al., 2006). Research by Dawes, Maslin, & Munro (2014) recruited sixteen patients to participate in a focus group related to their hearing aids. The scholars found that there were a variety of experiences other young adults had that were like my own experience. A participant in their study described their first exposure to new sound as being a "bombardment of noise." This description is consistent with the overwhelming reaction I had in my first moments of using hearing aids. There was incessant clicking and other sounds that made me feel trapped in a glass case of sound. Participants also reported having to learn to get acclimated to sounds they once could not hear. They shared their animosity of having to readjust to sound when they hadn't worn their hearing aids for a short period (Dawes, Maslin, & Munro, 2014). I could simply not handle the noises when I first got hearing aids. After two years of use, I still have moments when I am frightened of a sound that I don't recognize.

Unfortunately, having a hearing loss is not only a physical issue, but also can have psychosocial implications. Research by Kricos (2006) suggests that counseling can be helpful for those who have self-confidence issues as a result of their loss. People who have a hearing impairment often manage stigma that is attached to using hearing aids. There may be a degree of embarrassment that comes from wearing hearing aids because they are regarded as a disability and have potential to cause the user to feel incompetent (Dawes, Maslin, & Munro, 2014). Some also have an issue accepting their hearing loss. Dawes, Maslin, and Munro (2014) discovered that a pre-condition to getting used to hearing aids is realizing that they have difficulty hearing. Those who are diagnosed may be reluctant to accept that they have a problem. Throughout my narratives of hearing loss, I've constantly been called into question by medical practitioners and others noting that I don't sound the part. This also contributed to my difficulty in trying hearing aids. I felt as though my hearing was normal despite years of testing to prove that I was not. The use of hearing aids can affirm the presence of a hearing loss to help people increase their acceptance of their disability (Dawes, Maslin, & Munro, 2014).

CONCLUSION

Clinical trials have demonstrated that hearing aids can enhance overall quality of life, and improve communication (Weinstein, 2013, Mulrow & Agular, 1990). However, many in the United States still live without hearing aids (Blustein & Weinstein, 2016). As aforementioned, hearing aids are not only expensive, but there is a stigma that may come with the use of hearing aids. Additionally, users must account for an adjustment period to using the hearing aids. In my experience, I went over two decades without wearing hearing aids I was consistently told I needed. Some of it was a result of the stigma

I faced at school, the other half was my parent's inability to afford hearing aids that would have cost them over $6,000. The years I spent without hearing aids led to a decline in my mental health, self-esteem, and quality of life. Additionally, communication with medical practitioners became increasingly more demanding as I attempted to navigate the biomedical world with insufficient resources. Being hearing impaired is a disability; however, there is often a lack of regard and education for facilitating more effective modes of communication for the hearing impaired. Many medical practitioners may not adjust well to their hearing-impaired patients simply because they have not been trained or given tools to help them in these situations. It is also difficult to acquire hearing aids and other surgical procedures that could improve a person's ability to hear. To this day I still am terrified to admit that my hearing impairment has changed my life, not always for the better. I am still confronted with a world where the hearing-impaired and deaf community almost feels like an afterthought.

REFERENCES

Adams, T. E., Jones, S. H., & Ellis, C. (2015). *Autoethnography: Understanding qualitative research.* New York: Oxford University Press.

Arlinger, S. (2003). Negative consequences of uncorrected hearing loss: A review. *International Journal of Audiology, 42*(2), 2S17–2S20.

Blustein, J., & Weinstein, B. E. (2016). Opening the market for lower cost hearing aids: Regulatory change can improve the health of older Americans. *American Journal of Public Health, 106*(6), 1032–1035. doi: 10.2105/AJPH.2016.303176.

Brooks, D. N. (1989). *Adult aural rehabilitation.* London: Chapman and Hall.

Chisolm, T. H., Johnson, C. E., Danhauer, J. L., Portz, L. J., Abrams, H. B., Lesner, S., McCarthy, P. A., & Newman, C. W. (2007). A systematic review of health-related quality of life and hearing aids: Final report of the American Academy of Audiology Task Force On the Health-Related Quality of Life Benefits of Amplification in Adults. *Journal Academy of Audiology, 18*(2), 151–183.

Cole, D. A., Maxwell, S. E., Martin, J. M., Peeke, L. G., Seroczynski, A. D., et al. (2001). The development of multiple domains of child and adolescent self-concept: A cohortsequential longitudinal design. *Child Development, 72*, 1723–1746.

Davis, A., Smith, P., Ferguson, M., Stephens, D., & Gianopoulos, I. (2007). Acceptability, benefit and costs of early screening for hearing disability: A study of potential screening testsand models. *Health Technology Assess, 11*(42), 1–294.

Dawes, P., Maslin, M., & Munro, K. J. (2014). 'Getting used to' hearing aids from the perspective of adult hearing-aid users. *International Journal Of Audiology, 53*(12), 861–870. doi: 10.3109/14992027.2014.938782.

Denzin, N. K. (2014). *Interpretive autoethnography* (2nd ed.). Los Angeles: Sage Publishing.

Dillon, H. (2012). *Hearing aids.* Sydney: Boomerang Press.

Ellis, C. (2004). *The ethnographic I: A methodological novel about autoethnography.* Walnut Creek, CA: AltaMira Press.

Goggins, S., & Day, J. (2009). Pilot study: Efficacy of recalling adult hearing-aid users for reassessment after three years within a publicly-funded audiology service. *International Journal of Audiology, 48*, 204–210.

Hallam, R., Ashton, P., Sherbourne, K., & Gailey, L. (2006). Acquired profound hearing loss: Mental health and other characteristics of a large sample. *International Journal Audiology, 45*, 715–723.

Harter, S. (2006). *Self-processes and developmental psychopathology.* In D. Cicchietti & D. J. Cohen (Eds.), *Developmental psychopathology* (pp. 370–418). Hoboken, NJ: Wiley & Sons.

Hartley, D., Rochtchina, E., Newall, P., Golding, M., & Mitchell P. (2010). Use of hearing aids and assistive listening devices in an older Australian population. *Journal of American Academic of Audiology, 21*, 642–653.

Hearing Loss Association of America. (2018). Retrieved October 5, 2018, from: https://www.hearingloss.org/hearing-help/hearing-loss-basics/symptoms-diagnosing/.

Heron, R., & Wharrad, H. (2000). Prevalence and nursing staff awareness of hearing impairment in older hospital patients. *Journal of Clinical Nursing, 9*(6), 834–841.

Hétu, R. (1996). The stigma attached to hearing impairment. *Scandinavian Audiology Supplement, 4*, 12–24.

Hines, J. (2000). Communication problems of hearing-impaired patients. *Nursing Standard (through 2013), 14*(19), 33–37. Retrieved from: https://libcatalog.atu.edu:443/login?url=https://libcatalog.atu.edu:2409/docview/219794173?accountid=8364.

Hougaard, S., & Ruf, S. (2011). EuroTrak 1: A consumer survey about hearing aids in Germany, France, and the UK. *Hearing Review, 18,* 12–28.

Jones, E. M., & White, A. J. (1990). Mental health and acquired hearing impairment: A review. *British Journal Audiology, 24*, 3–9.

Kramer, S. E., Kapteyn, T. S., Kuik, D. J., & Deeg, D. J. (2002). The association of hearing impairment and chronic diseases with psychosocial health status in older age. *Journal of Aging Health 14*(11), 122–137.

Kricos, P. B. (2006). Audiologic management of older adults with hearing loss and compromised cognitive/psychoacoustic processing capabilities. *Trends Amplif, 10*, 1–28.

Mackenzie, I., & Smith, A. (2009). Deafness – the neglected and hidden disability. *Annals of Tropical Medicine and Parasitology, 103*, 565–571.

McCormack, A., & Fortnum, H. (2013). Why do people fitted with hearing aids not wear them? *International Journal of Audiology, 52*(5), 360–368. doi: 10.3109/14992027.2013.769066.

McShea, L. (2015). Managing hearing loss in primary care. *Learning Disability Practice (2014+), 18*(10), 18. doi: 10.7748/ldp.18.10.18.s19.

Mick, P., Foley, D. M., & Lin, F. R. (2014). Hearing loss is associated with poorer ratings of patient–physician communication and healthcare quality. *J Am Geriatr Soc, 62*(11), 2207–2209.

Monzani, D., Galeazzi, G. M., Genovese, E., Marrara, A., & Martini, A. (2008). Psychosocial profile and social behavior of working adults with mild tomoderate hearing loss. *Acta Otorhinolaryngol Ital, 28*, 61–66.

Mueller, H. G., & Powers, T. A. (2001). Consideration of auditory acclimatization in the prescriptive fitting of hearing aids. *Seminars in Hearing, 22,* 103–124.

Mulrow, C. D., & Aguilar, C. (1990). Quality-of-life changes and hearing impairment: A randomized trial. *Ann Intern Med, 113*(3), 188–194.

Munro, K. J. (2008). Reorganization of the adult auditory system: Perceptual and physiological evidence from monaural fitting of hearing aids. *Trends Amplif, 12,* 254–271.

National Institute on Deafness and Other Communication Disorders. (2017). Retrieved October 5, 2018, from: https://www.nidcd.nih.gov/.

Palmer, C. V., Bentler, R. A., & Mueller, H. G. (2006). Amplification with digital noise reduction and the perception of annoying and aversive sounds. *Trends Amplif, 20,* 95–104.

Popelka, M. M., Cruickshanks, K. J., Wiley, T. L., Tweed, T. S., Klein, B. E., et al. (1998). Low prevalence of hearing-aid use among older adults with hearing loss: The Epidemiology of Hearing Loss Study. *Journal of the American Geriatrics Society, 46,* 1075–1078.

Ronai, C. (1992). Multiple reflections of child sex abuse: An argument for a layered account. *Journal of Contemporary Ethnography, 23,* 395–426.

Slaven, A. (2003). Communication and the hearing-impaired patient. *Nursing Standard, 18*(12), 39+. Retrieved from: http://libcatalog.atu.edu:2189/apps/doc/A1122 46701/AONE?u=aktechuniv&sid=AONE&xid=8cfd1afa.

Stephanie, C. P. M. T., Rieffe, C., Netten, A. P., Briaire, J. J., Soede, W., Kouwenberg, M., & Frijns, J. H. M. (2014). Self-esteem in hearing-impaired children: The influence of communication, education, and audiological characteristics. *PLoS One, 9*(4). doi: 10.1371/journal.pone.0094521.

Verma, L., Sanju, H. K., Scaria, B., Awasthi, M., Ravichandran, A., Kaki, A., & Rathna Prakash, S. G. (2017). A comparative study on hearing aid benefits of digital hearing aid use (BTE) from six months to two years. *International Archives of Otorhinolaryngology, 21*(3), 224–231. doi: 10.1055/s-0036-1592117.

Wayner, D. S., & Abrahamson, J. (2001). *Learning to hear again* (2nd ed.). Latham: Hear Again Publishing.

Weinstein, B. E. (2013). *Geriatric audiology* (2nd ed.). New York, NY: Theime Medical Publishers.

Part III

NARRATING PATIENTHOOD: INTERSECTIONS OF COMMUNICATION AND THE PERSONAL, RELATIONAL, PROFESSIONAL, AND CULTURAL

Chapter 10

From Consumer to Community-Based Researcher

Lessons from the PLHIV Stigma Index

Andrew Spieldenner, Laurel Sprague,
Ari Hampton, Meta Smith-Davis, Dwight Peavy,
Ann D. Bagchi, Barb Cardell, Vanessa Johnson,
Gina Brown, and Russell Brewer

The HIV epidemic has transformed the American health-care system in criti-cally important ways. When AIDS first appeared in the United States in 1981, the medical and scientific community had no treatment options and little knowledge about what was causing the immune breakdown. Even after HIV was first identified in 1984, viable HIV treatment would not be available for at least a decade (1995). Within this time, people living with HIV organized as a community to effect change in organizations, government institutions, and media (Brier, 2009). With the emergence of activist groups such as the AIDS Coalition To Unleash Power (ACT UP) and nonprofit community-based organizations such as Gay Men's Health Crisis, the HIV epidemic also paved the way for other patient-led health movements such as those focused on breast cancer (Rabkin et al., 2018).

People living with HIV movements started as peer-networks—often as support groups where people diagnosed with HIV could connect with others, sharing treatment news, medical advice, and information on which organiza-tions and medical providers were helpful and which to avoid (Adelman and Frey, 1997). The HIV activist movement was led by people living with HIV, and engaged in advocacy at federal and local levels with elected officials, health departments and other government agencies, the courts, and media. This activism took many forms: from street protests, to political funerals, to letter writing campaigns, to kiss-ins. Some of these groups built community organizations to provide HIV services such as outreach and education, linkages to medical care, housing and other social services, and, in some cases, direct clinical care (Brier, 2009; Rabkin et al., 2018).

The medical community was not prepared for HIV, and had little to offer at the start. Research could not move fast enough to get needed results, and the hospitals and doctors in the early epicenters were overwhelmed by patients with the disease. With HIV, it was not just the lack of medical options that presented challenges for health-care providers, but the demographic of those with HIV including people who inject drugs, sex workers, people of color, immigrants, and gay men. The social discrimination against these identities further complicated healthcare, as medical providers had to cope with their fear of the mysterious illness alongside their own values about sex, sexual orientation, drugs, immigrants, and race (Rabkin et al., 2018). Research was also hampered by political inaction and lack of will (Brier, 2009). Even more than individual fear of infection, structural stigma shaped the response, so much so that HIV-related stigma remains prevalent after so many years.

Since medical providers struggled with knowledge about the disease, people living with HIV became experts in their own care. Through peer-education and partnerships with medical doctors, people living with HIV sought out new ways of coping with the disease, developed markers for health and illness, and explored options that integrated multiple kinds of medicines and treatments (Rabkin et al., 2018; Spieldenner, 2017). The shift in the doctor-patient relationship—where people living with HIV were considered partners in their own health—was the result of community organizing and empowerment movements, including the women's health movement of the 1970s.

HIV community organizing and empowerment movements also impacted governmental agencies and research. The decades-long protests to legislators made HIV a priority in urban America and some key states, as HIV advocates and organizations built relationships with elected officials and heads of agencies. Activism eventually led the federal Food and Drug Administration to fast track drug development, despite inaction from other federal agencies including the president. Behavioral and social science research organizations began to build specific HIV divisions, as more and more researchers studied—and received funding—to examine HIV and its myriad issues (Brier, 2009; Ramirez-Valles, 2011). Much of this research was conducted in collaboration with HIV organizations and groups of people living with HIV. While these empowerment movements have had critical successes, they have waned as HIV services shift to a more clinic-based model, often casting people living with HIV as "consumers" of services rather than integral community partners (Guta, Murray, & Gagnon, 2016).

The stigma associated with HIV began early and remains to this day. While the first evidence of stigma included health-care, housing, and employment discrimination, it also entered the interpersonal and community sphere, as those living with HIV were actively excluded from families, dating, and public positions (Brier, 2009; Global Network of People with AIDS, n.d.). While HIV-related stigma may have changed as science and community norms shift, it remains a pervasive force in marginalizing people living with HIV. HIV-related stigma has been associated with lapses in medical care, mental health challenges, and treatment nonadherence (Ramirez-Valles, 2011; Sprague, Simon and Sprague, 2011).

In this chapter, we examine how one community-based participatory research (CBPR) initiative on HIV stigma impacts the people that implement it (Rabkin et al., 2018). We will describe the PLHIV Stigma Index, and explore the discourses around "consumer" and "community researcher" in the HIV epidemic of the United States. We will explore our own experiences in the implementation sites in Detroit, MI; New Orleans and Baton Rouge, LA; and New Jersey. We engage in critical narrative self-reflection. As such, most of us identify as people living with HIV and people of color, and will indicate our positionalities through our quotes. At some point in our lives, those of us living with HIV have accessed social and clinical services through HIV organizations and other publicly funded agencies.

THE PLHIV STIGMA INDEX

In 2008, a partnership of UNAIDS, the International Community of Women living with HIV (ICW), the International Planned Parenthood Federation, and the Global Network of People Living with HIV (GNP+) developed the PLHIV Stigma Index as a CBPR initiative to document experiences of stigma of people living with HIV and to intervene in stigma at the country level (Global Network of People with AIDS, n.d.). GNP+, an international nongovernmental organization comprised of networks of people living with HIV, currently leads the management of the PLHIV Stigma Index project on behalf of an international partnership comprised of GNP+, ICW, and UNAIDS. GNP+ collaborates with other civil society groups and networks of people most affected by HIV, including gay and bisexual men, people who use drugs, sex workers, and transgender people, to address health disparities in HIV globally.

As a CBPR initiative, the PLHIV Stigma Index involves people living with HIV at every level of development. The PLHIV Stigma Index involves a partnership between a network of people living with HIV and a research partner, usually engaging public health offices and other civil society organizations as well. GNP+ can provide technical assistance and the actual research tool to the partnership, but country efforts are resourced locally or through global funders, such as the Global Fund to Fight AIDS, TB, and malaria or the President's Emergency Plan for AIDS Relief (PEPFAR). Research partners work with the network of people living with HIV to develop a sampling strategy and to clean and analyze the data. Findings are then interpreted within the local context, bringing researchers and people living with HIV together, and used to design and implement anti-stigma initiatives at the local and national level. As of 2017, over 100,000 people living with HIV have been part of the PLHIV Stigma Index in over 90 countries. Groups of people living with HIV chose to conduct the PLHIV Stigma Index in the United States, with meetings beginning in 2014.

Several key challenges emerged. The United States is more racially heterogeneous than other countries that have implemented the HIV Stigma Index, so issues of race and historical racism were not explored in the tool adequately. In addition, the tool was first developed prior to two key paradigms currently in HIV: the treatment cascade and treatment as prevention. The treatment cascade provided an HIV care continuum that indicated how and where people fell in and out of medical care. The mathematical model has been used widely by health departments and government agencies to better understand where to bolster and resource efforts in their jurisdictions. Similarly, treatment as prevention emerges from the understanding that viral suppression reduces transmission rates to nil. While the international partnership was committed to updating the PLHIV Stigma Index, a process completed in early 2018, the US Implementation Committee committed to the PLHIV Stigma Index while resourcing was available. To address some of the challenges and to better adapt the tool for the United States, a group of people living with and affected by HIV from diverse backgrounds and experiences worked together to identify and add new questions and additional response options. As a result, racial and ethnic demographic questions were added as well as a new set of questions on experiences of people living with HIV who had been incarcerated. In addition, a module was included with questions about barriers to testing and treatment. This module was developed initially for use in PLHIV Stigma Index implementations in Eastern and Central Europe and Central Asia, and was based on open-ended responses from people living with HIV who were interviewed as part of PLHIV Stigma Index implementations in Southern, Eastern, and Western Africa.

We will use a narrative approach to this study. As a group, we have responded to a core set of questions about the PLHIV Stigma Index process and its impact on us, as well as in our observations in the implementation in Detroit, Baton Rouge, New Orleans, and across New Jersey. Narrative approaches work well in managing multiple viewpoints, kinds of knowledge and voices (Kellett, 2017). With CBPR, researchers and community groups engage each other in dynamic and often complex ways. Every CBPR project has varying roles for researchers and community partners; in the case of the PLHIV Stigma Index, the community partner is centered in determining sampling, recruiting participants, collecting and cleaning data, participating in data interpretation, and developing and implementing resulting stigma interventions. Through our narratives, we will examine the dynamics of the PLHIV Stigma Index that transform people living with HIV from "consumers" to "community-based researchers/leaders." We will look specifically at intersectionality, regarding economics and other forms of diversity, and the ways that a sense of community can be built through the PLHIV Stigma Index.

When we speak of intersectionality, we are utilizing the framework developed by Crenshaw (1991) to describe how each person has multiple kinds of identities, some of which are characterized by social advantages and ascribed social value and some of which are characterized by social disadvantage and prejudice. Multiple kinds of identities that are socially devalued can coexist in one person, thus leading to several multiple experiences and different kinds of structural oppressions (e.g., racism, homophobia, sexism, transphobia, etc.). In our framework, we see how the community of people living with HIV often exists at an intersection of identities that face additional hardships that interact to create new levels of entangled stigma and discrimination. Where a gay man of color living with HIV faces an intersection of racism and homophobia alongside HIV-related stigma. In addition, he may also have mental health issues, substance use history, experience with the criminal justice system, experience poverty, be erratically housed, and/or be from another country: all leading to ways of being marginalized or unseen in healthcare and other areas.

DEFINING "CONSUMER"

Language and discourse around HIV have been the center of multiple struggles for community groups, service organizations, public health, law enforcement, media, and governments. As early as 1983, the People with AIDS Coalition asserted that language was political, and had to come from the community. As such, their bill of rights, the Denver Principles, begins "we condemn attempts to label us as 'victims', a term that implies defeat, and we are only occasionally 'patients', a term that implies passivity, helplessness, and dependence upon the care of others" (People with AIDS Coalition, 1983). HIV movements since have used this motto as an organizing principle, particularly when marginalized. Gay men, people of trans* experience, people of color, women living with HIV, immigrants, people who use drugs, and sex workers have all challenged organizations, conferences, policies and initiatives that utilized dehumanizing language or descriptions. While these battles have resulted in changes in policy and public discourse, new forms of marginalizing language continue to emerge and require challenges to this day.

In the HIV industry, people with HIV are now often referred to as "consumers" in both common organizational terminology as well as in descriptions of jobs (e.g., Consumer Peer Navigator), initiatives (e.g., Consumer Outreach), and leadership opportunities (e.g., Consumer Advisory Board). The notion of a "consumer" draws up questions about *who* is consuming *what*. It offers a vision that people living with HIV are eating the services provided, like insects in a field of vegetables, or a virus burning through a body's resources. It does not speak to principles of self-determination and empowerment; rather, it perpetuates an image of a passive, greedy and mindless need and of capitalistic structures in which the productive produce and the others consume.

The position of "consumer" is strongly felt within the HIV industry. When HIV organizations hire people living with HIV, the positions are often as line staff or "peer" support staff for HIV organizations. These positions often have little to no decision-making power at the institutional level. While people living with HIV have unique knowledge about the local HIV epidemic, this is rarely consulted in developing programs, policy or evaluation initiatives.

> People living with HIV are predominantly seen as clients for service organizations rather than as critical agents in their own lives and as valued experts in the HIV response. When people living with HIV are brought into places to speak or hired as case managers, they are often treated as exceptional or tokenistic and are expected to act as individuals rather than as part of a group or community— Laurel, White lesbian woman living with HIV, Detroit.

After over two decades of living with HIV, Laurel has been a "consumer," a "researcher," and an "advocate." She has seen how the role of people living with HIV is minimized in the field.

While HIV organizations might seem like odd places to uncover HIV-related stigma, people living with HIV are often vulnerable in these spaces. Whether obtaining medical care or social services, the relationship in many of these organizations tends toward patronage. The HIV organization positions itself as benevolent, and the person living with HIV is positioned as consumer. To obtain services, people are often asked to conduct themselves with propriety, taking on the "good patient" role that listens to authority, appreciates all forms of help, and does not ask questions. Where this might work in other populations, often people living with HIV are marginalized not just from HIV, but also from the circumstances surrounding HIV acquisition such as sexuality, substance use, poverty, and mental health issues. In addition, many people living with HIV have experiences of self and peer empowerment processes and have learned to expect to be treated as equals by service providers. Together, these do not produce the congenial "good patient" mode that most clinics require.

> Participating in the project highlighted the stigma we have against one another—even in a "safe space" like HIV-centered service agencies. People realized that they stigmatize others and how they judge "how people should conduct themselves." These attitudes may not always be expressed openly, but the feelings are there.—Dwight, African American gay man living with HIV, New Jersey.

Dwight is discussing a version of the politics of respectability that happens in HIV clinics. Higgenbotham (1993) conceptualized the politics of respectability to describe black women organizing in the black church in the early 1900s—where a critique of the American failure to live up to its liberal promises was accompanied by behavior codes reminiscent of middle-class white values. Enacting dominant social norms in interactions—including middle-class white notions of propriety and manners—is a way of embodying the possibility of taking social capital. In a similar way, many HIV clinics expect patients to act in ways that are "respectable"—showing up on time, being docile in the clinic space, agreeing to treatments, and adhering to drug regimens. When people show up with trauma, markedly from the structural and interpersonal violence that many people living with HIV experience both before and after diagnosis, and its aftermath, including as mental health suffering or increased substance use, these guidelines of respectability are violated, and clinics exert disciplinary forces on people living with HIV, including barriers to transgender hormones, lack of respect and compassion in the clinic space, dismissal of concerns about side effects, exerting pressure for people to disclose their HIV status without regard for their safety or need for privacy, and delays in social support services.

Ari acknowledges these power differentials in the HIV service space. The stigma prevalent in the wider society emerges in the workplace in specific ways.

> A lot of PLWH [People Living with HIV] were still being discriminated or stigmatized not just by the community but also in certain professional setting[s] as well.—Ari, mixed-race gay man living with HIV, Detroit.

Ari's assessment of the workplace is echoed by Barb. Rather than overt stigma, often people living with HIV are limited in the roles permitted in organizations.

> Many of the [interviewers] were engaged as case managers or other support staff at community-based organizations but had never considered their own expertise

in living with HIV.—Barb, White heterosexual woman living with HIV, New Jersey and Detroit.

Both Ari and Barb are talking about the limits that the HIV workspace gives to people living with HIV. In the professional setting, people living with HIV are relegated to service or support roles, rather than tapped into for the expertise they have with living with HIV. In addition, people living with HIV often internalize this message, leading to their underestimating their capacity to inform or guide HIV planning, programming, and initiatives.

This staffing gets played out in other ways, such as who gets reimbursed for what kinds of labor. Dwight points out the tension that is present in HIV advocacy.

> There is generally an "us versus them" feeling, whereby providers are compensated for the time they spend in HIV advocacy efforts, but [people living with HIV] are not (e.g. providers may be paid members of the Planning Council but consumers generally are not).—Dwight, African American gay man living with HIV, New Jersey.

While HIV advocacy circles want people living with HIV to be involved, this involvement is unpaid for variety of reasons including the lack of salaried position at an HIV organization, rules about reimbursements within HIV Planning Councils, and a dearth of funding for advocacy roles in the HIV field, as well as a sense that people who are already employed should be compensated for their time while those unemployed or with personal experience ought to give of their experience without remuneration. HIV advocacy efforts have been central to battling structural level HIV-related stigma, however, the lack of people living with HIV able to be at those tables highlights deep economic disparities, including among those living with HIV, with the most economically advantaged, and their concerns, being also the most likely to be included in decision-making bodies.

Intersectionality: Economic Justice

In all three sites, economic justice emerged consistently in our narratives. From paying people living with HIV for participating to acknowledging the unpaid labor people living with HIV do, we each found that part of the PLHIV Stigma Index intervention had to center economic justice. Laurel describes the surprise when looking at the data from the first site.

> The one thing that really did leap to the forefront of the characteristics of people living with HIV when we started to look at the data, though, was how incredibly

economically vulnerable people were, especially, but not only, young people living with HIV. We did not seek out people to interview based on different economic statuses. When the numbers came back, without even doing outreach around poverty, we had really high proportions of people who were currently or recently homeless and had insufficient food to eat. Further, when we analyzed people's experiences of stigma based on their economic vulnerability, we found that those with the most experiences of stigma were those who were the most economically fragile.—Laurel, White lesbian living with HIV, Detroit.

While we expected economics to play a role, we did not anticipate the amount of erratic housing, unemployment, and poverty. By conducting the interviews, we learned more about how economics impacts the local HIV community.

Maintaining steady income was a challenge across the sites. Sprague, Simon, and Sprague (2011) describe a range of challenges that people living with HIV face in employment. For some, employment was difficult due to anticipated stigma, forced disclosure of HIV status, exclusion in the workplace due to HIV status, and job termination. In addition, people living with HIV experience social marginalization based on other identities such as gay and trans* identity, being part of a community of color, as well as experience with substance use, mental health challenges, and incarceration. The structural violence against these identities can exclude or limit educational opportunities too.

The PLHIV Stigma Index became an intervention in economic justice in each site, at least while the PLHIV Stigma Index was being conducted. Locally, people living with HIV were trained in recruitment, interviewing, and quality assurance skills. Interviewers were paid for the interview and for quality-checking the questionnaires. Barb talks about the challenges in ongoing employment with a project that is finite and time sensitive.

The skills are transferable but ongoing employment is not supported ... The economic partnership gave validity and importance to the work. This move away from "perma-volunteerism" was empowering but would like to have other projects for them to be engaged and employed with.—Barb, White heterosexual woman living with HIV, Detroit and New Jersey.

Paying for labor becomes evidence of its value. People living with HIV engaged with the PLHIV Stigma Index are reminded of their critical and essential place in understanding the local HIV community.

As people living with HIV become engaged with the PLHIV Stigma Index, they begin to transform from a passive role into a more confident space with their local HIV community. This new capacity was reflected in action plans and in the sense of community brought on by the PLHIV Stigma Index locally. Meta describes this transformation as a success.

> Well if you think having a forum where [people living with HIV] can share their truth as well as their struggles with other [people living with HIV] and then compensate them monetarily; well I'd call that a success every day of the week.—Meta, African American woman living with HIV, Louisiana.

While economic justice became an apparent need, it further reflected how much more there was to discover about the HIV community. Poverty became part of understanding how intersectional stigmas operate, how some privileges can marginalize or obscure different stigma experiences around race, sexuality, gender identity, ability, immigration status, language, and social capital. Even as familiar as we might have thought we were with other people living with HIV, the process of the PLHIV Stigma Index—in its systemic collection of data—revealed the diversity of the local HIV community. These differences caused us to think more deeply about who gets involved in these processes, and who continues to be left out. In Louisiana, for example, we recognized that we did not have sufficient youth voices. Also, given how we recruited individuals for the study, most were in HIV care.

Intersectionality: Diversity of the HIV Community

We are a diverse group of people living with HIV and allies, and the PLHIV Stigma Index illuminated how varied local HIV communities are. In all three sites, the stories of immigrants living with HIV were hardest to obtain. Some places struggled to meaningfully include other groups including youth, people who have been incarcerated, and people of transgender experience. Through the PLHIV Stigma Index, community members began to see how limited their actual reach in the local HIV community was. In this way, the PLHIV Stigma Index increased the knowledge about intersectional stigmas and exclusion within the HIV community. A key principle of the PLHIV Stigma Index is inclusion, given the diversity of people and experiences.

At the start though, community participants were resistant to understanding this diversity. As people living with HIV—and often as people of color living with HIV, community participants did not acknowledge challenges in reaching other parts of the HIV community.

> While presentations raised awareness about the degree of stigma and the impact of stigma ... I saw very little understanding of what it means to be a person living with HIV let alone motivation to create space for understanding cultural markers and nuances of each population segment within the HIV community.—Vanessa, African American heterosexual woman living with HIV, Louisiana.

Early on, Vanessa saw how entrenched people were in their beliefs about the HIV community. For many, they had always thought of themselves as the face of diversity in the HIV community, without critical self-reflection on who they know, and why they did not have different kinds of people living with HIV in their social circles.

Reaching beyond this first group became pivotal to each research site. In some cases, this meant bringing on new interviewers. In others, it meant expanding the resources dedicated to outreach. In all the sites, those people living with HIV involved in the interviews acknowledged this need to do more, to reach past their own comfortable boundaries.

> The challenges were few, but they did make a difference. One challenge was finding way[s] to create more diversity by trying to get folks out of our own circles.—Meta, African American woman living with HIV, Louisiana.

As Meta describes, when the challenge of diversity emerged, the groups worked to find solutions. The first step toward this was to raise the consciousness of people living with HIV about the limits of their own personal networks in relationship to the wider community of people living with HIV.

While the PLHIV Stigma Index intends to bring people living with HIV together to work on HIV stigma in the local community, it can remain difficult to bring in those with various experiences that are not necessarily visible—such as a history with substance use, sex work, and/or incarceration. Further, people who have these histories are often marked with multiple concurrent health concerns, which can lead to limited health-care options, a dearth of adequate support, and reduced quality of life for a person living with HIV (Brewer et al., 2014). These experiences are stigmatized, and people often prefer to keep these hidden. It remains a challenge to support people with these experiences to be involved.

While in Detroit, youth were a primary focus of steering committee, recruitment and interviewers, this was not held across all sites. Youth remained an important but inadequately included population in two of the sites, who struggled to bring in young people living with HIV involved as interviewers and steering committee members.

> The only demographic we didn't have, was an interviewer between 18–24 years old. To me the challenges were in identifying a large pool of 18–24 year olds. I think their experience with stigma may be a little different than that of older people.—Gina, African American woman living with HIV.

Each site strategized differently. One brought in a young interviewer later in the PLHIV Stigma Index, others focused on youth organizations. They realized that young people organized differently in HIV, and do not necessarily become active in the HIV community until later.

The community actions increased service provider and researcher awareness of the extensive diversity of the local HIV community. By coming together and bringing forward the intersectional challenges that other people living with HIV face, then more plans were developed to bring in more people living with HIV, especially those that are out of the health-care system.

> The sample we obtained was somewhat biased towards those already engaged in care, so the study likely missed many people experiencing the wors[t] levels of stigma. This has given us a renewed sense of importance to conduct additional outreach and research going forward.—Ann, HIV-negative White heterosexual woman.

Ann's comments reflect a larger community commitment toward engagement and inclusivity. More, she acknowledges that these efforts are necessary to reduce HIV stigma, as well as to increase the HIV knowledge base.

BECOMING COMMUNITY RESEARCHERS

We are employing the language of "researcher" here rather than "activist" for two reasons: the hierarchy in public health between researcher and activist roles; and the acknowledgment that our actions in the PLHIV Stigma Index—recruiting, collecting and analyzing data, and sharing these findings with community—is the foundation of good CBPR (Phillips et al., 2018). The PLHIV Stigma Index increases dignity for people living with HIV who have the experience at least one time of being the central actors in research for and about them and on behalf of their communities, and having their knowledge and expertise not only recognized and valued but central for the entire project. In this way, the people living with HIV involved understood that the hierarchy that is often found in HIV: researchers and government being the most resourced at the top, then HIV organizations, then the people living with HIV who are viewed as consumers. In implementing the PLHIV Stigma Index, the researchers initially involved learned to let go of preconceived structures associated with "research" and trust in the voices and power of the research coordinators and the networks of people living with HIV.

When we started to identify as part of a community research team, each of us felt connected, and part of leading a process to meaningfully involve people living with HIV in HIV stigma reduction. No matter how we started in this process, the PLHIV Stigma Index gave credence to our experiences as credible and valuable toward changing our local communities. Some of this growth came from noticing microaggressions from HIV service providers.

> I have had many of the interviewers reach out to me to "gut check" a passive aggressive statement from an [AIDS Service Organization] Executive Director, brainstorm responses for a call to action and ask for resources to support their legislative agendas.—Barb, White heterosexual woman living with HIV, Detroit and New Jersey.

As people noticed these microaggressions, they took back power and developed their own agendas.

For many, at the start, there was a sentiment that, as people living with HIV, our skills were not enough. In the process of training, collecting data, analyzing and producing local stigma plans, there was a recognition of how essential the view and voices of people living with HIV are in this process.

> I went into this feeling a lot underqualified and because of this project, I came out the other side feeling more confident, motivated, compassionate, and determined. The ways that it impacted me personally, it did the same thing professionally. My work is done with a deeper sense of what folks are feeling and not saying, it makes my work even more important and meaningful than ever.— Meta, African American woman living with HIV, Louisiana.

The development of this sense of self that was emboldened by community connection enriched the lives of people living with HIV who were involved in the PLHIV Stigma Index implementation.

Over and over, people created a foundation that involved their own experiences, the knowledge about the local community of people living with HIV, and the skills they gained. People who were interviewers or on the steering committees created new programs and started giving presentations through the community, including public health and health-care settings, academic settings, and with veterans. New programs were developed by the interviewers and steering committee members to support young people living with HIV to gain life skills, employment skills, and advocacy skills. People learned to write presentations, write grants, manage programs, and speak publicly—not through training programs but through direct action.

The PLHIV Stigma Index had other impacts, particularly with people who were new to HIV advocacy and people who had been involved but had withdrawn from HIV advocacy due to burnout or other challenges. Several youth engaged the PLHIV Stigma Index process in Detroit, who later went on to do HIV prevention work. At one site, a trans* woman started a trans-lead organization. People who had left the field also found new reasons to reengage.

I think giving people the power to utilize their voices gave them a confidence like many never seen before. Telling stories that are all too often neglected or stigmatized as traumatic banter, have all too often silenced many of us. This process broke those chains and gave them freedom for most of the participants to re-engage themselves back into care, get back on meds and/or use their voices to advocate for other people living with HIV."—Ari, mixed-race gay man living with HIV, Detroit.

In each site, people living with HIV renewed their sense of community. They recognized its contours, its varied needs, and its power in moving the HIV response forward.

CONCLUSION

This chapter summarizes our own experiences through the various imple-mentation sites of the PLHIV Stigma Index in the United States. Some of us came to the table as researchers with doctorate degrees; others were work-ing in line-staff positions at HIV service organizations or independent HIV advocates. Through this process we gained new perspectives on the diversity of the HIV community, including the many ways that economics impacts our quality of life and experiences with HIV stigma. The PLHIV Stigma Index helped people move from being static recipients to fully engaged members of their community, full of ideas and energy and passion. We saw people recognize and become frustrated at the poor quality and limited options some of their community-based organizations have provided them. We met people living with HIV who are ready to take over planning councils, question AIDS Service Organizations without people living with HIV in governance or staff leadership positions, and refuse to sit on a Consumer Advisory Board without a meaningful voice and impact on programs.

The PLHIV Stigma Index is a valuable tool in the HIV field. It brings together people living with HIV across their diversity and starts/renews the process of building a community. Through the PLHIV Stigma Index, the community can look at stigma in different domains. HIV-related stigma is not just a big cloud—vague and unassailable. The local community sees the concrete ways that HIV-related stigma can be defined and analyzed and intervened.

In our case, we saw the deep enmeshment of intersecting stigmas. HIV is one part of the identity that has multiple stigmas. As a community of people living with HIV, we must understand how these intersecting stigmas further disenfranchise parts of our community, and look at ways to work together to enfranchise them. While we have incorporated sexuality, gender, and race in most HIV community discussions, we need to see how the HIV identity is complicated by a history of substance use, mental health, sex work, immigration, incarceration, and/or poverty.

This chapter documents our own journey from "consumer" to "community researcher" through our work with the PLHIV Stigma Index. This process expanded conversations about stigma, connected communities in dialogue, and enlarged the role of people living with HIV as leaders in their local communities. Our vision of the HIV community moving forward is to build platforms where people living with HIV are central and irreplaceable parts of the discussion, where leadership is built and accountable to the larger community, where we wrestle and constantly expand who is included in the discussion.

REFERENCES

Adelman, M. B., & Frey, L. R. (1997). *The fragile community: Living together with AIDS*. Mahwah, NJ: Lawrence Erlbaum Associates Publishers.

Brewer, R. A., Magnus, M., Kuo, I., Wang, L., Liu, T.-Y., & Mayer, K. (2014). The high prevalence of incarceration history among Black men who have sex with men in the United States: Associations and implications. *American Journal of Public Health, 104*(3), 448–454.

Brier, J. (2009). *Infectious ideas: U.S. political responses to the AIDS crisis*. Chapel Hill: University of North Carolina Press.

Crenshaw, K. (1991). Mapping the margins: Intersectionality, identity politics, and violence against women of color. *Stanford Law Review, 43*(6), 1241–1299.

Fisher, R. (2005). Social action community organizing: Proliferation, persistence, roots, and prospects. In M. Minkler (Ed.), *Community organizing and community building for health* (pp. 51–65). New Brunswick, NJ: Rutgers University Press.

Global Network of People with AIDS. (n.d.). The people living with HIV Stigma Index. Accessed July 7, 2018 at: http://www.stigmaindex.org/.

Guta, A., Murray, S. J., & Gagnon, M. (2016). HIV, viral suppression and new technologies of surveillance and control. *Body & Society, 22*(2), 82–107.

Higgenbotham, E. B. (1993). *Righteous discontent: The women's movement in the Black Baptist Church, 1880–1920*. Cambridge, MA: Harvard University Press.

Kellett, P. M. (2017). *Patienthood and communication: A personal narrative of eye disease and vision loss*. New York, NY: Peter Lang Publishing.

People with AIDS Coalition. (1983). *The Denver principles*. Accessed July 5, 2018 at: http://www.actupny.org/documents/Denver.html.

Phillips, L., Olesen, B. R., Scheffmann-Petersen, M., & Nordentoft, H. M. (2018). De-romanticising dialogue in collaborative health care research: A critical, reflexive approach to tensions in an action research project's initial phase. *Qualitative Research in Medicine & Healthcare, 2*, 1–13.

Rabkin, J. G., McElhiney, M. C., Harrington, M., & Horn, T. (2018). Trauma and growth: Impact of AIDS activism. *AIDS Research and Treatment*. doi: 10.1155/2018/9696725.

Ramirez-Valles, J. (2011). *Campeñeros: Latino activists in the face of AIDS*. Urbana, Chicago and Springfield: University of Illinois Press.

Spieldenner, A. R. (2017). Infectious sex?: An autoethnographic exploration of HIV prevention. *QED: A Journal in LGBTQ Worldmaking, 4*(1), 121–129.

Sprague, L., Simon, S., & Sprague, C. (2011). Employment discrimination and HIV stigma: Survey results from civil society organisations and people living with HIV in Africa. *African Journal of AIDS Research, 10*(Suppl), 311–324.

Chapter 11

The Gendered Nature of Generosity in Post-Hysterectomy "Dear Honey" Letters

Jill Yamasaki

Dear Honey

This is probably the best chance I have of leading a normal life. Apparently staining the bed, my clothes, etc. is not normal. Apparently bleeding three weeks out of four is not normal. Apparently not being able to conceive when there are no justifiable reasons is not normal. Certainly, all these symptoms have affected my state of mind terribly, so they must be affecting our marriage. I don't want this to happen to me. I don't like what is happening to me. I'm trying hard not to panic. I'm trying to stay calm and rational. I don't want anyone to see how I really feel. I don't want to admit how I really feel. I'm really sorry (really) that this is happening to us. I can't seem to be able to keep it from affecting you, though I try really hard. I just want everything to go back to the way it was. (KS)

Hysterectomy—removal of the uterus—is one of the most frequently performed surgical procedures and, following Caesarean section, the second most common surgery for women (Moore, Steiner, Davis, Stocks, & Barrett, 2016). Approximately 500,000 women[1] in the United States undergo a hysterectomy each year, with many of these surgeries also involving removal of the cervix, fallopian tubes, and/or ovaries (Moore et al., 2016). In most cases, as KS describes in her letter to her husband, hysterectomies are performed to relieve the profound pain, discomfort, and inconvenience brought on by benign conditions such as endometriosis, uterine fibroids, abnormal uterine bleeding, and uterine prolapse (American College of Obstetricians and Gynecologists, 2017). While not life threatening, these gynecological issues often interfere significantly with normal everyday functioning and greatly impede quality of life, general well-being, and psychological health. Social and intimate relationships may be disrupted, as well. For many women, including KS, symptoms like pronounced depression or fatigue, lost fertility, and sexual dysfunction mark the pre- and post-hysterectomy illness experience as something "that is happening to *us*."

The decision to undergo hysterectomy usually comes after considerable time spent weighing the lived burden of distressing symptoms against the benefits and risks of surgery (Williams & Clark, 2000). Following a hysterectomy, some women—citing relief and a return to normal activity—note pronounced improvement in their health status, subjective well-being, and quality of life (Cabness, 2010; Majumdar & Saleh, 2012; Markovic, Manderson, & Warren, 2008; Rannestad, 2005). For others, a hysterectomy brings unexpected new issues, including post-surgical pain, surgical menopause, grief, and even resentment (Cabness, 2010; Flory, Bissonnette, & Binik, 2005; Root, 2015; Williams & Clark, 2000). Regardless of outcome, research highlights commonalities related to the hysterectomy experience that have particular import for this chapter. First, the prospect of losing her uterus and/ or ovaries stimulates reflection for a woman regarding her nuanced understandings of the impact of surgery on her personal perceptions of gender identity (Elson, 2004; Fredericks, 2013). Second, partners can play a significant role—often more so than other family members or friends—in a woman's recovery and adjustment to hysterectomy (Askew & Zam, 2013; Rannestad, 2005). Women in stable, supportive relationships are more likely to cope better with the effects of surgery, while pre-hysterectomy relationship problems tend to predict further negative issues after surgery (Askew & Zam, 2013; Lalos & Lalos, 1996; Rannestad, 2005; Williams & Clark, 2000). Given that even a woman's *perception* of her partner's level of support, understanding, and/or adjustment can be influential, scholars call for more research regarding the surgery's effects on—or because of—partners and intimate relationships to widen understandings of the hysterectomy experience overall (Askew & Zam, 2013; Williams & Clark, 2000).

To that end, I draw from Frank's (2004) work on narrative, illness, and generosity to examine how women make sense of their partners' care and support post-hysterectomy. Frank (2004) describes generosity in the caregiving relationship as offering consolation in times of inevitable loss. In this chapter, I focus on Dear Honey letters posted by women on HysterSisters, an online community for women of all ages seeking information and support for gynecological diagnoses, treatment options, and surgical recovery. While most threads contain women-to-women posts, the Dear Honey forum restricts replies and is designed instead for members to write letters to their partners[2] regarding the care and support they have or have not received through their illness journey. My analysis of these Dear Honey letters illustrates how women story generosity in relation to gendered familial responsibilities and roles at home, with promises of consolation to helpful partners and expectations of consolation from those who aren't.

GENDERED ILLNESS: EMBODIMENT AND IDENTITY

Illness is a subjective experience constructed at the crossroads of biology and culture (Kleinman, 1988; Morris, 1998). While people may share the same diagnosed disease (or, in this case, undergo the same surgical procedure), social and cultural prescriptions personalize and contextualize each person's unique illness experience (Yamasaki, Geist-Martin, & Sharf, 2016). Gender identities are similarly constructed in complicated interactions between the material body and society: "It is crucial to bear in mind that an individual develops her sense of identity from perceptions received through her body and expresses her identity through her body" (Elson, 2004, p. 11). Taken together, the way women experience illness "is very much dependent on broader social constructions of gender in society" (DasGupta & Hurts, 2007, p. 2), with lived accounts of illness, diagnosis, and treatment reflecting cultural complexities of women's bodies, experiences of sexuality and reproduction, and roles as professional and family caregivers (DasGupta & Hurts, 2007; Elson, 2004).

Hysterectomy—and the stigmatizing symptoms (e.g., heavy bleeding, depression, infertility, sexual dysfunction) of most conditions that prompt it—compels women to examine and articulate what it means to be a female in relation to their physical body (Elson, 2004; Fredericks, 2013). For some women, reproductive organs symbolize an important part of their female identities, making the surgery a source of great loss and biographical disruption. Other women feel initial loss after surgery but, over time, can reclaim their gender identities through biographical work that helps them redefine their ideas of womanhood. Still others find that hysterectomy strengthens their identities as women, citing a return to desired social roles and freedom from the constraints that necessitated surgery (Elson, 2004). Elson's (2003, 2004) seminal work on hysterectomy and gender identity further reveals a "hormonal hierarchy" in which the ovaries—and not the uterus—bear greater symbolic meaning regarding gender identity. According to Elson (2003), most respondents associate hysterectomy with loss of their ability to bear children but more closely identify oophorectomy (removal of one or both ovaries) with loss of their femaleness (i.e., hormonal balance and sex drive) and femininity (i.e., ability to display sexual attractiveness). As a social construction, this hormonal hierarchy serves to affirm normative gender status for respondents "according to how closely they measure up to the two-ovary norm following surgery" (Elson, 2003, p. 765). Ultimately, respondents who retained one or both ovaries worked to identify themselves with "biologically normal" women and to distance themselves from the outgroup of women who no longer had ovaries and were thus pitied or stigmatized as "less than" (Elson, 2003, 2004).

Gender also influences the way care during illness is perceived, provided, and experienced. Husbands and wives endure unique stresses and possess different abilities when caring for a chronically ill spouse. Research shows that differences in dyadic care work reflect a repertoire of gender-based skills, resources, and expectations resulting from different norms of masculinity and femininity prescribed by a particular culture at a particular point in time (Hong & Coogle, 2016; Russell, 2007; Ussher, Sandoval, Perz, Wong, & Butow, 2013). It is often expected that people performing care work draw upon these repertoires to affirm normative gender identities (Calasanti & King, 2007); however, individuals must also cross these gender boundaries when caring for opposite-sex spouses. Male caregivers demonstrate role flexibility, for example, when they take on their wives' gendered activities such as doing housework, running errands, engaging in childcare, arranging and participating in appointments, helping with personal care, and providing emotional support (Shannon, 2015; Ussher et al., 2013).

Calasanti and Bowen (2006) contend that two types of care work, in particular, cross gender boundaries. First, married caregivers must assume the tasks usually handled by their spouses. Although couples negotiate the division of labor in different ways, a persistent gender gap exists, with women performing most daily domestic work, such as cooking and cleaning, while men do more episodic, automotive, or outdoor work (Calasanti & Bowen, 2006; Revenson, Abraido-Lanza, Majerovitz, & Jordan, 2005). Second, caregivers may need to find ways to help maintain the care recipient's gender identity (Calasanti & Bowen, 2006). Following hysterectomy, women often seek to assuage insecurities by demonstrating to others that they are undoubtedly very feminine, and therefore still female, through impression management strategies such as self-care, dress, hair, and make-up (Elson, 2004). Social reactions and other people's perceptions of them as female, particularly from intimate partners, are central for both confirming and reinforcing this identity. Research with couples following a hysterectomy shows husbands generally (1) display role flexibility by assuming long-established familial patterns of activity and (2) manage their partners' female identities by assuming the role of caretaker, showing love and acceptance in spite of emotional or physical changes, and accepting new limits such as cessation of fertility (Askew & Zam, 2013; Butt & Chesla, 2007; Gates, 1988). Ultimately, such research suggests that the nature of the relationship may be more important than gender in determining caregiving decisions (Calasanti & King, 2007), with committed couples better equipped to engage in mutual care characterized by reciprocity, flexibility, sensitivity, and concern for the other (Askew & Zam, 2013; Butt & Chesla, 2007; Revenson et al., 2005; Shannon, 2015).

NARRATIVE, GENEROSITY, AND CONSOLATION

Illness is a call for stories (Frank, 1995)—stories told, stories heard, and stories constructed in dialogic ways. Such stories offer coherence to "wounded storytellers" (Frank, 1995), whose lives have been disrupted by illness and possibility to those who bear witness (Sharf, Harter, Yamasaki, & Haidet, 2011). When people think *with* stories—rather than thinking *about* stories— they imaginatively attend to the lived experiences of others. Doing so helps individuals examine and better understand their own lives, as well as give voice to and offer empathy for the suffering of others (Brody, 2003; Frank, 1995; Morris, 2001). These moral acts comprise the generosity often missing from medical treatment but needed for hospitable healing (Arber & Gallagher, 2009; Carmack, Bouchelle, Rawlins, Bennet, Hill, & Oriol, 2017).

Frank (2004) conceptualizes care as "an occasion when people discover what each can be in relationship with the other" (p. 4). He calls for "*guests* (those needing care) and *hosts* (those temporarily in a position to offer care)" (p. 11, italics in original) to increase the generosity and gratitude gracing those relations through dialogue (space to come together), alterity (kinship despite difference), face (the obligation to be who the vulnerable other needs), justice (help for those in need), and joy (pleasure in helping others). This generosity begins in welcome with an offer of consolation for guests who are suffering. Frank (2004) describes consolation as comfort when loss occurs or is inevitable, including one person's promise not to abandon another or a promise that the present suffering will someday turn (p. 4). Providing that comfort depends on a person's capacity to imagine and understand situations from another's perspective. This moral imagination (Arber & Gallagher, 2009) helps caregivers recognize, acknowledge, reflect upon, and react to the difficulties experienced by those in need of care (p. 3). From this perspective, men generously attend to the needs of their partners pre- and post-hysterectomy— including care work that crosses gender boundaries—and women then reciprocally share their experiences (in this case, online in a specific supportive community) in an act of care for those facing similar issues. Indeed, Frank (2004) claims the renewal of generosity requires envisioning care for suffering "as one in which we all participate together, each doing his or her part that would be impossible without others doing their parts" (p. 10).

HysterSisters (www.hystersisters.com) is a website designed to offer women-to-women hysterectomy support from gynecological diagnosis to treatment (including alternatives to hysterectomy) to surgery recovery. With almost 473,000 registered members, the site offers both informational and emotional support through articles, resources, helpful products, and a community message board where members share their experiences and seek advice or comfort from others. Prior research suggests that members report high levels of perceived social support at home, including from intimate partners, and visit HysterSisters primarily for informational support, particularly concerning preparation and recovery issues (Bunde, Suls, Martin, & Barnett, 2006, 2007). Indeed, the site acknowledges that men want to help their partners and encourage them to handle the hysterectomy journey with an abundance of understanding and loving care (Wood, 2005). To that end, HysterSisters devotes a section of the website to "Mister HysterSisters" with help, hints, and information for the patient's family, as well as the Dear Honey forum where members are urged to write letters to their loved ones. According to the website, Dear Honey letters "help the lurking husbands who visit our site, looking for ways to help their wives during this time: pre-op and post-op and beyond." The forum does not permit replies and recommends letter writers "be specific about your physical and emotional needs and how they [family members] can help. Be thankful and grateful too!"

To understand how women story generosity and consolation throughout the hysterectomy journey in relation to gendered responsibilities and roles at home, I examined all Dear Honey letters posted in the eponymous forum as of Spring 2018. Of the 433 posts, I focused solely on the 357 that were written specifically to intimate partners rather than to mothers, children, siblings, or general family. Narrative theorizing and principles of dialogic narrative analysis guided my close readings of those 357 letters (see Charon, 2006). While I focused primarily on content to identify thematic patterns related to gendered roles and responsibilities (see Riessman, 2008), I also considered the storytelling context (i.e., the relational hysterectomy experience) in relation to those patterns. A number of questions informed my thinking during this process: (1) What sorts of actions or developments does the setting suggest and/or require? (2) How are the past and future envisioned in light of present circumstances? (3) What subjectivities/identities are called into being by stories? and (4) What worldviews are reflected in stories? (Yamasaki, Sharf, & Harter, 2014, pp. 105–106). Ultimately, my analysis centered on the mode of storytelling—Dear Honey letters—and the collective story of generosity and consolation that emerged from this dialogical affiliation (Frank, 2010, 2012). I offer two readings of this collective story, using examples from the individual letters, throughout the remainder of the chapter.

"YOU'RE ALWAYS THERE FOR ME"

The predominant story told throughout the individual Dear Honey letters is one of appreciation. Most of those letters (295) offer praise and gratitude to partners for being supportive, caring, and loving throughout the hysterectomy experience—a finding that is consistent with prior research (Askew & Zam, 2013; Rannestad, 2005; Williams & Clark, 2000). In this story, women highlight generous partners who care for them with hospitality and joy by imaginatively responding to their gendered physical, emotional, and task-related needs. This care then prompts a reciprocal gratitude with promised acts of consolation in return.

For many of these women, their partners' generosity begins in dialogue. They describe joining together with partners who not only recognize their suffering but continually respond in welcome (Frank, 2004):

> From the very first day I heard that a hysterectomy may help my pain, you were there for me. You not only stayed, you did research and talked to doctors and went to countless appointments with me. You talked to everyone you knew, and you helped me know that I was not crazy—just hormonal. You called off work just to stay with me and take me to the doctors. You went to countless ER visits because we didn't know what was wrong. You were the one who found the ever-so-wonderful progesterone cream and made me order it. You were the one who talked to my doctor and told him your concerns and made the appointment.

As TT describes, and other women echo, partners help assuage the over-whelming chaos associated with and culminating in a hysterectomy through advocacy, research, and a constant, calming presence at appointments and at home. "You have been there through all the appointments as we learned I'd be having a hysterectomy and might have cancer," writes LC. "I know you know WAY more about my anatomy then you ever wanted to, but I love that you have been involved in the discussions." According to CO, "I will never forget all of the research and late-night Internet journeys we have taken together, or you have taken for me, to find information because I couldn't do it alone." Some women even thank their partners for turning to HysterSisters as a resource. "Thank you for getting the Mister HysterSister book and being ready!" exclaims LM. "For your constant care and understanding! For getting it!" PD writes, "You set up a Google sheet to track our appointments and information and named it HystLists, which totally made me giggle. And you had me send you the URL for Mister HysterSisters even after you made fun of the name." Other women express appreciation for their partners' careful attention during the appointments. "You took your time and really listened to the nurse to get it right," writes VG, while JN recounts, "After the surgery when I was really emotional and would cry, you would hold me in your arms and say things like 'Don't feel bad, it's ok, the doctor said you would be a little emotional.'"

Frank (2004) conceptualizes alterity as kinship despite difference in a relationship of otherness (p. 115). Throughout the Dear Honey letters, this moral ideal is likened to partnership in the face of adversity. While their stories of suffering may overlap with their partners' and with other women's similar experiences, these women carry the weight of their gendered illness in myriad ways. They specifically recognize the ways their partners join with them through dialogue in the midst of this chaos. "When we knew I needed to have the surgery, you held my hand and said, 'We'll get through it together,'" writes HP. "We did and we have ... I couldn't have done it without you." EQ similarly details her husband as "a pillar of physical, emotional, and spiritual strength ... As you always say, we are a team." Another woman, MW, remembers these same sentiments shared repeatedly with each new diagnosis. "When we found out about the endometriosis, you said we will get through this, we're in this together," she writes. "When I had my hysterectomy, before I could express my fears, you put your loving arms around me and said, 'Don't worry. We will be just fine. We'll get through it together.'"

Other women describe the chaos of problematic symptoms, multiple diagnoses, and various procedures, including hysterectomy, as a journey taken with their partner. According to SD, "This has been a journey for us, and we are going to get through it." Similarly, MI thanks her partner "for all the love, support, and understanding you have shown. I'm truly blessed having you to share this journey, and I know I could have never made it without you by my side through all the various female problems I've endured over the past eight years." Many women quote their partners, writing, "like you've always said, 'it's you and me against the world!'" As BR explains, "You dealt with high-risk pregnancies and babies while holding down two jobs so I could stay home with our children. Now this! We have no family support. It has always been me and you against the world."

Coming together in generosity obliges the caregiver to be who the suffering, vulnerable other person needs him to be (Frank, 2004). As Calasanti and Bowen (2006) note, gendered care work requires that male partners demonstrate role flexibility in assuming household tasks and in maintaining their partners' gender identities. All of the Dear Honey letters comprising this story of appreciation acknowledge the male caregivers' willingness to handle domestic and familial responsibilities; perhaps more importantly, many of these women also express gratitude to their partners for continuing to see them as desirable, whole women. Doing so requires a recognition of the woman's fears and needs, followed by an appropriate response. For example, BL writes:

> The best thing that you have done for me is to reassure me that I am not a failure as a woman or a wife. That I am still a woman with just a little less parts. Your attention, your time, cuddling with me, the extra hugs and kisses. The sexual innuendos. The touching and the comments—have meant the world to me. They reassure me when nothing else has that I am still attractive to you. That you still want me, that you still need me. These things above all else have helped me through my recovery.

Other women describe similar reassurances in response to their insecurities and feelings of loss. JM writes, "Thank you for reminding me that I'm still a beautiful woman who is absolutely no less without my baby-making parts," while SP says, "You make me feel pretty when I'm feeling my ugliest." The collective letters detail various ways their partners have made these women feel beautiful, desired, and "enough" when they feel "less than." "Not once have you ever been upset with me or disappointed in my not being able to give you a child," writes DO. "You amaze me. Your only concern is for my health and well-being." JA says, "I feel less of a woman because I no longer have all my parts. In my eyes, you deserve so much more than what I am, but you tell me no matter what that I am beautiful and always will be." HK appreciates her husband for making her feel more important than the "what-ifs of more children." She writes, "You have never made me feel less for not having more babies for you. Instead, you make me feel needed and special just for being your wife."

Relatedly, the women often draw on gendered ideals of masculinity when recounting the care provided for them. They thank their partners for being their guardian angel, their champion, their Prince Charming, their king, their everything, and their source of strength. For example, PM writes:

> Not only are you the love of my life, but you have been my source of strength through this ordeal. You have taken such good care of me and made me feel so loved through everything. Your attitude of accepting nothing less than total recovery for me, even when we were afraid we were facing a malignancy and chemo, was what kept the fear at bay. I knew I could face anything as long as you were by my side and holding my hand. Your arms have been my haven, and I am so grateful that they are there for me every day. Thank you for your strength, for your support, and most of all, for your love. You are my heart, and I love you with all of that heart. Thank you for everything.

Other women detail similar strength from hospitable partners, whom they characterize in a variety of ways. Some women, like AH, claim their partners are "knights in shining armor." She writes, "You have done things the last few days that were uncomfortable and embarrassing, and yet I felt completely at ease knowing you were willing to do it for me. I could never have done this without you! You are my knight in shining armor and so much more." Other women deem their partners superheroes for being there for them. "People say that having a hysterectomy changes everything, but not for me—it was your love," writes SS. "Your love saved me. Utterly and frankly. We are only 28 and you have stepped up to the plate and brought me through this like some sort of Superman." Several women equate their partners as metaphorical rocks, providing a solid foundation during chaotic suffering. "Thank you for being my rock through the cancer scares and the mammograms and all the craziness that we have dealt with the past few months," writes GE, while TW similarly recounts, "You hold me while I cry, you listen while I vent, you wait on me when I don't feel well, and you lift me up whenever there is need. You are my rock and my forever best friend."

Central to Frank's (2004) call for generosity are reciprocal increases in gratitude and a mutual joy in helping others. The Dear Honey letters comprising the story of appreciation collectively offer a promise that the present suffering will turn as generous consolation to hospitable partners. These women recount their partners' willingness to care for them despite their avowed side effects of hysterectomy and/or prior gynecological issues—"no matter how witchy or whiny I get"; "my hot mess hormones"; "I'm moody and I cry a lot"; "I'm a very difficult, moody, irritable person to live with"—and seek to return the favor in years to come:

> All I can say is I will get better and we will have a "normal" life again. I will become more of the person you married and hopefully be deserving of all you've done for me. We will have fun and do the things together we love once again. I'm looking forward to being a good wife and mother again. I want to grow old with you and share more memories. I will never regret a moment we spend together. I love you and will never take all you do and all you are for granted.

Like RZ, these women promise "a new chapter in our lives" and "good times in front of us once this horrible period in our life is over." Many of them look forward to renewed intimacy, as well. "I can't wait to be the wife you married and to please you the way you should be pleased during lovemaking," writes NT, while MU exclaims, "I can't wait until I get clearance from the doctor to be intimate again." GI writes, rather cheekily, "Double up on those vitamins! I should be recovered by spring, and this will be the best summer we've ever had. I look forward to spoiling and adoring you." Ultimately, these women look forward to resuming their loving relationships made stronger through mutual joy and a "renewable capacity to give" (Frank, 2004, p. 2). "You're always there for me," writes TH. "You are my one true love, and I will always be there for you."

"IT'S NOT ABOUT YOU"

The second story told in the remaining sixty-two Dear Honey letters is a counter-narrative written to partners who, at best, "don't get it," and, at worst, spark feelings of apathy, disgust, betrayal, and abandonment. In this story, women seek the generosity of partners who will care for them physically, emotionally, and authentically. When this care does not materialize as desired, these women demand consolation in the form of action, patience, flexibility, and support, with permanent repercussions to the relationship as an inevitable consequence—or as consolation bestowed upon themselves.

Calasanti and Bowen (2006) claim that care work crosses gender boundaries when husbands assume the household tasks usually handled by their wives. For many women, this type of care is either absent or a source of great stress during their recovery. "The house will not suddenly grow arms and clean itself," writes BK in aggravation. "If you see that there are 3 loads of laundry, dirty toilets, tubs that need scrubbed, dishes in the sink, floors that need mopped or vacuumed, numerous trash cans that need to be emptied, or beds that need made ... then why on earth should I have to ask!!!!!" Other women cleaned and prepared food prior to surgery or enlisted the help of friends or other family members so their partners would have fewer tasks to assume. One of these women, SQ, is nonetheless aggravated with her partner's behavior. In her letter, she flips earlier positive sentiments of caregiving partners as superheroes:

> I am so grateful you have been there for me and took time off work to help me. I tell you every day I'm grateful. I say thank you for every little task you do, but PLEASSSEEE stop throwing in my face comments like "it's a good thing you're not single" and "oh, I'm sure your ex wouldn't have done all this for you" to feed your insecurities or ego. I love you; we're married. You're right I'm not single; otherwise, I would have had to make other arrangements. Prior to my surgery I did ALL the cooking and cleaning. All of it. I prepped all our food so you would only have to heat up things. My daughter came to clean. So, once again, thank you for being there, but please stop acting like you're a superhero. I just had a hysterectomy. I had two blood transfusions and another surgery after almost bleeding out. If anyone is a superhero, it's me.

While some men, like SQ's partner, seek praise for helping with daily household tasks, others begrudgingly assume the work with complaints, sarcastic jokes, and arguments. "I just underwent major medical surgery," writes AK. "Please stop treating me like I'm milking it. Get off your ass and actually help." WW uses the same expression to share similar sentiments: "Seriously? You are accusing me, even 'jokingly,' of milking my situation to get more help from you?" BF writes that she would rather risk further surgery by doing more than she should around the house than fight with her unhelpful partner:

> Everyone tells me to slow down, rest, to stop what I am doing, but they don't understand the fight that would cause if I did. I don't want to fight with you. My hormones are driving me nuts as it is. So I sacrifice my health. I have officially

hurt myself and extended my road to recovery. You have your own medical problems with your knees, I get that, but I need more help than I am getting. You will never truly see the damage that has been caused until I am back in surgery trying to get it fixed. I am to my breaking point and don't know what to do. A little piece of me dies every time I have to do something I'm not supposed to.

Conversely, some women praise their husbands for handling the household tasks but, at the same time, lament this singular focus. In these letters, women desire help in maintaining their gender identity post-hysterectomy from husbands who will pamper and care for them. "Right now, I am weak, I am sad, I feel ugly, I feel like less than a woman," explains GB. "I need you to tell me I'm pretty. I need you to hold me without me asking. I need you to understand that I'm mourning the children I will never have. This would be a good time for flowers. It would be a good time to play with my hair." YG offers similar strategies for her husband:

> You do all the "man" things, like a good husband. ... However, I have to say a little sensitivity and romance would be nice during this very difficult time in my life ... It's not too late. Maybe you could draw me a bath and light a scented candle now that I have the all-clear for a bath. Maybe you could pick me up a funny card or a small trinket the next time you run into town. Maybe you could prepare a romantic dinner for just the two of us. Buy me a gift certificate to the salon so I can feel feminine again. There are so many ways you could show me the support and love I need right now. Please open your eyes!

Other women seek understanding and nurturing from partners who will validate their feelings rather than dismiss their concerns. "All I want from you is understanding," writes SY. "You can't understand that I hurt! Please just take some of our responsibilities away from me, talk nice to me, and for God's sake hug me when I'm crying instead of saying, in a gruff voice, 'what's wrong with you?'" Similarly, LC writes, "This isn't a problem I need to you to fix or diagnose. I need you to just be patient and understand my emotional state is very fragile." AA struggles with a partner who minimizes her physical recovery and emotional pain:

> I'm afraid you will begin to resent my selfishness in trying to recover at my pace. I'm having a hard time dealing with you minimizing what I say, think, and do in regards to this situation. Yes, you have supported me in this, but you have also downplayed my feelings, emotions, and comments in reference to it. I am afraid you'll feel differently about me as a woman when I am recovered. I need you to support me, be there for me and not be so judgmental of how I handle what is happening to my body. Please allow me the dignity to mourn the loss and fear the unknown whether it is rational or not.

Still others feel their partners' resentment or fear becoming burdensome during their long recovery. "You've never ONCE asked me how I am feeling, or fussed over me, or made me feel pampered," writes AG. "I know you don't see any stitches, but I had major surgery and it takes time to recover. I feel your resentment when I am laying on the couch or getting some rest. Your anger is palpable ... and the stress from your attitude is hampering my recovery." DDG implores her partner to "be my advocate rather than making me feel like a burden," and SS explains to her husband that "fighting with you about all of this is just exhausting me more and making my healing process slower." When her husband teases her for taking an afternoon nap, PZ responds with sarcasm. "Really? How nice for me to have a total hysterectomy and be in the midst of a painful and tiring recovery," she writes. "I would rather be doing a million other things than taking a nap because I don't feel good. I did not choose this surgery. It chose me when my body betrayed me." Ultimately, these women claim their partners "just don't get it," as NR illustrates in her letter:

I'm scared and broken and weak, and I can't handle it. Be patient with me. You have been wonderful, but you just don't get it. My uterus is gone!! The first home my babies resided in is gone!! I feel lost!!! I cannot help that I want to be superwoman ... the one who nursed a baby while changing another, the one who was together even after two toddlers and a newborn tried so hard to drive her crazy. You remember her??? I miss her—the one who went back to school at night—the one who followed her dream and became the nurse she was destined to be—well, now she is broken and weak and I cannot handle it. What if I can't be her anymore? The fight has been drained. Will I ever be "alright" again??? Be patient with me—you have been wonderful—but you just don't get it.

Patience, particularly regarding sex and intimacy, is an issue of contention for many of the women co-constructing this story. "No, I don't care how long you'll have to go without sex while I'm recovering," writes BX. "Yes, I know you're (somewhat) joking and you think you're lightening the mood, but you're not. You're just making me mad and making a bad situation worse. So, knock it off. It's not about you." SK is similarly annoyed with her partner:

Okay, I know we haven't had sex in three months. I'm well aware of this fact, and I can point to the exact day on the calendar when we were last intimate. It's only been just shy of three weeks since my hysterectomy ... I don't want to hear you ask me EVERY DAY when the five-week waiting period is up. Give me a break!! I'm as anxious as you to find out if my parts still work, especially since they had to take my cervix. I'm worried about never having an orgasm again, and you can't wait to get in there and fish around. Thanks, but I don't need that kind of pressure!! Back off. Leave me to heal.

The anxiety expressed by SK is repeated by other women in their letters, as well. The hysterectomy left some of them embarrassed by their bodies and worried about potential pain or sexual issues. "Why would you want to have sex with someone who looks like me? My body is embarrassing," writes JT. "You say you love me no matter what, but my mind has a hard time believing that. I'm so afraid that I'm going to lose you because of my problem ... Deep down inside I'm hurting and aching with the way I feel about me." SM's letter demonstrates similar embarrassment, this time stemming from physical pain. "It's not that I don't want sex ... It's that it hurts," she writes. "I'm afraid to even start because halfway through all I can think about is pain, regret, & how much I wish it was over ... Do you know how embarrassing that is? Do you know how much anxiety that causes, especially during sex?" Regardless of reason, the women collectively express sadness, frustration, and anger that their partners are pushing them for intimacy, effectively prioritizing the man's ongoing sexual needs over the woman's immediate need to heal. As LQ writes:

> This does not mean I don't love you. It means I had to make a life-changing decision that I didn't want to have to make, and I'm still healing emotionally and physically and I NEED MY SPACE. Hell, I can't even cry about this in front of you because you get upset. It's MY body, it was MY uterus, and I'm allowed to grieve. Get over it and let me have my time.

Unlike the first story in which women promise consolation to generous partners, the letters comprising this second story reveal inevitable consequences stemming from their partners' lack of generosity. Nonetheless, in doing so, the women offer some consolation to their partners by acknowledging first what they have done or do well. "I love you. I appreciate you being at the hospital during surgery. I appreciate that you're handling the bills while I'm worried about money," writes VQ before shifting in tone. "When I am, how you treated me now—when I am at my lowest—will probably always color how I see you." PF is similarly resolute in her letter. "You're here for me physically, but I'm going through this alone," she writes. "If this is the way our marriage is going to be—as much as it breaks my heart to say it—I don't want it." Ultimately, some women, like SI, determine divorce is a justified consolation chosen for themselves:

> You could understand why I want someone I feel I can count on to be there for me—especially as we get older. Even though I am very strong and independent—it matters. I'm sorry this has been so hard for you and you don't have a clue what I have gone through and what a major life event this is. I love you, but I love myself enough to realize I have to heal and recuperate and get on with my life.

CONCLUSION

Taken together, the two stories comprised of individual Dear Honey letters collectively construct the relational and gendered care women desire, need, and receive (or don't) throughout the hysterectomy experience. LT's unaddressed letter captures the nuanced nature of this surgery and recovery:

> Please understand that a hysterectomy is a major procedure that is hard on all women and very debilitating to some. We are losing major female organs. A lot of us are left feeling empty, lost, alone, and very scared, especially when our "partner" is not emotionally supportive. (How would you like to lose your testicles?) It causes not only physical pain but a deep emotional hurt as well. As the physical wounds heal, you need to understand we are having to find who we are all over again. Some of us do very well and heal physically and emotionally in a very short time. Others take more time or try to rush the process because we feel we have to for various reasons. Men, please do not be afraid to do "women's" work. Don't be afraid to tell your "partner" that you are there for her and that it is ok to grieve or hurt. Don't try to rush her. Hold her tight and let her cry. Let her know it is ok if she just wants to sleep some days. Do not use harsh words or tone of voice. She is very emotionally fragile right now and it takes so very little to break her. Please just take good care of her in this time of need.

Through their letters, the women on HysterSisters utilize a frame of generosity and consolation to make sense of the support they perceive from their intimate partners. When these men imaginatively attend to their partners' gendered suffering with a spirit of hospitality, women respond in gratitude with promises of reciprocity. Given the significant role of intimate partners throughout the healing process—and the relational nature of gynecological issues for both partners—these understandings are vital for determining who the patient and caregiver can be for one another during lived experiences of illness. After all, stories of generosity "can show what is possible for any of us at any time. That is their consolation" (Frank, 2004, p. 9).

NOTES

1. According to the American College of Obstetrics and Gynecologists (2017), overall hysterectomy rates are highest among women ages 40–44 and 45–49, followed by women ages 35–39 and 50–54. The primary diagnosis for women ages 35–54 is uterine fibroids, while the most common diagnosis for women ages 55 or older is either uterine prolapse or cancer.

2. The term *partner*, in this chapter, refers to men and boyfriends, a choice made based on the available data collected but one that nevertheless perpetuates a

heteronormative perspective identified in other research (Solbraekke & Bondevik, 2015). The effects of hysterectomies on lesbian partners are under-reported (Askew & Zam, 2013), an absence that AX also notes in her Dear Honey letter: "Your loving support, both emotional and physical, has been wonderful during this time ... HysterSisters has been a great help too. I only wish that they were more aware that not everybody who is partnered has a husband, and welcome them also. Thank you, my loving wife, for helping me after my hysterectomy."

REFERENCES

American College of Obstetricians and Gynecologists. (2017). Choosing the route of hysterectomy for benign disease: Committee Opinion No. 701. *Obstetrics & Gynecology, 129,* e155–e159.

Arber, A., & Gallagher, A. (2009). Generosity and the moral imagination in the practice of teamwork. *Nursing Ethics, 16,* 775–785.

Askew, J. C., & Zam, M. (2013). In sickness and in health: The effects of hysterectomy on women's partners and intimate relationships. *Journal of Couple & Relationship Therapy, 12,* 58–72.

Brody, H. (2003). *Stories of sickness* (2nd ed.). New York, NY: Oxford University Press.

Bunde, M., Suls, J., Martin, R., & Barnett, K. (2006). Hystersisters online: Social support and social comparison among hysterectomy patients on the Internet. *Annals of Behavioral Medicine, 31,* 271–278.

Bunde, M., Suls, J., Martin, R., & Barnett, K. (2007). Online hysterectomy support: Characteristics of website experiences. *CyberPsychology & Behavior, 10,* 80–85.

Butt, F. S., & Chesla, C. (2007). Relational patterns of couples living with chronic pelvic pain from endometriosis. *Qualitative Health Research, 17,* 571–585.

Cabness, J. (2010). The psychosocial dimensions of hysterectomy: Private places and the inner spaces of women at midlife. *Social Work in Health Care, 49,* 211–226.

Calasanti, T., & Bowen, M. E. (2006). Spousal caregiving and crossing gender boundaries: Maintaining gender identities. *Journal of Aging Studies, 20,* 253–263.

Calasanti, T., & King, N. (2007). Taking "women's work" "like a man": Husbands' experiences of care work. *The Gerontologist, 47,* 516–517.

Carmack, H. J., Bouchelle, Z., Rawlins, Y., Bennet, J., Hill, C., & Oriol, N. E. (2017). Mobilizing a narrative of generosity: Patient experiences on an urban mobile health clinic. *Communication Quarterly, 65,* 419–435.

Charon, R. (2006). *Narrative medicine: Honoring the stories of illness.* New York, NY: Oxford University Press.

DasGupta, S., & Hurst, M. (2007). The gendered nature of illness. In S. DasGupta & M. Hurst (Eds.), *Stories of illness and healing: Women write their bodies* (pp. 1–7). Kent, OH: The Kent State University Press.

Elson, J. (2003). Hormonal hierarchy: Hysterectomy and stratified stigma. *Gender and Society, 17,* 750–770.

Elson, J. (2004). *Am I still a woman? Hysterectomy and gender identity.* Philadelphia, PA: Temple University Press.

Flory, N., Bissonnette, F., & Binik, Y. M. (2005). Psychosocial effects of hysterectomy: Literature review. *Journal of Psychosomatic Research, 59,* 117–129.

Frank, A. W. (1995). *The wounded storyteller: Body, illness, and ethics.* Chicago, IL: The University of Chicago Press.

Frank, A. W. (2004). *The renewal of generosity: Illness, medicine, and how to live.* Chicago, IL: The University of Chicago Press.

Frank, A. W. (2010). *Letting stories breathe: A socio-narratology.* Chicago, IL: The University of Chicago Press.

Frank, A. W. (2012). Practicing dialogical narrative analysis. In J. A. Holstein & J. F. Gubrium (Eds.), *Varieties of narrative analysis* (pp. 33–52). Thousand Oaks, CA: Sage.

Fredericks, E. (2013). A qualitative study of women's decisions not to have a hysterectomy. *The Qualitative Report, 18,* 1–12.

Gates, M. (1988). Caring behaviors experienced by couples during a hysterectomy. In M. M. Leininger (Ed.), *Care, discovery and uses in clinical and community nursing* (pp. 71–85). Detroit, MI: Wayne State University Press.

Hong, S.-C., & Coogle, C. L. (2016). Spousal caregiving for partners with dementia: A deductive literature review testing Calasanti's gendered view of care work. *Journal of Applied Gerontology, 35,* 759–787.

Kleinman, A. (1988). *The illness narratives: Suffering, healing, and the human condition.* New York, NY: Basic Books.

Lalos, A., & Lalos, O. (1996). The partner's view about hysterectomy. *Journal of Psychosomatic Obstetrics & Gynecology, 17,* 119–124.

Majumdar, A., & Saleh, S. (2012). Psychological aspects of hysterectomy & postoperative care. In A. Al-Hendy (Ed.), *Hysterectomy* (pp. 365–393). Rijeka, Croatia: InTech.

Markovic, M., Manderson, L., & Warren, N. (2008). Pragmatic narratives of hysterectomy among Australian women. *Sex Roles, 58,* 467–476.

Moore, B. J., Steiner, C. A., Davis, P. H., Stocks, C., & Barrett, M. L. (2016). *Trends in hysterectomies and oophorectomies in hospital inpatient and ambulatory settings, 2005–2013. HCUP Statistical Brief #214.* Rockville, MD: Agency for Healthcare Research and Quality.

Morris, D. B. (1998). *Illness and culture in the postmodern age.* Berkeley, CA: University of California Press.

Morris, D. B. (2001). Narrative, ethics, and pain: Thinking *with* stories. *Narrative, 9,* 55–77.

Rannestad, T. (2005). Hysterectomy: Effects on quality of life and psychological aspects. *Best Practices & Research Clinical Obstetrics and Gynaecology, 19,* 419–430.

Revenson, T. A., Abraido-Lanza, A. F., Majerovitz, S. D., & Jordan, C. (2005). Couples coping with chronic illness: What's gender got to do with it? In T. A. Revenson, K. Kayser, & G. Bodenmann (Eds.), *Couples coping with stress:*

Emerging perspectives on dyadic coping (pp. 137–156). Washington, DC: American Psychological Association.

Riessman, C. K. (2008). *Narrative methods for the human sciences*. Thousand Oaks, CA: Sage.

Root, E. (2015). The empty woman: Dealing with sadness and loss after a hysterectomy. In R. E. Silverman & J. Baglia (Eds.), *Communicating pregnancy loss: Narrative as a method for change* (pp. 180–194). New York, NY: Peter Lang.

Russell, R. (2007). Men doing "women's work:" Elderly men caregivers and the gendered construction of care work. *The Journal of Men's Studies, 15*, 1–18.

Shannon, C. S. (2015). 'I was trapped at home': Men's experiences with leisure while giving care to partners during a breast cancer experience. *Leisure Sciences, 37*, 125–141.

Sharf, B. F., Harter, L. M., Yamasaki, J., & Haidet, P. (2011). Narrative turns epic: Continuing developments in health narrative scholarship. In T. L. Thompson, R. Parrott, & J. F. Nussbaum (Eds.), *Handbook of health communication* (2nd ed., pp. 36–51). New York, NY: Routledge.

Solbraekke, K. N., & Bondevik, H. (2015). Absent organs–present selves: Exploring embodiment and gender identity in young Norwegian women's accounts of hysterectomy. *International Journal of Qualitative Studies on Health and Well-being, 10*. doi: 10.3402/qhw.v10.26720.

Ussher, J. M., Sandoval, M., Perz, J., Wong, W. K. T., & Butow, P. (2013). The gendered construction and experience of difficulties and rewards in cancer care. *Qualitative Health Research, 23*, 900–915.

Williams, R. D., & Clark, A. J. (2000). A qualitative study of women's hysterectomy experience. *Journal of Women's Health & Gender-Based Medicine, 9*(Supp. 2), S15–S25.

Wood, E. H. (2005). Hyster sisters: Comfort and support for hysterectomy patients and families. *Journal of Consumer Health on the Internet, 9*, 55–58.

Yamasaki, J., Geist-Martin, P., & Sharf, B. F. (2016). *Storied health and illness: Communicating personal, cultural, and political complexities*. Long Grove, IL: Waveland Press.

Yamasaki, J., Sharf, B. F., & Harter, L. M. (2014). Narrative inquiry: Attitude, acts, artifacts, and analysis. In B. B. Whaley (Ed.), *Research methods in health communication: Principles and application* (pp. 99–118). New York, NY: Routledge.

Chapter 12

The Narrative Journey and Decision-Making Process of Plastic Surgery Patienthood

Ashley M. Archiopoli

The decision to undergo elective surgery is rarely taken lightly. Elective plastic surgery consumers usually choose plastic surgery for reasons tied to biopsychosocial processes such as self-esteem, body image, or physical discomfort (Crerand, Infield, & Sarwer, 2007; Haas, Champion, & Secor, 2008; Milothridis, Pavlidis, Haidich, & Panagopoulou, 2016; Solvi et al., 2009; Zwier, 2014). While processes related to physical, emotional, and social function serve as motivating factors, plastic surgery patients must carefully consider the decision to pursue surgery considering a series of factors including the risks versus rewards, issues of identity, and access to appropriately certified and professional surgeons. Thus, it is essential for plastic surgery patients to be informed consumers, seeking out information about their chosen procedure beyond their consultation with a plastic surgeon. In the digital age many choose to do so online, taking advantage of the strong-tie/weak-tie network (Wright, Johnson, Bernard, & Averbeck, 2011); online social support networks are particularly useful for those who lack a strong-tie network and/or those that wish to engage anonymously online (Wright et al., 2011).

The Internet has provided a space for weak-tie support to flourish. Further, advantages of online support include access to multiple perspectives—specifically those with firsthand experience, anonymity and the associated reduction of stigma, similarity to other users, and convenience among other advantages (Wright et al., 2011). One such weak-tie network is the online gathering space for aesthetic and plastic surgery consumers, RealSelf.com. This chapter advances two ideals: first, the unique experience of plastic surgery patients as agents moving through the plastic surgery decision-making process; and second, the importance of community for plastic surgery patients, specifically the role that online social support communities such as RealSelf.com have on enhancing the plastic surgery patient experience.

According to the American Society of Plastic Surgeons (2018), 1,790,832 cosmetic surgical procedures were performed in 2017, a 1 percent increase from 2016. In contrast, 15.7 million cosmetic minimally invasive procedures were performed—a 2 percent increase from 2016. Three of the top-five surgical procedures in 2017 were performed on the body, while the top minimally invasive procedures were on the face (American Society of Plastic Surgeons, 2018). Demand for surgical procedures continues to rise; thus, it is critical to understand and discuss the plastic surgery patient experience. This chapter will focus on plastic surgery as opposed to other types of cosmetic procedures; this decision was made due to the serious nature of surgery and the informational and psychological needs of patients prior to and after their chosen procedure(s).

ESTABLISHING CREDIBILITY

Six months before my thirtieth birthday, I walked into a plastic surgeon's office seeking a breast augmentation consultation. This consultation had been many years in the making—about fourteen to be precise. Prior to this appointment I spoke with a few close friends about their own breast augmentations and consulted the website RealSelf.com. Over the years between my initial interest and following through with the surgery I had varying dispositions toward plastic surgery that ranged from viewing it as an unnecessary alteration to a choice that, I, as an agent became committed to. After a pleasant consultation in which my chosen provider answered all my questions, I decided to move forward with the operation. I scheduled a date just a few weeks from the initial consultation taking a "now or never" attitude. Throughout those weeks leading up to the surgery I grappled with various issues of plastic surgery patienthood, "will I like the change?" "what if something goes wrong?" "will I wake up from anesthesia?" "what will recovery feel like?" "how long will recovery take?" "what about revision?" "can I exercise the same way as before?" "when can I resume my exercise regime again?"

While my friends served as a great source of support they were not always available when a nagging question popped into my head. Then, I turned to RealSelf.com, the community was there as an informational source that allayed my fears and helped me feel confident in my decision. Engaging with the community provided a richness of the experience as a plastic surgery patient that could not be found any other way. Two years and beyond I reflect on my decision with assurance it was the right decision for me. As an insider, a plastic surgery patient, I write to highlight the voices of women and men who choose plastic surgery. Much of the present literature on the topic is written from an outsider perspective that theorizes on individual choice.

While I do not speak for all plastic surgery patients, I speak from my own knowledge, experience, and vested interest in the health and well-being of plastic surgery patients. In this chapter I theorize on the decision-making process for a plastic surgery patient constituted through the literature, my own experiences, and the RealSelf.com community. This begins with a grounding in previous research on plastic surgery.

PLASTIC SURGERY PERSPECTIVES

Studies of plastic surgery can be found in a range of disciplines from medicine and nursing with a focus on screening and caring for patients (Crerand et al., 2007; Furnham & Levitas, 2012; Haas et al., 2008; Milothridis et al., 2016; Montemurro, Porcnik, Hedén, & Otte, 2015; Ubbink, Santema, & Lapid, 2016) as well as marketing to, or interacting with patients (Camp & Mills, 2012; Domanski & Cavale, 2012), psychology (Greenberg, Blashill, Ragan, & Fang, 2016; Günel & Omurlu, 2015; Panayi, 2015; Tam, Ng, Kim, Yeung, & Cheung, 2012), cultural studies (Fraser, 2003; Sarkar, 2015), and communication and media studies (Denadai, Araujo, Samartine Junior, Denadai, & Raposo-Amaral, 2015; Domanski & Cavale, 2012; Markey & Markey, 2010; Park & Allgayer, 2018; Wen, Chia, & Hao, 2015). All these foci offer insight into plastic surgery. While these studies highlight important aspects of plastic surgery, many of these sources fail to speak from the insider perspective, that of the patient. Further, few provide a richness around the plastic surgery decision-making process. In a study of breast augmentation (BA) patients, Walden, Panagopoulous, and Shrader (2010) concluded that the Internet is a key informational source for patients aged twenty to fifty, and further that in the decision-making process BA patients are independent and private thinkers. The following proposes a model for understanding the plastic surgery decision-making process that honors the agency of plastic surgery patients.

PLASTIC SURGERY PATIENT
DECISION-MAKING PROCESS

There are many perspectives that can be taken to understand the process of choosing plastic surgery. I argue that like theories of behavior change, the decision to undergo plastic surgery is a behavior that is unique to the plastic surgery patient perspective. Thus, I advance a four-step decision-making model for plastic surgery patients (1) interest/motivation, (2) reality testing, (3) surgery and recovery, (4) evaluation and identity management. The first stage is the interest stage. Much of the literature on plastic surgery focuses here, examining the characteristics of those with interest in plastic surgery.

Interest/Motivation for Plastic Surgery

Individuals are motivated to seek plastic surgery for a variety of reasons that may range from psychosocial factors to discomfort in one's body. Many studies have examined predictors of plastic surgery to better understand individuals whom choose plastic surgery. Solvi et al. (2009) evaluated fourteen women aged nineteen to forty-six seeking breast augmentation and discovered various psychosocial motivators. Their study found that the primary drive was femininity, generated by six factors: dissatisfaction with their appearance, body ideal, self-esteem, comments of others, clothes, and sexuality. Further, they found five motivating factors identified as the media, physicians, romantic partners, previous breast augmentation patients, and finances. The authors conclude that these findings would be helpful to aid in communication with patients as well as understand patient motives and the growing popularity of plastic surgery. Similarly, Crerand et al. (2007) found that dissatisfaction with one's body image, as well as the size and shape of their breasts, served as primary motivators for BA. Another study examined motivating factors for women seeking labial reduction surgery, the research-ers found that patients were motivated by emotional and functional issues, citing that online reviews featured more references to emotional issues, while plastic surgeon websites referenced functional issues more frequently (Zwier, 2014).

In their systematic review of interest in cosmetic surgery, Milothridis et al. (2016) reviewed twelve studies and found a series of contributing factors to one's interest in plastic surgery. Their findings indicate individual character-istics such as BMI, general health status, issues with interpersonal relation-ships, and high body orientation impact one's interest. The authors discuss the psychopathology and indicate that issues such as body dysmorphic dis-order should be heavily screened. To further this point, Panayi (2015) found in a systematic review of the prevalence of body dysmorphic disorder (BDD) among plastic surgery patients that BDD rates range from 2.9 percent to 53.6 percent of the population. However, the author believed that these estimates may be overstated due to self-report and or essentializing the distinct con-cepts of BDD and general dissatisfaction with one's appearance (Panayi, 2015). The study conducted by Milothridis et al. (2016) is limited as it only assessed mere interest in plastic surgery, not the actual experience of plastic surgery patients. This ignores critical decision points of financing and fear of the procedure—both of which are essential aspects of the decision-making process. Similarly, Sood, Quintal, and Phau (2017) used the theory of planned behavior to predict young consumers' intention to engage in cosmetic procedures, but failed to consider extant variables that influence decision-making, moving from intention to follow-through. This is where the next stages in the plastic surgery patient decision-making model are key to understanding additional variables in the decision-making process. Plastic surgery patients then make a move from the interest/motivation stage to the reality testing stage. In doing so, many go online to informational marketplaces such as RealSelf. com to learn more.

In my own case, I decided to seek plastic surgery for many of the same bio-psychosocial reasons discussed above. I was unsatisfied with my body shape, clothes did not fit me properly, and my body felt disproportionate. These were thoughts and feelings I had over several years, but never moved forward due to various blocks such as lower levels of interest in the surgery at points in time, concerns over payment and timing, and fears associated with the actual process of surgery. Thus, the reality testing stage is a vital stage in the plastic surgery decision-making model.

Reality Testing

Once interest in a procedure has been piqued, a patient moves into the next stage of reality testing. In this stage, individuals who have developed interest in plastic surgery move beyond the ideation and takes next steps in learning about what the surgery means to them. Though I had the interest and motivation in plastic surgery for many years, it took the alignment of high-interest, intimately understanding the process of the procedure, financial readiness, fit with my schedule, and community to move forward. Though these aspects all aligned I still grappled with distress and anxieties associated with the surgery such as fear of "going under" or anesthetic as well as concerns that I would not like the outcome. Considering these experiences, I propose that the reality testing stage includes developing literacy in plastic surgery and one's chosen procedure(s), evaluating and meeting for consultations with plastic surgeons, determining cost and payment of the procedure, length of the procedure and recovery, scheduling, and developing a supportive community. While these are presented in a linear fashion here, they may not be experienced this way. This section will explore each of these, and place emphasis on the role that online sources have in the reality testing stage.

In this stage of the decision-making process many go online, seeking more information from sites such as Real Patient Ratings or RealSelf.com. These sites can be used as an entry point to this reality testing stage. According to Montemurro et al. (2015) 95 percent of plastic surgery patients seek information about their chosen procedure online and 46 percent used social media. However, the study also found that 85 percent of plastic surgeons felt that social media created unrealistic expectations for outcomes, while at the same time 45 percent found that patient use of social media made consultations easier. This analysis pays attention to RealSelf.com as a popular peer-to-peer informational marketplace, and how each of the aspects of the reality testing stage are represented in community member interactions.

Understanding RealSelf

At its most basic, RealSelf.com is an online space for individuals to ask and answer questions, comments, concerns, and so on, related to various plastic surgery or cosmetic procedures. The site provides three avenues of exploration for consumers. The first is research, where consumers can read reviews on treatments from members. These reviews may include photos, costs, and general opinions on the procedure. This includes 250 procedures categorized into body, face and skin, and smile (RealSelf.com, 2018a). From "A to Z" these are abdominal etching to zoom whitening (RealSelf.com, 2018e). Another way to view this is through their most popular treatments; the top three are breast augmentation, Brazilian butt lift, and breast reduction (RealSelf.com, 2018a). The second is access to RealSelf community of doctors in which one can reach out for their professional opinion. And the third is to find a doctor, where consumers can search for board-certified medical professionals registered with RealSelf.com.

While consumers use the site in their decision-making process, providers use the site as a marketing tool in which they can claim and maintain their account. The site works to build its provider network by boasting 9.9 million visitors each month as well as 5 million referrals to provider sites (RealSelf.com, 2018d). They may also become more active on the site to achieve varying levels of distinction. These range from distinguished member by answering at least fifty consumer questions to Top Doctor in which they have received positive consumer feedback on their given advice (less than 10 percent of the RealSelf community) to the RealSelf 100, the highest distinction of consumer dedication and satisfaction (RealSelf.com, 2018d).

In "About" section, the site is self-described as "RealSelf is the leading and most trusted source for people considering an elective cosmetic treatment. More than ten years ago, we built RealSelf as the destination for people to learn about cosmetic procedures, share their experiences, and connect with top providers. Today there are more cosmetic treatment options than ever before—from Botox to laser hair removal, microneedling to CoolSculpting. That's why RealSelf provides unbiased information about cosmetic procedures and the doctors and clinicians who perform them" (RealSelf.com, 2018b, para 1–2).

In their careers section, their mission is developed further as "At RealSelf, you'll build innovative products that empower people with the unbiased information they need to make confident medical and aesthetic choices" (RealSelf.com, 2018c, para 1). Clicking through to their LinkedIn profile from the careers section reveals the same strategic message found on their website, but also additional information about the culture of the organization, "As stewards of our community, we live by values that align us with our members' interests and enable us to deliver on our mission: to bring confidence to every important health and beauty decision" (RealSelf LinkedIn, 2018, para 3).

The site has seen some publicity with features in various online publications, each taking a different perspective. In Moss (2014), an article published through Business Insider, the author provides an overview of the website providing basic instruction on how the site is used and moderated. Another article posted by Pando (Griffith, 2013), a blog for tech startups, detailed the ingenuity of the site. Griffith (2013) described the model of RealSelf as "find a market that thrives on its lack of transparency and make it transparent" (para 2). The author continues to reveal more about the business model (Griffith, 2013, para 10):

> RealSelf isn't trying to be booster for the plastic surgery industry. In fact, many in the industry view it as disruptive. Prices are listed, which means patients are armed with more information when shopping around. In fact, that's the whole goal of RealSelf: giving people as much information as possible about a procedure. In many cases, reviews convince users not to get a procedure done. For example, the Lifestyle Lift, a facelift alternative that advertises heavily on late night infomercials (um, red flag?), is so poorly reviewed that, after browsing the site's horror stories, it's unlikely anyone would want to sign up for it. "That's why we're a media company, not a pay-per-lead company," Seery [CEO of RealSelf.com] says. "That would set us on the wrong side of this."

Jezebel (Shade, 2015) had another take. The author places a negative bend on the topic, and associates use of the online social community as related to aspects of workplace discrimination due to physical appearance as well as a source of never-ending body consciousness. While Shade (2015) provides one perspective on the topic, and those sentiments were echoed or built upon by commenters, another group of commenters provides alternative experiences that highlight the necessity of such procedures post-children, pain from aging, or simply fulfilling the desire to feel confident about oneself.

Navigating the Site

On the homepage of RealSelf.com the eye is immediately drawn to the words, "find the right cosmetic surgery or treatment," from there the user can navigate to "find a doctor" or informational pages specific to treatments useful to "research and review." Selecting the "Research Treatments" click-through takes the user to a list of treatments that can be organized in different ways. Initially, this list is organized by the number of reviews with breast augmentation leading with an impressive 28,583 reviews followed by tummy tuck at 24,710 the top-ten reviewed procedures can be found in Table 12.1. Treatments may also be sorted by treatment area: nose, face, eyes, mouth, and so forth as well as average cost, and finally by "Worth It" rating. Clicking through the most highly reviewed procedure, breast augmentation, provides insight in the information available about each procedure. At the top are quick links to reviews, cost, photos, providers, Q&A, guides, videos, and forum. Below on the page is a brief definition of the procedure, the average cost, and followed by community reviews many of which include photos and video.

Like the treatments page, the reviews can be sorted in a variety of ways: best match, recent, nearby, and comments. Results can also be narrowed by ratings (worth it, not worth it, or don't know), or key words contained within the review or other aspects of the procedure. At this point it is important to note that the rating given to a procedure is author generated—meaning the individual whom is providing the review of the procedure provides their own assessment if the procedure was in their opinion "worth it"—meaning the rewards outweighed the risks within the frame of their own experience. In their evaluation of RealSelf.com, Domanski and Cavale (2012) concluded that the "worth it" rating was influenced by price, expectations, and outcomes of the procedure. Table 12.2 displays the top ten procedures when sorted by worth.

Regardless of the way that individual enter the site, they typically have a specific procedure in mind, and will use the informational marketplace in

Table 12.1   Top Ten Reported Procedures

Procedure (Avg. Cost)	Rating	Number of Reviews
Breast Augmentation ($6,450)	98% Worth It	28,583
Tummy Tuck ($8,150)	96% Worth It	24,710
Brazilian Butt Lift ($6,525)	91% Worth It	22,515
Rhinoplasty ($7,475)	90% Worth It	14,755
Mommy Makeover ($12,375)	97% Worth It	11,692
Breast Implants ($6,325)	97% Worth It	10,356
Breast Reduction ($7,250)	97% Worth It	10,051
Botox ($550)	95% Worth It	9,838
Liposuction ($6025)	88% Worth It	6,986
Breast Lift with Implants ($8,775)	95% Worth It	6,298

Table 12.2   Top Ten Procedures by Reported "Worth"

Procedure (Avg. Cost)	Rating	Number of Reviews
Collagen Injection ($775)	100% Worth It	45
Photofacial ($450)	100% Worth It	171
Pulse Dye Laser ($725)	100% Worth It	27
Glycolic Peel ($125)	100% Worth It	88
Acne Surgery ($2,100)	82% Worth It	37
Calf Implant ($7,450)	100% Worth It	55
Teeth Whitening ($425)	100% Worth It	113
Dermaplaning ($125)	100% Worth It	15
Deep FX ($2,750)	81% Worth It	45
Pearl Laser ($1,450)	100% Worth It	73

their reality testing process. While all aspects of the reality testing stage can be found within the pages of RealSelf.com, patients most likely begin with developing plastic surgery literacy and the consultation aspects.

Plastic Surgery Literacy

To be health literate means that an individual has the skills and capacity to make decisions that will positively influence their health outcomes (World Health Organization, 1998a), then to develop plastic surgery literacy is to have the ability to properly evaluate and assess surgeons and procedures, within one's own physical, mental, and social health. Plastic surgery literacy can develop through a variety of means: interpersonal interactions with those that have completed a procedure, as well as engagement with traditional media, for example, television shows like Nip/Tuck, Botched, or even the Real Housewives series, and social media sites where one can engage with celebrity surgeons such as Dr. Miami or Dr. Schulman, both popularized through SnapChat. Engagement with these media might work to develop interest, but also provide information. Montemurro et al. (2015) found that most of plastic surgery patients seek information about their chosen procedure prior to their consultation with a surgeon. Similarly, Hoppe, Ahuja, Ingargiola, and Granick (2013) found that the Internet is an important educational tool for plastic surgery patients, but it does not replace the role of the consultation. Sites such as RealSelf provide the consumer with information that is key to the first stage of reality testing: basic descriptions of the procedure, cost, and connection to providers in one's area. This is where my own search began, I used to site to familiarize myself with the basics of the procedure and research board-certified plastic surgeons.

Consultation

Once a patient has begun focused research on their procedure, their next step is to set up a consultation with their chosen provider(s). The consultation acts as a solidifying process and is key to creating a well-informed patient (Hoppe et al., 2013; Lazar & Deneuve, 2013; Montemurro et al., 2015). Much of the literature focuses on the role of the patient consultation, and the role that the surgeon must play in evaluating the patients desired outcome and screen for possible negative factors such as body dysmorphic disorder (BDD) (Greenberg et al., 2016; Panayi, 2015). Additional literature details the process of consultation, and the role that the surgeon plays in making the procedure desirable by holding excess fat or highlighting various areas of the body (Mirivel, 2008). Many choose to consult with multiple surgeons before committing to the procedure, though once an individual chooses their surgeon they are typically asked to secure the surgery date with a deposit. While, one may have shown interest in plastic surgery moving forward with the act of meeting with a plastic surgeon adds a certain level of commitment to the process. In my own experience, once I chose my surgeon, using my aforementioned "now or never" attitude, I scheduled and put down the deposit. But this was far from the end of the reality testing stage—this merely held me accountable to the decision.

Feasibility Measures

Another aspect of reality testing is coordination and scheduling of the procedure itself. There are three aspects of feasibility that must be assessed. The first is cost and payment as these are critical decision points. This is exemplified throughout interactions on RealSelf.com, for example, on a review on Brazilian butt lift (BBL) provided by BigBootyTinyWaist, we see similar interactions among users. In her original post she details her desire to seek out the surgery as such, "I am married and my husband supports me 100% with this, infact hes paying for it, he says an unhappy wife equals an unhappy home which equals an unhappy him. I have 2 beautiful children but unfortunately, they have taken all my beauty from me. I used to model before I had kids all up until my 2nd child 1 year ago and boy has she done a job on my body. Ive been anxiously waiting for the time to come." In response a commenter shares a similar story, "My husband is also paying for mine and giving me his support. I also have two kids a boy 2yrs and a 1 yr old girl ... They did a work on my body lol i used to dance and now i am a little insecure about my body so i really want the work done so i cn get back to work." In this exchange there is also mention of the financial aspect from both parties. Similarly, user EnjoyingLife on a tummy tuck review provided information about her surgery, including a fee breakdown. In a later post she details the deposit made to her surgeon, and that the deposit goes toward the surgery, but it is not refundable.

Plastic surgery can be costly, which means that an individual must budget for the procedure or find a way to finance the procedure. From there, once an individual has secured this aspect they must consider the time and scheduling of the procedure that aligns with the surgeon's calendar and their own; considering the amount of time the procedure will take and more specifically, how long it will take them to recover from the surgery and how this aligns with other life obligations. It is important that these feasibility measures align for the plastic surgery patient to move forward with the process. The first three aspects of reality testing can be cumbersome to complete on one's own, which is why the next aspect of reality testing, finding a supportive community is critical to the process. Personally, knowing I had moved through these feasibility measures prior to meeting for my consultation, I then looked for community to ease my fears moving forward.

Supportive Community

Those seeking online social support are often seeking connections they are not able to make in their everyday life. The weak-tie/strong-tie theory (Wright et al., 2011) establishes that individuals looking for social support online may benefit from the characteristics of online support that draw together individuals with like interests as well as the mobility and reach of the Internet. RealSelf.com promotes itself as a community first. This is evidenced by the language used throughout the site to reference community. For example, reviews are headed as "Community Reviews & Photos," this language sets the framework for interaction on the site. Throughout the site the term community is used by moderators as well as users to describe the online gathering space. In the reviews, it is clear to see how community develops among the users, specifically around a procedure, as these individuals are like-minded in the sense they are seeking the same procedure and are moving through the decision-making process together.

There are two primary ways that peers can engage one another on the site. The first is through reviews. Sorting through reviews one can seek out a review from someone who lives within proximity, has seen their chosen provider, is the same height and weight, or is considering the same approach to the procedure, and so on. From there, peers can engage by commenting on each other's reviews or indicating that a review was helpful by using a heart symbol. The review itself serves as a gathering point for users to convene. Each review develops its own sub-community, and within these communities the reviewer or original poster becomes the peer expert. The phenomenon of peer expert is used to describe users who have been through the procedure and their lessons from the experience. Individuals who serve as peer experts gain the status by providing their review, often including detailed accounts of their experience through numerous posts that include photos or video. This action establishes credibility for the reviewer, and credibility continues to develop through the users' additional interactions with commentators. The peer expert is revered as a source for different types of support. Firstly, informational support as RealSelf is primarily an informational marketplace—user interactions generally surround questions or concerns directly related to the procedure or recovery. This provides a functional purpose for both the patient and providers as many plastic surgery websites lack in terms of readability (Ricci, Vargas, Chuang, Lin, & Lee, 2015).

Messages exchanged can also be informational such as which surgical approach is best, postoperative care and recovery, or how to navigate interpersonal interactions around the surgery. The second type of support common on RealSelf is emotional support. Seeking out surgery can be an emotional process, one that those that have not experienced it or come from a different worldview may not be able to share, but because individuals engaged on this site have shared interests or experiences they are able to understand the emotional aspects tied to the surgery more acutely.

On reviews, commenters thank the original poster by stating, "thank you for posting your journey" or "your post and pictures have really helped me, and you are very informative." Given the serious nature of plastic surgery; those seeking plastic surgery must satisfy their needs for informational, social, and psychological support. This is best represented by the term "journey" that is used throughout reviews and comments to refer to one's surgery experience. For example, the breast augmentation review with the most comments on RealSelf.com was created by Anna 1989 in 2014 and the latest review and comments were posted in 2017. Her review details her experience with breast augmentation with more than 60 original posts, including 437 photos, two videos, 3,873 comments, and 71 endorsements for helpfulness.

Commenters support the original poster by providing compliments such as "perfect" or "nice job." Others thank the original poster for their review and photos, "thank you so much for sharing your pics." Images are critical to reviews, the top reviews for procedures such as breast augmentation, Brazilian butt lift, tummy tuck, and calf implants all feature photos. The photos serve a function that allows peers to not only hear about the experience but make an evaluation of the work to see if it aligns with their own conception of "worth it." On various reviews commenters state things such as one review for a tummy tuck, "thank you so much for sharing your pics." On another review for breast augmentation many commenters state things such as, "my wish boobs" or "showing my plastic surgeon your pic." Peer experts' photos and videos can be used to instill confidence in the individual seeking the procedure.

The second way peers engage is through forums. Each procedure features a variety of monitored topics that are either site-generated or user-generated. Forum topics include check-in for individuals going through surgery during the same month, soliciting concerns about recovery, or other questions, comments, concerns related to the procedure and beyond. Forums can be used to provide a sense of confidence in the procedure and community. For example, each month a moderator develops a forum for individuals seeking the procedure at that time. Once a patient is properly prepared, or their surgery date arrives, they move into the next stage, surgery and recovery.

Leading up to my surgery I spent hours scouring the site—reading reviews, reading forums. Looking at images of my surgeon's previous work. Reading about the safety of anesthesia, running through every possible scenario in my head. Then surgery day arrived, my mom came into town to accompany me to the surgery and take care of me after. Honestly, I was a nervous wreck. As time approached, I prepared for the surgery at home washing with a special antibacterial soap, laid out my medications and loose-fitting clothing for my return and recovery. Then I drove to the surgery center with my mom. I felt nervous, but ready, and supported.

Surgery and Recovery

Once a plastic surgery patient has determined that plastic surgery is the right choice for them, they then follow-through on the surgery and in turn go through the recovery process. Generally, the surgery portion can be completed in one day. In my case, the nurses prepped me for surgery and I met one final time with the surgeon. The surgeon, nurses, and I reviewed the plan once more, and it was time. The surgery took less than one hour, but the recovery took much longer. My mom stayed with me the first week of recovery. Generally, my recovery was smooth. There was pain as expected, but after a week or so it subsided. From there I had to be patient as my body healed, and I could resume regular activity. Specifically, exercise is an important part of my daily life. During recovery, the patient must be diligent in understanding the effect the surgery will have on their day-to-day life during recovery, and beyond. This may include taking time off work, securing someone to care for the patient while they recover, and other accommodations for short-term limited mobility.

In a study about day surgery patients postoperative three themes emerged: (1) preparation for surgery and recovery at home, (2) physical and emotional implications of recovery, (3) responsibility of the individual to care for oneself (Berg, Kjellgren, & Årestedt, 2016). The authors concluded that developing clear expectations for recovery and self-care can be the key to improving day surgery. The post-surgery period can be a strange time as one is healing and adjusting, while also experiencing the first stages of evaluation and identity management. During this stage in the process, users at RealSelf.com may use the review section to connect with their community. For example, they may post updates of their recovery and healing process.

At first it may be difficult to see past the images of disembodied body parts; but taking a closer look at the user comments reveals the impact of the review and the usefulness of the images. Further, while images of body parts may evoke sexual thoughts, the RealSelf community helps to remove the sexualized nature, and allows for objective discussion of these topics in a way that other spaces may not. While, I never wrote a review myself, or even commented on a review, I still spent hours browsing the site, and felt a sense of community even from my spectator role. RealSelf provides a space for individuals to engage in this conversation in a safe, non-threatening environment. It can also be theorized that sharing the reviews and images at stages throughout the process, for example, pre-operative, postoperative, and weeks beyond with a community of people with genuine interest creates a sense of belonging. I knew that my offline community had little interest in engaging the topic with me to the degree that I desired. Where one's own strong-tie network may tire, those in the weak-tie network or online community provide a space for individuals to engage in the topic, discussing their recent surgery and the intricacies of the healing process with an audience that also has vested interest due to their own or anticipated experiences.

Evaluation and Identity Management

The final stage of the decision-making process is evaluation and identity management. At this point the patient is healed and is now in the process of adjusting to the impact of the surgery and evaluating the value of the surgery against their frame of reference. At this point an individual may indicate that they are satisfied with their surgery or they may not be satisfied, either way, this leads to issues of identity management and quality of life. For example, one user, bobinhood, on a rhinoplasty review, detailed her experience—lamenting the impact the surgery had on her smile, and how this led to uncertainty about the value of the surgery. She indicated that she changed her "worth it" to a "don't know" at that point. In a later post, she explained the four ways the rhinoplasty changed her life including the ways she interacts with others, finding herself smiling more post-surgery, thinking less about the appearance of her nose or trying to hide it, and how she is treated in interpersonal relationships, romantic and non-romantic. She concludes, "In general, I've just had a more positive attitude and outlook on life since my surgery, and in many ways it has changed my life for the better. I must not forget that." In her post she alludes to the impact of the surgery on her quality of life.

Quality of Life

In reading the literature, the pursuit of a higher quality of life is the underlying motivating factor. Quality of life is defined by the World Health Organization

(1998b) as "an individual's perception of their position in life in the context of the culture and value systems in which they live and in relation to their goals, expectations, standards and concerns. It is a broad ranging concept incorporating in a complex way the person's physical health, psychological state, level of independence, social relationships, personal beliefs and their relationship to salient features of the environment" (p. 3). In line with motivating factors for seeking plastic surgery, individuals seeking plastic surgery do so in order to improve their quality of life. Generally, studies have found that plastic surgery leads to greater self-reported quality of life (Adams, 2010) in a variety of procedures such as BA (Kalaaji, Bergsmark Bjertness, Nordahl, & Olafsen, 2013), rhinoplasty (Günel & Omurlu, 2015), and breast reduction which is consistently cited as the cosmetic procedure with the highest rate of satisfaction and improvement of quality of life (Adams, 2010; Milothridis et al., 2016).

In accord with the literature, I do feel an enhanced quality of life after my procedure. My original motivators of dissatisfaction with my body shape, clothes not fitting me properly, and feeling that my body was out of proportion were satisfied with the surgery. I am pleased with the results of my surgery, and I see the ways it has enhanced my life. Though, it is important that this section include a discussion of other aspects post-surgery in terms of identity management. In particular for me as an academic I pause even writing these words—afraid of criticism I might receive from my contemporaries for my decision-making process. I hesitated to include my own story in this chapter for fear that this identity as a plastic surgery patient conflicts with my identity as an academic and a scholar. However, I determined that this chapter would gain richness of quality and authenticity by including my experiences.

Plastic surgery prompts an examination of the management of intersecting identities such as woman, man, feminist, professional, parent, or athlete and how decision points around plastic surgery can work to enhance or detract from those identities through a process of framing and negotiating said identities. Specifically examining their meaning, for example, a woman seeking plastic surgery to restore her body after children manage any physical discomforts that arose post-childbirth, a reclamation of womanhood (through her chosen procedures), and the feminist choice to freely determine if plastic surgery is her desired course of action. In moving through this process, the plastic surgery patient may experience the dialectical tension between secrecy and openness/sharing. For example, my own thought process on the subject shared above. A plastic surgery patient must learn to navigate the way they discuss plastic surgery, making critical decisions about how they share in their offline lives. Some may choose to be more secretive with their surgery to keep it private, while others might choose to share in interpersonal circles or anonymously online. The evaluation and identity management stage can theoretically be an ongoing process as we are continually negotiating our identities; further in the case of some plastic surgery patients they may need to seek revision, which may prompt the entire process over again.

CONCLUSION

The purpose of this chapter is to advance an insider's perspective on the plastic surgery decision-making process. In the decision-making process, the plastic surgery patient moves through a four-stage process from interest/motivation, through reality testing, surgery and recovery, and finally evaluation and identity management. This decision-making model is meant to recognize the range of factors that influence one's decision to undertake plastic surgery. Though some aspects of the process may be generalized such as the predictors for interest in plastic surgery or one's satisfaction with the outcome, there are a series of other factors that have a considerable impact on the experience, such as one's comfort with the procedure, their support community, their chosen surgeon, the aesthetic outcome in relation to their own value system or the "worth" of the procedure, and the impact the procedure has had on their quality of life.

Health communicators have a special role to play in the process of information seeking and delivery for plastic surgery patients. As the popularity of plastic surgery continues to grow, health communicators can assist in the ways that information about plastic surgery is sought, disseminated, and discussed among plastic surgery patients. In doing this, health communicators can work to ensure that these patients are moving forward with procedures in the safest forms possible through a decision-making process that includes a diligent assessment of available information about their chosen procedure as well as an assessment of their own values and how they align with the chosen procedure and perceived outcomes.

REFERENCES

Adams, J. (2010). Motivational narratives and assessments of the body after cosmetic surgery. *Qualitative Health Research, 20*(6), 755–767.

American Society of Plastic Surgeons. (2018). 2017 national plastic surgery statistics [Press release]. Retrieved from https://www.plasticsurgery.org/news/press-releases/new-statistics-reveal-the-shape-of-plastic-surgery.

Berg, K., Kjellgren, K., & Årestedt, K. (2016). Postoperative recovery from the perspective of day surgery patients: A phenomenographic study. *Day Surgery Australia, 15*(1), 14–23.

Camp, S. M., & Mills, D. C. (2012). *The marriage of plastic surgery and social media: A relationship to last a lifetime.* Blackwell Publishing Ltd Oxford, UK.

Crerand, C. E., Infield, A. L., & Sarwer, D. B. (2007). Psychological considerations in cosmetic breast augmentation. *Plast Surg Nurs, 27*(3), 146–154. doi: 10.1097/01. PSN.0000290284.49982.0c.

Denadai, R., Araujo, K. M., Samartine Junior, H., Denadai, R., & Raposo-Amaral, C. E. (2015). Aesthetic surgery reality television shows: Do they influence public perception of the scope of plastic surgery? *Aesthetic Plastic Surgery, 39*(6), 1000–1009. doi: 10.1007/s00266-015-0577-6.

Domanski, M. C., & Cavale, N. (2012). Self-reported "worth it" rating of aesthetic surgery in social media. *Aesthetic Plastic Surgery, 36*(6), 1292–1295.

Fraser, S. (2003). The agent within: Agency repertoires in medical discourse on cosmetic surgery. *Australian Feminist Studies, 18*(40), 27–44.

Furnham, A., & Levitas, J. (2012). Factors that motivate people to undergo cosmetic surgery. *Canadian Journal of Plastic Surgery, 20*(4), 47–50.

Greenberg, J. L., Blashill, A. J., Ragan, J., & Fang, A. (2016). Cognitive behavioral therapy for body dysmorphic disorder. In Timothy J. Petersen, Susan Sprich, & Sabine Wilhelm. *The Massachusetts general hospital handbook of cognitive behavioral therapy* (pp. 141–153). Springer.

Griffith, E. (2013). Meet RealSelf: The profitable, under-the-radar plastic surgery site. Retrieved from https://pando.com/2013/01/23/realself-makes-plastic-surgery-transparent/.

Günel, C., & Omurlu, I. K. (2015). The effect of rhinoplasty on psychosocial distress level and quality of life. *European Archives of Oto-Rhino-Laryngology, 272*(8), 1931–1935.

Haas, C. F., Champion, A., & Secor, D. (2008). Motivating factors for seeking cosmetic surgery: A synthesis of the literature. *Plast Surg Nurs, 28*(4), 177–182. doi: 10.1097/PSN.0b013e31818ea832.

Hoppe, I. C., Ahuja, N. K., Ingargiola, M. J., & Granick, M. S. (2013). A survey of patient comprehension of readily accessible online educational material regarding plastic surgery procedures. *Aesthetic Surgery Journal, 33*(3), 436–442.

Kalaaji, A., Bergsmark Bjertness, C., Nordahl, C., & Olafsen, K. (2013). Survey of breast implant patients: Characteristics, depression rate, and quality of life. *Aesthetic Surgery Journal, 33*(2), 252–257.

Lazar, C. C., & Deneuve, S. (2013). Patients' perceptions of cosmetic surgery at a time of globalization, medical consumerism, and mass media culture: A French experience. *Aesthetic Surgery Journal, 33*(6), 878–885.

Markey, C. N., & Markey, P. M. (2010). A correlational and experimental examination of reality television viewing and interest in cosmetic surgery. *Body Image, 7*(2), 165–171.

Milothridis, P., Pavlidis, L., Haidich, A. B., & Panagopoulou, E. (2016). A systematic review of the factors predicting the interest in cosmetic plastic surgery. *Indian J Plast Surg, 49*(3), 397–402. doi: 10.4103/0970-0358.197224.

Mirivel, J. C. (2008). The physical examination in cosmetic surgery: Communication strategies to promote the desirability of surgery. *Health Communication, 23*(2), 153–170.

Montemurro, P., Porcnik, A., Hedén, P., & Otte, M. (2015). The influence of social media and easily accessible online information on the aesthetic plastic surgery practice: Literature review and our own experience. *Aesthetic Plastic Surgery, 39*(2), 270–277.

Moss, C. (2014). 'RealSelf' is like a social network for people who want cosmetic surgery. Retrieved from http://www.businessinsider.com/realself-for-cosmetic-su rgery-2014-2.

Panayi, A. (2015). The prevalence of body dysmorphic disorder in patients undergo-ing cosmetic surgery: A systematic review. *Psychiatria Danubina, 27*(1), 438–444.

Park, S.-Y., & Allgayer, S. (2018). Cosmetic surgery advertising exposure, attitudes toward the surgery and surgeons, and perceptions of the advertisement features. *Journal of Communication in Healthcare, 11*(1), 69.

RealSelf LinkedIn. (2018). Retrieved from https://www.linkedin.com/company/re alself-com/.

RealSelf.com. (2018a). Retrieved from realself.com.

RealSelf.com. (2018b). About. Retrieved from https://atwork.realself.com/.

RealSelf.com. (2018c). Careers. Retrieved from https://atwork.realself.com/careers/.

RealSelf.com. (2018d). Claim profile. Retrieved from https://www.realself.com/dr/ claimprofile.

RealSelf.com. (2018e). Topics. Retrieved from https://www.realself.com/topics.

Ricci, J. A., Vargas, C. R., Chuang, D. J., Lin, S. J., & Lee, B. T. (2015). Readability assessment of online patient resources for breast augmentation surgery. *Plastic and Reconstructive Surgery, 135*(6), 1573–1579.

Sarkar, S. (2015). Playing with boundaries: Posthuman digital narratives in RealSelf. com. *Rupkatha Journal on Interdisciplinary Studies in Humanities, 7*(1), 82–90.

Shade, C. (2015). How do you know if your butt lift was 'worth it'? just ask RealSelf. com. Retrieved from https://jezebel.com/how-do-you-know-if-your-butt-lift-w as-worth-it-just-1724524208.

Solvi, A., Foss, K., von Soest, T., E Roald, H., C Skolleborg, K., & Holte, A. (2009). Motivational factors and psychological processes in cosmetic breast augmentation surgery. *Journal of Plastic and Aesthetic Surgery, 63*(4), 673–680. doi: 10.1016/j. bjps.2009.01.024.

Sood, A., Quintal, V., & Phau, I. (2017). Keeping up with the Kardashians: Consum-ers' intention to engage in cosmetic surgery. *Journal of Promotion Management, 23*(2), 185–206.

Tam, K.-P., Ng, H. K.-S., Kim, Y.-H., Yeung, V. W.-L., & Cheung, F. Y.-L. (2012). Attitudes toward cosmetic surgery patients: The role of culture and social contact. *The Journal of Social Psychology, 152*(4), 458–479.

Ubbink, D. T., Santema, T. B., & Lapid, O. (2016). Shared decision-making in cosmetic medicine and aesthetic surgery. *Aesthetic Surgery Journal, 36*(1), NP14–NP19. doi: 10.1093/asj/sjv107.

Walden, J. L., Panagopoulous, G., & Shrader, S. W. (2010). Contemporary decision making and perception in patients undergoing cosmetic breast augmentation. *Aesthetic Surgery Journal, 30*(3), 395–403. doi: 10.1177/1090820X10374101.

Wen, N., Chia, S. C., & Hao, X. (2015). What do social media say about makeovers? A content analysis of cosmetic surgery videos and viewers' responses on YouTube. *Health Communication, 30*(9), 933–942.

World Health Organization. (1998a). Health promotion glossary. http://www.who.int/healthpromotion/about/HPG/en/.

World Health Organization. (1998b). World health organization quality of life. http://www.who.int/healthpromotion/about/HPG/en/

Wright, K. B., Johnson, A. J., Bernard, D. R., & Averbeck, J. (2011). Promises and pitfalls for individuals coping with health concerns. *The Routledge Handbook of Health Communication*, 349, 349–362.

Zwier, S. (2014). "What motivates her": Motivations for considering labial reduction surgery as recounted on women's online communities and surgeons' websites. *Sexual Medicine, 2*(1), 16–23.

Chapter 13

Narrative Sense-Making in Systemic Lupus Erythematosus

Katherine M. Castle and Jody Koenig Kellas

Systemic lupus erythematosus (SLE) is a chronic, inflammatory multi-system autoimmune disease that is life limiting and potentially life threatening, affecting more than 1 million Americans (Wallace, 2008, p. 3), primarily women (Aberer, 2010; Wallace, 2008). The disease is characterized by a failure of the immune system to differentiate between antigens and the body's own cells and tissues, resulting in the body essentially attacking itself. SLE is often misunderstood and misdiagnosed because it presents in such varied ways (Aberer, 2010; Wallace, 2008), complicating the way women and their families make sense of the disease.

Good family communication, and the social support and coping resources it provides (Pecchioni, Overton, & Thompson, 2015), is clearly linked to positive health outcomes in chronically ill individuals (Rosland, Heisler, & Pettit, 2012). On the other hand, the strained family relationships so often associated with an SLE diagnosis (Roper Survey, 2011) can impede the process of sense-making in SLE given that families are central sites for sense-making (Pecchioni & Keeley, 2011). The way individuals and families make sense of illness shapes patient orientations toward their condition (Villagran & Sparks, 2010), their ability to cope with the illness (Frank, 2013), and their willingness and ability to comply with medical directives (DiMatteo, 2003). Thus, family sense-making processes are of central concern to the health and well-being of women struggling with SLE and are the central foci of this chapter.

NARRATIVE SENSE-MAKING

Sense-making about illness is often narrative in nature (Kleinmann, 1988; Sharf & Vanderford, 2003) given that humans are inherently storytellers

(Fisher, 1987). Bruner (2004) asserts that formal structures for experience are laid down early in the discourse of family life and these formal structures, or narratives, persist despite the changing circumstances that characterize the illness experience. These narratives are therefore constructed in, and have implications for, family communication and are primary resources for sense-making (Koenig Kellas & Kranstuber Horstman, 2015). Thus, they are valuable in studying the transitions associated with negotiating an illness like SLE in a family context (Holmberg, Orbuch, & Veroff, 2004).

Although SLE has been studied from a narrative perspective by Mendelson (2006, 2009), this work is ethnographic with a focus on gaining an in-depth description of what daily life is like for women living with SLE. Specifically, Mendelson's (2006) analysis of women's stories of lupus revealed that the central phenomenon is that they live socially and medically complex lives characterized by uncertainty, shifts in identity, and financial burden. Further, in a case study analysis of the same data set, Mendelson (2009) found that the narratives of women with SLE were predominantly focused on seeking a diagnosis. Mendelson (2009) ultimately concluded that the absence of a diagnosis held women's identity construction in abeyance, inhibiting the development of a coherent narrative and impeding the sense-making process.

Here, we are interested in the ways women with SLE communicate to make sense of their experience with SLE. Thus, we collected women's stories—primary vehicles of communicated sense-making—about their illness identity as it intersects with communication in their family. We show that narrative identity (re)construction and narrative coping are continuous, emergent processes that occur in light of, and despite, diagnosis—given that the experience of illness begins with the onset of symptoms and often precedes a diagnosis (Charmaz, 2000). Identity (re)construction is fundamentally a process of communicated sense-making (Koenig Kellas & Kranstuber Horstman, 2015) that, along with coping processes, affects and reflects family communication and health and well-being in illness. This chapter builds from and extends Mendelson's (2006, 2009) findings in exploring both the *narrative* and *communicative* nature and implications of sense-making in families affected by SLE.

COMMUNICATED NARRATIVE SENSE-MAKING

Situated as a type of communicated sense-making (CSM) in Koenig Kellas and Kranstuber Horstman's (2015) model, communicated *narrative* sense-making (CNSM) highlights the centrality of storytelling in sense-making processes associated with the fundamental narrative functions of coping, socialization, and identity (re)construction (see also Koenig Kellas & Trees,

2013). CNSM theory (Koenig Kellas, 2018) positions narrative as a central sense-making process in families and empirically links these processes to health and well-being. In order to highlight the communicated nature of narrative sense-making, CNSM theory focuses on one of three heuristics, including retrospective storytelling (the content of family stories/storytelling), interactional storytelling (storytelling processes), and translational storytelling (applications and interventions) (Koenig Kellas, 2018; Koenig Kellas & Kranstuber Horstman, 2015). The current study falls within the purview of retrospective storytelling which focuses on the lasting effects of the (family) stories we hear and tell. CNSM's Proposition 1 states that *The content of retrospective storytelling reveals individual, relational, and intergenerational meaning-making, values, and beliefs.* In other words, the stories that we hear and tell reveal much about what matters to storytellers and story listeners in a given historical, relational, and affective moment. The current study tests this proposition by focusing on the content of illness narratives affecting and reflecting the sense-making processes of women with SLE. Specifically, we examined the articulation of their illness story as well as through their recollections of family communication and stories important to their illness experience. Retrospective storytelling about significant family events—such as illness—allows narrators to construct identity, and cope, in light of difficulty. Stories illustrate the meaning women have assigned to SLE both as it pertains to their own and their family's identity.

The communicative nature of narratives is at the heart of CNSM (Koenig Kellas, 2005), suggesting that they result from collaboratively constructed storytelling interactions (Koenig Kellas & Trees, 2006) and/or the interactions between storytellers and story listeners (sunwolf, Frey, & Keranan, 2005). However, as demonstrated and guided by Frank (1995, 2010) and McAdams (1993), narratives are primarily conceptualized and studied as psychological constructs (Koenig Kellas, Trees, Schrodt, LeClair-Underberg, & Willer, 2010). As Koenig Kellas (2015) argues, it is vital that we better understand the communicated nature of narratives. One way we can do this is to understand and study the ways in which communication affects and reflects our personal narratives (Eisenberg, 2001). Thus, guided by CNSM, this study positions retrospective storytelling as a means by which women narrate their SLE experience, position their own identity in relation to SLE, and make sense of the ways in which the family communication affects and reflects the narrative coping process.

In addition to acting as a call for research on the links between communicated narratives and psychosocial well-being, CNSM is also a framework for organizing the impact of extant research and theorizing on our understanding of these links (Koenig Kellas & Kranstuber Horstman, 2015). In other words, we can understand the ways in which the stories people tell and hear have a lasting impact in affecting and reflecting their sense-making. In line with this approach, and in order to understand the power of identity construction and coping in the process of retrospectively narrating SLE, we further draw from Frank's (2013) approach to illness narratives and McAdams's (1993) theory of narrative identity to examine SLE narratives.

FRANK'S TYPOLOGY OF ILLNESS NARRATIVES

In his foundational work, Frank (1995, 2013) delineated six illness narrative types. These have come to serve as a foundation for understanding the various cultural narratives available to, and adopted by, people coping with illness. Frank's illness narratives serve as master narratives, of sorts, from which individuals draw and place their own personal stories of illness. Despite their widespread use in understandings of health and illness narratives, research has yet to apply this typology to an illness context like SLE, and explore how the narrative types emerge in communication about and through the chronic illness experience. We anticipated that four of Frank's six narrative types have the potential to inform the experience of SLE: restitution, chaos, quest, and life as normal[1]. The *restitution* narrative is the dominant biomedical narrative of illness, with the triumph of medicine as the main plot of the story. In this narrative, the person gets sick, seeks treatment from a medical provider who helps return the patient to good health. It is a story of recovery through medical intervention.

The *chaos* narrative is characterized by an absence of control, cohesion, and discernible narrative order. It is told, as it is experienced, by the ill person. Often, those working within this narrative frame seem to relate their experiences as one difficulty after another (i.e., "this happened, and then this happened, and then this, and then this"), with no apparent sense of reflection or meaning-making. These are difficult narratives to articulate and to witness because listeners often do not wish to acknowledge this particular experience of illness.

The *quest* narrative is comprised of stories that meet illness head on, accept suffering, and seek to use it to gain something from the experience of illness. In this narrative, suffering is the mechanism through which the teller becomes the hero. The goal is not to be restored, but to make sense of the illness and the self after the illness in a way that is beneficial to others.

In *life-as-normal* narratives life continues as normal so that illness-related changes to relationships can be minimized. The illness is either excluded or minimized in these stories, and normality is viewed as a good story for the moment. The life-as-normal narrative is what Frank (2013) refers to as a narrative in abeyance, or one waiting to be told.

Frank's illness narrative types have the potential to shed light on the way that women with SLE make sense of the illness. At the same time, although they speak to the plot of the story, they do not necessarily speak to the way the storyteller evaluates their illness narrative. The evaluation of a narrative is central to narrative sense-making (Labov & Waletzky, 1967), thus, the way a story is told is as important as the story itself (Frank, 2010; Koenig Kellas, 2018; McAdams, 1993). It is therefore important to consider not just the plotline, but also the way the storyteller affectively frames the narrative. One way to examine this is through an analysis of the tone of the narrative as it is presented by the narrator.

NARRATIVE TONE

Along with coping, CNSM (Koenig Kellas & Kranstuber Horstman, 2015) positions identity construction as a primary function in narrating difficulty. McAdams (1993) presents narrative identity as the communicative construction of a personal myth that serves as a "patterned integration of our remembered past, perceived present, and anticipated future" (p. 12). He posits that ideally, one's life is a coherent story that accounts for all of our experiences and orders them in a sequence that promotes this cohesiveness. Illness, however, represents a disruption to this coherent story and often contributes to the emergence of an incoherent account of the self (Charmaz, 1983, 1995, 2000). Thus, narrative sense-making not only facilitates coping, but serves to (re)construct a sense of self in the face of illness. In turn, identity (re) construction throughout the experience of illness is central to coping with it (Charmaz, 2000).

Narrative tone is central to narrative identity (re)construction, and thus, coping with illness, and refers to the overall emotion or attitude of the narrative that someone tells, whether it is positive and optimistic or negative and pessimistic. It is expressed in both the content of the story and the manner in which the story is told (McAdams, 1993, 1996). McAdams (1993) asserts that the tone of an individual's narrative reflects the presence or absence of dispositional optimism, which is a general expectation for good rather than bad outcomes to occur in any given situation. A redemptive narrative is characterized by stories told in a way in which bad events that occur are expected to give way to a good outcome. This kind of positive tone displays the presence of dispositional optimism. A contaminated narrative is characterized by stories that are told in which bad events are expected to remain bad or get worse (McAdams, Reynolds, Lewis, Patten, & Bowman, 2001). This is a negative tone that reveals an absence of dispositional optimism. Some narratives do not convey a strong positive or negative tone and can therefore be considered ambivalent (Koenig Kellas, Baxter, LeClair-Underberg, Thatcher, Rouston, Normand, & Braithwaite, 2014).

Dispositional optimism has been linked to positive effects on coping with illness (McAdams, 1993). Thus, the tone imbued in the way women talk about their illness experience will reveal important information about the ways in which they cope with the illness and how they have incorporated it into their overall identity as they (re)construct it throughout illness. For example, as a narrative type, Frank's (2013) restitution narrative of striving for restoration to the pre-illness state could be redemptive (e.g., characterized by hope for recovery), contaminated (e.g., characterized by the expectation of inevitable failure), or ambivalent (e.g., told without a great deal of affect). Narrative tone, then, provides an important nuance to the analysis of illness narrative types in that it lends insight into the narrator's affect regarding the illness experience. Thus, we argue that an analysis that includes attention to both the distinct illness narrative type (i.e., Frank's 2013 typology) and narrative tone (i.e., McAdams 1993 narrative tone) comprises distinct and identifiable *illness narrative plotlines* that guide the sense-making process of women with SLE. In essence, as suggested in the first proposition of CNSM, we argue that these illness narrative plotlines animate the meanings, values, and beliefs emergent in narrative sense-making. Thus, we asked:

RQ: How do illness narrative types and narrative tone combine in narrative plotlines to characterize the stories of women with SLE?

METHODS

Participants and Recruitment

After securing IRB approval, participants were recruited from online support groups, the Lupus Foundation of America, physician referrals, and from the researchers' personal network using snowball sampling techniques. Snowball sampling is particularly useful when trying to access populations that are not easily identifiable (Noy, 2006), like those struggling with SLE.

The sample for this study included twenty-eight women ranging in age from thirty-six to seventy-for ($M = 57.00$, $SD = 11.22$). The majority of participants ($n = 24$, 89%) identified as Caucasian. One participant (4%) identified as a mixture between African American and African Indian, one (4%) identified as Mexican, one (4%) identified as Italian American, and another (4%) identified as Jewish American. Participants varied in the number of years since symptoms began, with one reporting "since childhood" and the remaining twenty-seven participants ranging between four and sixty years ago ($M = 22.41$ $SD = 13.54$). Similarly, they varied in their time since diagnosis, with diagnosis ranging between one and half and thirty-three years ago (*M* = 16.32 *SD* = 11.56).

We conducted the twenty-eight semi-structured interviews primarily over the phone based on interviewee preference and to manage the challenges presented by geographic distance. The first author asked participants to tell the story of their illness followed by questions about how they talked about the illness in their families, letting them define family (either nuclear or family of origin) as they responded to the questions in order to let the participants indicate what type of family communication was important to them. The interview ended with an opportunity for participants to add anything they deemed important.

Data Analysis

The 28 interviews included in this analysis lasted an average of 43 minutes (*M* = 43.23, *SD* = 14.01) and, upon transcription, resulted in 279 pages of single-spaced data. All participant names were changed to pseudonyms during the transcription process. Though we used MAXQDA, a qualitative data analysis software, to aid in our thematic analysis, each pseudonym was followed by the corresponding line number from the original transcript (e.g., *Nicole, 13–20*).

Coding

To answer the research question, we used MAXQDA to explicate and organize codes and themes within the data. Using this software, we first identified themes and subthemes (Braun & Clark, 2006) through a process of constant comparison (Corbin & Strauss, 2008) using Owen's (1984) criteria for repetitiveness (similar ideas), recurrence (same words or phrases), and forcefulness (vocal emphasis). Next, we recorded the MAXQDA text block numbers of relevant interviewee passages (Smith, 1995) for each theme identified in these data. We defined and refined themes (Braun & Clark, 2006) comparing each identified theme against the concepts identified in the data so that we could be sure the themes we identified represent the essence of the data (Braun & Clark, 2006; Smith, 1995).

Analysis of SLE Narrative Plotlines

The initial analysis involved analyzing participants' responses to the question "Can you tell me your illness story?" We found, however, that the stories of illness presented by the participants at the start of the interview were medicalized explanations of their illness (i.e., the stories only included diagnostic and treatment details). When we looked at the interview as a whole, it was characterized by considerably richer meaning-making relevant to the research question posed. Thus, to answer the research question in a way that reflected the participant experience of the illness, and similar to Frank's (2013) methods for identifying illness narrative types, we analyzed both the illness story and overall interview responses to ascertain the illness narrative types and tone.

The authors read through the first four transcripts individually, coding them for narrative type and tone. Specifically, each coder first individually identified which of Frank's (2013) narrative types were most predominantly reflected in each transcript. Second, each coder identified the overall tone of each transcript (i.e., redemptive, contaminated, or ambivalent), thus evaluating tone as a gestalt construct. The coders then came together in discussion, concurring on the coding of narrative type and tone across these initial transcripts. This, then served as a guide for subsequent analysis.

In order to further ensure the validity of the results, we conducted member checks by sending summation of the distilled SLE narrative plotlines to seventeen of the participants. We asked them to carefully review the findings to ensure that they resonated with their SLE experience in their family. We received a total of six responses (35% response rate) confirming the validity of the findings.

RESULTS

The research question in the current study asked how illness narrative types and narrative tone combine in narrative plotlines to characterize women's SLE experience. Results of the analyses indicate that six SLE narrative plotlines as characterized by Frank's (2013) illness narratives and McAdams's (1993) narrative tone emerged.

SLE Narrative Plotlines

In analyzing these data, it is clear that Frank's (2013) illness narratives are applicable in this population for this disease context, with the expected four of Frank's six narrative types emerging in the data (restitution narrative, the quest narrative, the chaos narrative, and life-as-normal narrative). As expected, each of the narrative types that emerged had a distinct narrative tone (McAdams, 1993). Thus, the analysis resulted in six SLE narrative plotlines constituted by combining Frank's illness narrative types and McAdams's affective tone into a typology of SLE plotlines. These include ambivalent life as normal, ambivalent chaos, ambivalent quest, contaminated life as normal, contaminated restitution, and redemptive quest (see Table 13.1). They are presented in their order of frequency.

Ambivalent Life-As-Normal Narrative Plotline

In total, ten (35%) of the twenty-eight participants demonstrated an *ambivalent life-as-normal narrative plotline*. This SLE narrative plotline is characterized by a desire to preserve normalcy in the family, though that sense of "normalcy" may look quite different to different people. This narrative plotline can be characterized by an acceptance of the "new normal" of lupus. Though they may recall chaotic periods of their illness, women with this narrative plotline have accepted that the illness is unpredictable and, while they do not articulate an anticipation of positive or negative outcomes (and are thus, ambivalent), they do articulate a matter-of-fact acceptance of the unpredictability of the disease:

> I mean I just never knew what it was going to throw my way. And over time I thought, well, I'm resilient, I'll just have to roll with whatever comes. But, you know that was a long path. (Nicole, 78–80)

Kara further exemplifies how acceptance characterizes this plotline:

> I mean my kids have grown up with it. My daughter was in middle school and my son was in middle school as well when I got really sick. My youngest was only 5 at the time. But he spent his Kindergarten year with me pretty much in bed and not able to breathe and his brother and sister helping him with

Table 13.1   Overview of Narrative Plotlines

SLE Narrative Plotline	Definition
Ambivalent Life As Normal	Preservation of the perception of normalcy. The underlying theme in this plotline is an acceptance of SLE and a desire to achieve or maintain what participants perceived to be a "normal" family life.
Ambivalent Chaos	A focus on daily struggle of SLE, little sense-making, disorganized, and primarily focused on difficulty.
Ambivalent Quest	Meeting the illness head on and positioning the life changes that result from illness as a productive transition in perception of self in their daily lives.
Contaminated Life As Normal	A desire to achieve a sense of normalcy though there is a felt discrepancy with others in what "normalcy" means in SLE.
Contaminated Restitution	A desire for restitution despite chronic complications.
Redemptive Quest	Meeting the illness head on and positioning the life changes that result from illness as a productive transition in perception of self in their daily lives coupled with active attempts to effect social change based on illness experience.

homework and doing that kind of stuff. They're great kids, they pulled together and they have a pretty good grasp on what's going on. Basically it sums up to I'm always gonna have pain. Lupus is never going to go away. And we just have to work around it. (Kara, 63–683)

Finally, some participants explain a desire to protect their family members' sense of normalcy, by protecting them from the implications of the illness. Tara explains how she avoids talking about her SLE in order to protect her daughter from worry:

Well I don't want my daughter to worry, so I pull back a little bit for her. She's just moved to Australia, so she went to college there so she just moved back and married her long term sweetheart and they're trying to get pregnant and I don't think the stress will be good for her, so now I'm holding back. So I don't stress her, so I'm holding back right or wrong. So it's what I'm judging is for her best interest. (Tara, 26)

In sum, the ambivalent life-as-normal narrative plotline is characterized by the contextualization of illness into everyday life in a way that these women feel preserves their perception of normalcy in their families. The underlying theme in this plotline is an acceptance of SLE and a desire to achieve or maintain what participants perceive to be a "normal" family life.

Ambivalent Chaos Narrative Plotline

Six (21%) of the twenty-eight participants exhibited the *ambivalent chaos narrative plotline* as dominant in their articulation of the illness experience. In Frank's (1995, 2013) chaos narrative, there is an absence of narrative order and reflection and a steadfast focus on the present difficulty of the illness. Thus, we characterize this plotline as belying an absence of order, a focus on the daily struggles of the disease, an overdetermination of difficulty, and no implicit or explicit expectation for positive or negative outcomes. Amy demonstrates the disorder that characterizes this plotline in her account of her experience:

So I have SLE lupus with the complication of vasculitis which means your capillaries tend to get inflamed. Any way he [my rhematologist] overdosed me with prednisone and when I would call him and say this is too much it made my metabolism go so high that I was taken down for three weeks, and I was bouncing off the walls. Essentially, it made me manic. And I kept calling his office and couldn't ever talk to him or his nurse. I think I did get one reply from his nurse where she said the doctor says you must take this medication or you're going to die. And I was working at kind of alternative medicine and I had gone by there and they told me I had to leave because I was making them nervous because my energy was so frantic. And I called my sister whose a nurse in Texas and I said, he won't talk to me, I'm bouncing off the walls, my brain is shorting out, I was losing time, I said what am I gonna do? And she said call your PCP [primary care physician] and so I did that and he said you need to check yourself into the ER so I went into the local hospital in [State] and so I went in with medically induced psychosis. Because I really was going into a fog and like I would put my food out and I'd come back later and I hadn't eaten it and I'd put my medication out and would come back later and it wouldn't be eaten. And one of my girlfriends was helping me out and called my family. I went into the psych unit where they reduced my prednisone. It was a wonderful program where you get counseling and all this and I went in there and was there over a weekend getting stabilized. (Amy, 27–43)

This excerpt exemplifies the characteristics of a chaos narrative. The focus is on the daily relational, physical, or mental struggle of the disease. Kaitlin explains:

So, you know, it's like I sometimes question myself, it's like WOW, can all this crap be really happening to me and I think no I'm not that kind of person, I'm a very strong person I'm not just gonna let something take over my mind. And but sometimes you do, I mean, I do, as a lupus patient I'm thinking man, am I really a hypochondriac, but everything's so real. And then, I was having muscle issues I notice that my muscles in my thighs were getting weaker, so I would do a biopsy and it was determined that it was kind of inconclusive. They thought maybe I had polymyothritis. It's a rare autoimmune disease where the body attacks the muscles. Which is basically what lupus does, your body attacks whatever it wants. Whatever organ it wants. (Kaitlin, 119–126)

As illustrated in both Amy and Kaitlin's narratives, the ambivalent chaos narrative plotline is defined as being predominantly disorganized, a focus on the daily struggle and hardships associated with SLE, an overdetermination of difficulty in that everything is presented as a struggle, and is lived primarily in the present with little reference to the past and no reference to the future. Despite a focus on difficulty, this plotline is ambivalent in nature because it is characterized by limited sense-making about SLE and thus, there is no expressed expectation for a positive or negative outcome.

Ambivalent Quest Narrative Plotline

Four (14%) of the twenty-eight participants most prominently demonstrated the *ambivalent quest narrative plotline*. We characterize the *ambivalent quest narrative plotline* as comprised of a matter-of-fact willingness to meet the illness head on, and an acceptance of both the suffering and illness-related changes. Unlike the previous two plotlines, the suffering in SLE is perceived as beneficial and it is used in service of others. Although, in accordance with Frank's (1995, 2013) quest narrative, the change that has already occurred due to the illness is itself perceived to be positive, there is no expressed expectation of future positive (or negative) outcomes of the illness, which is why these experiences were coded as ambivalent.

In this illness narrative plotline, the women and their families accepted that SLE had changed their lives and they used their experience to benefit others. Shannon explains how she became an SLE support group leader dedicated to helping family members better understand SLE. She introduces them to the Spoon Theory, a metaphor that helps to explain the limited and variable amount of energy SLE patients have access to each day:

> Spoon Theory is something that I would give every family member of anybody who has lupus. [Every family member] should read the spoon theory along with the lupus patient of course. Basically, it breaks it down real easily how we feel every-day. You could probably look it up on the internet, but in short, it's I wake up and say my energy is equated to spoons. And I have ten spoons today. I take a shower and I try to get myself together, now I've used up one spoon. And for each thing that I want to do depending on what it is, that's how many spoons it takes. So, as the day progresses, I might have to go to the store. I might have to run an errand or I might have to go to the doctor's and all those are going to cost me a certain number of spoons. So, by 4:00 I may or may not have any spoons left. And if I don't have any spoons left, that's it for the day. So the way it is told is really, really neat. I usually have at least 20 copies of it with me at my group that I facilitate with the Lupus Foundation of Florida is every month and I bring that with me and I make sure if anybody's new they get it and I also invite family members to the meeting and lot of people to bring family members and I make sure they get a copy and it really explains the fatigue part of lupus really well. (Shannon, 165–180)

Laura explains how her frustrations in managing SLE served as a catalyst for her similar involvement in helping others with the disease:

> The PCP [primary care physician] fellow wasn't taking me seriously at all. I think I had been in this car accident and I think he thought I was trying to build a case for the insurance company because I kept saying I feel sick, I ache all over, tired, and odd aches and pains and he just dismissed that. Between that and the next guy I saw it was frustrating. Very frustrating. And as a result of that I got very involved with the Lupus Foundation of America, now I guess there's lots of them, and I became president of the local chapter and did a lot of support groups and training seminars. (Laura, 52–58)

In sum, the ambivalent quest narrative type is characterized by meeting the illness head on and not only accepting the change imposed by the illness, but positioning the change as an important transition. Further, those whose SLE experience was characterized by this plotline take advantage of opportunities within their daily lives to assist others in their struggle with SLE.

Contaminated Life-As-Normal Narrative Plotline

Four (14%) of the twenty-eight participants exhibited the contaminated life-as-normal narrative type as dominant in their articulation of their SLE experience. We characterize *the contaminated life as normal narrative plotline* as being comprised of a desire to achieve or maintain a sense of normalcy, but contrary to the ambivalent life-as-normal plotline, these women perceived the existence of relational tension in their families about what "normal" should look like in the face of SLE. This tension may manifest as a perception that one person expects a return to the pre-illness state, while the other person accepts that as impossible. Evelyn, for example, explains how she and her husband have different ideas about how to live with SLE, and these differences create an uncomfortable tension for her:

> At one point, at one point, my husband did say. I was searching and searching and searching for something to help me. And he told me to stop. He said "This is what you have, it's not gonna get better and deal with it." And this was five years ago. So I was 46 and I said, I'm too young, and I gotta do this, nobody else will help me, so, it was very unsettling. (Evelyn, 69–72)

Thus, we characterize this narrative plotline as being comprised of avoidance and a feeling of being unsupported within the family. Melissa explains how she avoids talking about it because she perceives that her family prefers not to hear about the disease and its effects: "But I just think I probably don't talk about it they're just tired of hearing it" (Melissa, 157).

Dierdre explains that she and her family differ on what constitutes normal in SLE:

> Yes, and I've had experiences being invalidated or minimized. The symptoms being minimized. And you know, maybe the frustration on the part of others. It's not easy to describe to someone. It's not easy to describe to someone what it is. It's a disease LADEN with complexities and symptomology that mimics other things that have to be ruled out. But at the end of the day leaves me feeling unwell so often that I don't want to talk about with people because I don't want them to feel sorry for me. So, you know what I'm just gonna say I'm okay. (Dierdre, 110–115)

Ultimately, women who articulate contaminated life-as-normal stories have an overarching sense that they and their family members have different ideas about what life should look like with SLE.

Contaminated Restitution Narrative Plotline

Two (7%) of the twenty-eight participants demonstrate evidence of a *contaminated restitution narrative plotline* in their explanation of their illness experience. This narrative plotline was characterized by struggle for improvement in the disease despite an expectation for negative outcomes. In contaminated restitution, participants strive for a cure or improvement despite understanding the unlikelihood of improvement. Amber explains:

> So it changed my life completely. I had to quit working, I had to go on disability which was really hard for me. It still is hard. I keep thinking I might be able to go back, but I know I can't physically do it. So it's been life altering. (Amber, 47–49)

Thus, despite understanding the impossibility of restoration, these women continue to strive for restitution and resist allowing the illness to change their lives. Stephanie, a highly educated and driven person, explains the difficulty in accepting limitations in light of SLE:

> You know there's only so much energy I have at the beginning of the day and really sometimes I want to work and I can't work and I get up and sit at the computer and a whole day goes by and I haven't done anything. And I'm not having pains that day, but I'm just tired. That's the hardest fatigue because you can't see the fatigue, there's nothing to test for fatigue. And so that's the hardest thing and maybe the reason it's hard for me to communicate that as well is because I have a fear of being seen as lazy, just un-motivated. Because I've never been that way before, it's just REALLY really hard for me. (Stephanie, 208–215)

The fight for restitution that characterizes this illness narrative plotline may well exacerbate the compounding of physical and mental complications in chronic illness (Canary, 2008).

In this narrative plotline, women avoid talking about the disease in order to restore the sense of control they had over their lives pre-illness. Amber explains:

> Um, because I'd rather not talk about it. I feel like I don't want it to consume my whole life. And it has in so many ways and I feel like this is the only control I have left is to not talk about it all the time. (Amber, 128–130)

In this excerpt, Amber demonstrates how she chooses not to discuss the illness in her family in order to regain some control in her life, reminiscent of the restitution's narrative focus on restoration (Frank, 1995, 2013) as she attempts to restore some part of her life to her pre-illness sense of normal.

Thus, we characterize the contaminated restitution narrative type as focusing on restoration despite chronic complications and by avoidance in an attempt to regain control.

Redemptive Quest Narrative Plotline

Finally, two (7%) of the twenty-eight participants demonstrated the redemptive quest narrative plotline. The *redemptive quest narrative* plotline is a quest narrative in which the participants explicitly use their struggle with SLE to enact social change with an expectation that things will get better because of their suffering in illness. Bertha, for example, has used her suffering in SLE to educate others, including political leaders, about chronic illness in general and autoimmune diseases in particular. In fact, she has done so much of this work, that she was invited to the White House to talk about her experience with SLE:

> A good conversation [I had] was with senior staffer at the White House, and I brought my family to Washington D.C. and sat down and went to the White House to educate them, and you tell them what chronic illness is like and auto-immune disorders to show them what families go through. And it was a positive experience for my family because my kids felt like they were doing something actionable, and my husband felt like he was doing something that was action-able, I felt like I was doing something that was actionable and we felt like we were taking control. (Bertha, 158–163)

Elise used her experiences to publish a book aimed at educating patients with systemic lupus about the way the disease impacts their lives and goes on speaking engagements to educate patients, families, and medical professionals about systemic lupus:

> Yes, and my husband accompanies me and on speaking engagements when he can, when he can, he talks. Like I do my presentation, I've done it several times for family and friends of lupus and I usually get him to give his perspective and answer questions and he stays until I'm on it. He will read things and he just really tries to understand. (Elise, 81–84)

Thus, the redemptive quest narrative type is characterized by a willingness to meet the illness head on and an acceptance of the changes brought on by the illness as an important and meaningful life transition. However, what differentiates it from an ambivalent quest narrative is the desire to use their illness struggle to enact social change regarding SLE beyond her daily interactions (i.e., lobby for SLE awareness or author and publish a book about living with SLE).

SUMMARY

Distinct SLE narrative plotlines comprised of a combination of illness narrative types and narrative tone clearly emerged in these data. These plotlines differed in their primary focus (e.g., life-as-normal plotlines focused on normality, restitution focused on restoration, quest focused on making suffering meaningful, and chaos was focused on the struggle of the disease). They differed further in terms of their tone, or whether or not there was an expectation for a positive or negative outcome of the illness. Overall, the results suggest that the majority of women in our sample narrate their SLE in ambivalent terms, recognizing the complexities of lupus and the ups and downs it causes for them and their families.

DISCUSSION

The results reported in this study point to several important observations about CNSM in the experience of SLE. First, Frank's (2013) typology of personal illness narratives and McAdams's (1993) concept of narrative tone work together to illuminate narrative sense-making in SLE. Further, it was clear to us that SLE narrative plotlines reflect women's perceptions of their illness experience, suggesting a need to explore the implications of these plotlines. For example, future research should explore whether dominant SLE narrative plotlines are correlated with measures of physical, mental, and relational health and well-being.

Second, it was clear in these findings that family communication was intertwined in meaningful ways with the SLE narrative plotline that was most prevalent in these women's descriptions of their illness experience. For example, women whose stories were coded as *contaminated life as normal* had stories dominated by discrepancy in the way family members saw and talked about what "normalcy" meant for the family. Family communication is central to sense-making (Pecchioni & Keeley, 2011) and to health and well-being in illness (Rosland et al., 2012). Thus, the interaction of family communication and narrative sense-making should be explored in future research to better understand the ways in which family communication is shaped by and shapes the adoption of specific narrative plotlines in SLE. Specifically, given the clear importance of family communication in shaping identity in illness (Kleinmann, 1988), it is important that future research explore the ways in which family communication behaviors and dominant SLE narrative plotlines work together to shape sense-making about family identity in SLE.

Third, though Mendelson (2006) conceptualizes the time pre-diagnosis as a period of identity in abeyance, it is clear from these present data that the self is constantly emerging in and through experience. Consistent with Charmaz' (1995) assertion that identity (re)construction in illness begins with the onset of symptoms, these women narratively made sense of the experience of illness from the first indication that something was amiss. Thus, the results of this study support CNSM as a useful framework for understanding family sense-making in the context of illness, specifically, SLE. As the guiding theoretical framework, CNSM provided the space to identify patterns in the *process* of identity (re)construction across individual accounts of the traditionally idiosyncratic experience (Koenig Kellas, 2018; Koenig Kellas & Kranstuber Horstman, 2015).

Fourth, in line with CNSM Theory's (Koenig Kellas, 2018) Proposition 1, the narrative plotlines identified in the current study provide insight into individual, relational, and intergenerational meanings, values, and beliefs of women with SLE. There is a sense, for example, that most women in the study recognize and accept the ambivalence of SLE. For a small percentage of women, there was also a sense of purpose that emerged in their SLE stories. And, the stories in the current sample also revealed instances in which little sense-making was evident, instead trumped by the chaos of the illness experience. Using Frank's typology and McAdams's concept of tone, this study provides an example of one useful way research using CNSM theory to understand the link between illness stories and well-being might operationalize the positivity or overall tone of narratives. CNSM's Proposition 2 suggests a link between positive story framing and individual and relational well-being, but Koenig Kellas (2018) acknowledges the need for empirical sharpening of what positivity means. The current study brings at least one of those operationalizations into better focus and offers a guide for future research.

Fifth, as a chronic illness, patients working and living in the context of SLE make daily decisions that shape how well they are managing their disease process (Bodenheimer, Lorig, Holman, & Grumbach, 2002). Self-management behavior is critical to the success of chronic illness management (Telford, Kralik, & Koch, 2006), and so is of keen interest to physicians working with patients to manage this disease. Given the centrality of narratives in creating meaning in illness (Kleinman, 1988), and the importance narration has in helping individuals claim agency in their illness (Sharf & Vanderford, 2003), the findings of this study have the potential to help physicians support better self-management behavior in SLE. As physicians begin to understand the different narrative plotlines in SLE, they can achieve a more nuanced understanding of their patients' unique needs for support in their illness. Further, researchers can focus attention on understanding the conditions and communication behaviors that promote the emergence of specific plotlines. This translational potential reflects the third heuristic of CNSM (i.e., translational storytelling, Koenig Kellas, 2018) and provides researchers and practitioners with an exciting opportunity to engage CNSM in ways that benefit this under-studied population. Thus, future research should build on this study to fine-tune these distinctions and correlate them with outcomes specific to self-management and well-being in SLE.

The population for this study was primarily white women despite the fact that SLE is both more prevalent and more severe in African American, Hispanic, and Asian women (Wallace, 2008). Taken together, the extant research (e.g. Pecchioni & Keeley) and the findings from this study suggest the critical importance of family communication in sense-making in illness, though cultural and ethnic differences in family communication (Sillars, 1995) likely shape what behaviors enable/constrain sense-making. Thus, future research should examine family communication and narrative sense-making across ethnic and cultural contexts to ensure the populations most severely impacted by SLE are represented in the growing body of literature and, importantly, so they can benefit from interventions informed by this program of research.

Ultimately, in light of the growing evidence that social behaviors can improve patient health outcomes across illnesses (Shapiro, 2002), the findings of this study will serve as the basis for future research aimed at identifying both the conditions that promote the adoption of specific types of narrative plotlines in making sense of SLE and the implications for specific narrative plotlines for physical, mental, and relational health and well-being. Given the prevalence of SLE (Wallace, 2008), the difficulty SLE patients have communicating with their families (Roper Public Affairs Survey, 2011), and the importance of family communication to improved health outcomes in chronic illness (Rosland et al., 2011), this research trajectory will be undertaken in order to inform the development and implementation of much-needed interventions for families and medical providers living and working the context of SLE.

NOTE

1. We did not anticipate nor did we find two of Frank's six narrative types: The first is the broken narrative type, which refers to an illness narrative that must be narrated for a person, at least in part, by a relational partner due to memory loss or dementia. The second is the borrowed narrative type, which refers to an illness narrative that is drawn from larger social narratives, such as movies, because the person affected by the illness lacks the personal narrative resources from which to draw in making sense of the experience, as is often the case with children.

REFERENCES

Aberer, E. (2010). Epidemiologic, socioeconomic and psychosocial aspects of lupus eruthematosus. *Lupus, 19* (118–124). doi: 10.1177/0961203310370348.

Bodenheimer, T., Lorig, K., Holman, H., & Grumback, K. (2002). Patient self-management of chronic disease in primary care. *JAMA, 288,* 2469–2475. doi: 10.1001/jama.288.19.2469.

Braun,V., & Clarke, V. (2006). Using thematic analysis in psychology. *Qualitative Research in Psychology, 3,* 77–101.

Bruner, J. (2004). Life as narrative. *Social Research, 73,* 691–711.

Canary, H. E. (2008). Creating supportive connections: A decade of research on support for families of children with disabilities. *Health Communication, 23,* 413–426. doi: 10.1080/10410230802342085.

Charmaz, K. (1983). Loss of self: A fundamental form of suffering in the chronically ill. *Sociology of Health and Illness, 5,* 168–195.

Charmaz, K. (1995). The body, identity, and self: Adapting to impairment. *The Sociological Quarterly, 36,* 657–680.

Charmaz, K. (2000). Experiencing chronic illness. In G. L. Albrecht, R. Fitzpatrick, & S. C. Scrimshaw (Eds.), *The handbook of social studies in health medicine* (pp. 277–292). London, UK: Sage.

Corbin, J., & Strauss, A. (2008). *Basics of qualitative research.* Los Angeles, CA: Sage.

DiMatteo, R. (2003). Future directions in research on consumer-provider communication and adherence to cancer prevention and treatment. *Patient Education and Counseling, 50,* 23–26. doi: 10.1016/S0738-3991(03)00075-2.

Eisenberg, E. (2001). Building a mystery: Toward a new theory of communication and identity. *Journal of Communication, 51,* 534–552. doi: 10.1111/j.14602466.2001.tb02895.x.

Fisher, W. R. (1987). *Human communication as narration: Toward a philosophy of reason, value, and action.* Columbia, SC: University of South Carolina Press.

Frank, A. W. (1995). *The wounded storyteller: Body, illness, and ethics.* Chicago, IL: The University of Chicago Press.

Frank, A. W. (2010). *Letting stories breathe: A socio-narratology.* Chicago, IL: The University of Chicago Press.

Frank, A. W. (2013). *The wounded storyteller: Body, illness, and ethics.* Chicago, IL: The University of Chicago Press.

Holmberg, D., Orbuch, T. L., & Veroff, J. I. (2011). *Thrice told tales: Married couples tell their stories.* Mahway, NJ: Lawerence Earlbaum Associates.

Kleinman, A. (1983). *The illness narratives: Suffering, health, & the human condition.* New York, NY: Basic Books.

Koenig Kellas, J. (2005). Family ties: Communicating identity through jointly told family stories. *Communication Monographs, 72,* 365–389. doi: 10.1080/03637750500322453.

Koenig Kellas, J. (2018). Communicated narrative sense-making theory: Linking storytelling and well-being. In D. O. Braithwaite, E. A. Suter, & K. Floyd (Eds.),

Engaging theories in family communication: Multiple perspectives (pp. 62–74). New York, NY: Sage.

Koenig Kellas, J., & Keeley, M. P. (2005). Constructing life and death through final conversation narratives. In M. Harter, P. M. Japp, & C. S. Beck (Eds.), *Narratives, health, & healing: Communication theory, research, and practice* (pp. 365–390). Mahwah, NJ: Lawrence Earlbaum Associates.

Koenig Kellas, J., & Kranstuber Horstman, H. (2015). Communicated narrative sense making: Understanding family narratives, storytelling, and the construction of meaning through a communicative lens. In L. M. Turner & R. West (Eds.), *Sage handbook of family communication* (pp. 76–90). Thousand Oaks, CA: Sage.

Koenig Kellas, J., & Trees, A. R. (2006). Finding meaning in difficult family experiences: Sense-making and interaction processes in joint family storytelling. *Journal of Family Communication, 6*(1), 49–76. doi: 10.1207/s15327698jfc0601_4.

Koenig Kellas, J., & Trees, A. (2013). Family stories and storytelling: Windows into the family soul. In A. L. Vangelisti (Ed.), *Handbook of family communication* (2nd ed., pp. 391–406). Mahwah, NJ: Lawrence Erlbaum.

Koenig Kellas, J., Trees, A. R., Schrodt, P., LeClair-Underberg, C., & Willer, E. K. (2010). Exploring links between well-being and interactional sense-making in married couples' jointly told stories of stress. *Journal of Family Communication, 10,* 174–193. doi: 10.1080/15267431.2010.489217.

Labov, W., & Waletsky, J. (1967). Narrative analysis: Oral versions of personal experience. In J. Helm (Ed.), *Essays on the verbal and visual arts: Proceedings of the 1966 annual spring meeting of the American Ethnological Society* (pp. 83–97). Seattle: University of Washington Press.

McAdams, D. P. (1993). *Stories we live by: Personal myths and the making of the self.* New York, NY: Harper Collins.

McAdams, D. P. (1996). Personality, modernity, and the storied self: A contemporary framework for studying persons. *Psychological Inquiry, 7,* 295–321.

McAdams, D. P., Reynolds, J., Lewis, M. L., Patten, A., & Bowman, P. T. (2001). When bad things turn good and good things turn bad: Sequences of redemption and contamination in life narrative, and their relation to psychosocial adaptation in midlife adults and in students. *Personality and Social Psychology Bulletin, 27,* 472–483. doi: 10.1177/0146167201274008.

Mendelson, C. (2006). Managing a medically and social complex life: Women living with lupus. *Qualitative Health Research, 16,* 982–997. doi: 10.1177/1049732306290132.

Mendelson, C. (2009). Diagnosis: A liminal state for women living with lupus. *Health Care for Women International, 30,* 390–407. doi: 10.1080/07399330902785158.

Noy, C. (2006). Sampling knowledge: The hermeneutics of snowball sampling in qualitative research. *International Journal of Social Research Methodology, 11,* 327–344.

Owen, W. F. (1984). Interpretive themes in relational communication. *Quarterly Journal of Speech, 70,* 274–287. doi: 10.1080/00335638409383697.

Perchoni, L. L., & Keeley, M. P. (2011). Insights about health from family communication theories. In T. L. Thompson, R. Parrot, & J. F. Nussbaum's (Eds.), *The Routledge handbook of health communication* (pp. 277–389). New York, NY: Routledge.

Pecchioni, L. L., Overton, B. C., & Thompson, T. L. (2015). Families communicating about health. In L. H. Turner & R. L. West's (Eds.), *The family communication sourcebook* (pp. 226–240). Thousand Oaks, CA: Sage.

Roper Public Affairs and Corporate Communication. (2011). Lupus: A survey among SLE patients, physicians, and supporters. [Final report of data]. Retrieved from http://www.lupuscheck.com/pdf/TUiLRoperSurveyDownloadable.pdf.

Rosland, A., Heisler, M., & Piette, J. D. (2012). The impact of family behaviors and communication patterns on chronic illness outcomes: A systematic review. *Journal of Behavioral Medicine, 35,* 221–239. doi: 10.1007/s10865-011-9354-4.

Shapiro, E. (2002). Chronic illness as a family process: A social-developmental approach to promoting resilience. *Journal of Clinical Psychology, 58,* 1375–1384. doi: 10.1002/jclp.10085.

Sharf, B. F., & Vanderford, M. L. (2003). Illness narratives and the social construction of health. In T. L. Thompson, A. M. Dorsey, K. I. Miller, & R. Parrot's (Eds.), *Handbook of health communication.* Mahwah, NJ: Lawrence Earlbaum Associates.

Sillars, A. (1995). Communication and family culture. In M. A. Fitzpatrick & A. L. Vangelisti (Eds.), *Explaining family interaction* (pp. 375–399). Thousand Oaks, CA: Sage.

Smith, J. A. (1995). Semi-structured interviewing and qualitative analysis. In J. Am Smith, R. Harre, & L. Van Langenhove (Eds.), *Rethinking methods in psychology.* London, UK: Sage.

Sunwolf, Frey, L. W., & Keranen, L. (2005). Rx story prescriptions: Healing effects of storytelling and storylistening in the practice of medicine. In L. M. Harter, P. M. Japp, & C. S. Beck's (Eds.), *Narratives, health, and healing: Communication theory, research and practice* (pp. 237–258). Mahwah, NJ: Lawrence Earlbaum Associates, Publishers.

Telford, K., Kralik, D., & Koch, T. (2006). Acceptance and denial: Implications for people adapting to chronic illness: Literature Review. *Journal of Advanced Nursing, 55,* 457–464. doi: 10.1111/j.1365-2648.2006.03942.x.

Villagran, M. M., & Sparks, L. (2010). Social identity and health contexts. In H. Giles, S. Reid, & J. Harwood (Eds.), *The dynamics of intergroup communication.* New York, NY: Peter Lang.

Wallace, D. J. (2008). *The lupus book: A guide for patients and their families.* New York, NY: Oxford University Press.

Chapter 14

Healthy Mother, Healthy Baby

An Autoethnography to Challenge the Dominant Cultural Narrative of the Birthing Patient

Jennifer E. Ohs

Outcomes associated with maternity care in the United States have worsened substantially in the past two decades, while global health outcomes have improved (WHO, UNICEF, UNFPA, World Bank Group, and United Nations Population Division Maternal Mortality Estimation Inter-Agency Group, 2015; World Health Organization, 2015). The reasons for and potential solutions to the problem of increasing maternal mortality rate are beginning to surface in popular media (e.g., Casimir, 2018; Howard, 2018; Martin, 2018; PLOS, 2018) and research (e.g., Brown, 2018; Cohen, 2016; Davis, Hofferth, & Shenassa, 2014; Gage, Fang, O'Neill, & DiRenzio, 2013). Given the exigency of the issue, the cultural, organizational, and interpersonal influences on maternity care in the United States ought also be examined. Health communication scholarship has long pointed to the importance of such influences on health outcomes (e.g., Street, 2003). In the realm of maternal health, one influence of critical importance is the provider-patient encounter. As expectant mothers manage pregnancy-related uncertainty, interactions with providers influence their medical decisions, particularly during labor and delivery. These medical decisions are consequential for maternal health and have various long-term consequences (e.g., Cook & Loomis, 2012; National Academy of Sciences, 2013).

As a scholar of health communication whose area of specialization emphasizes health decisions, and as a woman who has had four birth experiences since the start of the twenty-first century in different medical settings in the United States, I offer an autoethnographic account of labor and delivery from an ecological perspective (Street, 2003). I narrate my experiences as a birthing patient, interacting with health-care professionals in various organizational health-care cultures. I am mindful of the dualistic nature of my identity as a health communication scholar and as a patient, integrating my "personal expertise" with "presentational expertise" (Foss & Foss, 1994). After offering my narrative, I challenge the dominant cultural narrative for birthing patients and discuss critical needs for research about provider-patient communication and uncertainty management during the birth experience, particularly related to provider-patient trust. My hope is that this analysis draws attention to the importance of considering the labor and delivery experience as fundamentally affected by the ecology in which it is situated, as well as social factors critical in maternal health care that have implications for advancing research in this area and improving maternity care in the United States.

MATERNAL CARE IN THE UNITED STATES

Health outcomes associated with maternal health care in the United States have declined in the recent years. From 2000 to 2014, the estimated maternal mortality rate per 100,000 births in the United States increased by 26.6 percent for forty-eight states and Washington, DC (MacDorman, Declercq, Cabral, & Morton, 2016). Only California showed a decline in mortality rate, whereas Texas had a sudden increase from 2011 to 2012. This stands in stark comparison to other nations. Between 1990 and 2015, the global maternal mortality rate (MMR) decreased by 44 percent, while in the United States, the MMR increased by 16.7 percent (WHO, UNICEF, UNFPA, World Bank Group, and United Nations Population Division Maternal Mortality Estimation Inter-Agency Group, 2015; World Health Organization, 2015). Not only is the United States behind other industrialized nations in providing high-quality maternity care and preventing maternal death, but the problem appears to be growing.

Factors impacting MMR are varied and complex. Undoubtedly, the trends in the United States are concerning. Particularly for a nation that boasts about its quality health care globally (Bush, 2001; Jacobson, 2012) and sees improving trends in other areas of health care (e.g., cancer treatment and care, American Society of Clinical Oncology, 2017; cardiac care, Jackson, 2017), maternity care performance comparatively should be better. The link between provider-patient communication and health outcomes (e.g., Brown, Stewart, & Ryan, 2003; Street, Makoul, Arora, & Epstein, 2009), particularly in the context of maternity care (Hunter, Berg, Lundgren, Olafsdottir, & Kirkham, 2008) suggests that an examination of how communicative and cultural elements contribute to quality maternal care is warranted.

Uncertainty plays a central role in pregnancy and childbirth (Matthias, 2009; Matthias & Babrow, 2007). Expectant mothers face uncertainty and anxiety (Gray, 2014) about their personal health during pregnancy, as well as the health of their offspring, when and how labor and delivery will proceed, and its outcomes (Matthias, 2010). In addition to experiencing uncertainty regarding the physiological process of childbirth, women face uncertainty about the procedures, rules, and cultures of a birthing place, such as a hospital or birth center (Kirkham, 1989). Women also manage uncertainty and stress of longer-range concerns associated with finances (Matthias, 2009) and child-care postpartum (Glazier, Elgar, Goel, & Holzapfel, 2004).

Labor and delivery are especially uncertain and unpredictable experiences (Parratt & Fahy, 2003), and medical providers experience uncertainty when caring for expectant mothers during childbirth (Matthias, 2010). While the outcomes of most childbirth experiences are healthy for mothers and their offspring, hundreds of thousands of births each year are not (World Health Organization, 2015). As such, the predominant view of childbirth is that it involves high risk and requires medical intervention to be successful (Hall, Tomkinson, & Klein, 2012; Rothman, 1991; Walsh & Newburn, 2002a, 2002b). This view has been criticized as a primary reason for the rise in unnecessary intrapartum interventions, particularly caesarean section deliveries (World Health Organization: Department of Reproductive Health and Research, 1997). The risk-averse approach to birthing is prominent across the globe, but is especially dominant in Western society (Cahill, 2001; Downe, Simpson, & Trafford, 2007; Hall et al., 2012). Viewing childbirth in terms of risk, a social construction oriented around threat (Adam & van Loon, 2000) has consequences for medical decisions and interventions. When risk is transformed into embodied danger, perceived threats can become tangible. Medical decisions based on the view of birthing as risky as opposed to natural, then, beget interventions to minimize perceived risks.

Health-care providers vary in how they view risks associated with childbirth (Hall et al., 2012) as well as birth-related uncertainty (Matthias, 2010) and decisions (Bylund, 2005; Matthias, 2010). While obstetricians adhere to a medicalized view of labor and delivery through a lens of risk, a midwifery model acknowledges uncertainty as a natural part of the birth process (Parratt & Fahy, 2003; Walsh & Newburn, 2002b) and encourages birth without intervention (Davis-Floyd & Davis, 1996; Parratt & Fahy, 2003). According to Matthias (2010), "With the obstetric belief that birth is risky comes the desire to exert greater control over these processes to minimize uncertainty. This, in turn, reduces a mother's decision-making power," (p. 208). On the other hand, Matthias found that midwives saw their role as a provider of information and education to mothers, enabling decision-making.

As they help patients manage uncertainty and provide information, providers influence a variety of health outcomes, such as empowering patients to make quality decisions and engage in effective self-care (e.g., Street et al., 2009). A shift to patient-centered care has been promoted in the twenty-first century that encourages providers to consider the needs, values, and expressed preferences of patients and to treat patients as informed decision makers in their care (e.g., Rathert, Wyrwich, & Boren, 2012). How this has manifested in maternity care, however, has yet to be systematically evaluated. Physician-patient care has traditionally been marked by a power differential that can silence the patient's voice (e.g., Beisecker, 1990; Fisher, 1993), and Pizzini's (1991) research demonstrated that the power differential in obstetric care manifested in particularly gendered ways: obstetricians exerted power by interrupting patients who demonstrated knowledge, reasserting their medical expertise and superiority.

An ecological perspective on provider-patient communication serves as an ideal foundation for examination of maternity care, particularly given the complexity associated with uncertainty management and medical decision-making during childbirth. Street (2003) proposes an ecological perspective on communication in medical encounters which considers the interaction between patients and health-care providers as situated within and affected by a variety of social contexts, including the political-legal, cultural, and organizational. In maternity care, examination of provider-patient interaction from an ecological perspective is especially informative. The dynamic between providers, expectant mothers, and the health-care organization has been shown to influence how birth is managed (e.g., Kingdon et al., 2009; Martin & Kasperski, 2010). Additionally, with the culture of risk-aversion and increased intervention in birthing practices, providers underestimate the influence of psychological, social, and cultural factors on their practice (Cherniak & Fisher, 2008). Given that provider-patient interactions have direct implications for subjective and objective dimensions of health and well-being (Street, 2003), exploring maternity care from an ecological perspective provides insight and meaning for the outcomes in this unique setting.

PATIENT NARRATIVE: AN AUTOETHNOGRAPHY

An autoethnographic approach is an ideal method from which to examine the patient experience from an ecological perspective. The autoethnographic method focuses on the autobiographical voice within a social context (Ellis, 1997; Ellis & Bochner, 2000; Reed-Danahay, 1997) that "reflects that intersection between culture, society, and politics" (Pinar, 1997, p. 86). Given the complexity of the patient experience in the larger cultural ecology, honoring the autobiographical voice in research offers a means of exploring the patient experience within the greater cultural context of medical care. Thus, I offer my self-narrative (Gergen & Gergen, 1997) as birthing mother on four occasions in different health organizations in order to extend understanding of the patient's position in the cultural context of birthing and how the dominant cultural context of medicine influences the birthing mother's patienthood. Throughout the account, my voice as a patient and my voice as a health communication scholar are evident. Sometimes the voices are distinct, and sometimes they are intertwined. Most evidently, they evolve as I grew personally and professionally. When I discovered I was pregnant with my first child, I had just completed my first year of doctoral study. My fourth child was born during the year I applied for tenure and promotion. The process of critical reflection involved documentation after each birth experience, journaling, discussions with other pregnant individuals, nurses, my providers, my husband and support persons, and reviewing over 400 pages of medical records from my birth experiences.

Consideration of the ecology of care in health practice can have implications for patient empowerment and, thus, care outcomes. By engaging an autoethnographic analysis on my birth experiences, I can offer understanding of the vital role that the greater ecology had on provider-patient interactions, trust, and uncertainty management during each experience. My hope is that future work can build from my observations and analysis to enhance provider-patient communication, improve birth experiences and outcomes, and stimulate shifts in the dominant cultural narrative of the birthing in the United States.

FIRST BIRTH: ASSUMPTION OF "TABULA RASA" DRIVES UNCERTAINTY MANAGEMENT

On Friday, January 16, 2004, I spent the morning diligently working on a manuscript I was completing for a professor I deeply respected. I was just over two weeks from my due date with my first child. I was determined to show that I could balance work and family, and that I was committed to a career in academe. I was uncertain and anxious about managing work after birth, so I wanted to work hard to complete as much as possible prior to my baby's arrival.

After an early morning of work, I left campus with just enough time to make it to a routine appointment with Jocelyn Bachner*, a Certified Nurse Midwife (CNM) with Center Medical and Associates in State College, PA.

---

* *All person's names, except those of immediate family members, have been changed. The names of health-care organizations in the St. Louis region were changed. Those in the State College area were not, given that they would readily be identified due to the limited number of practices in the area.*

Relieved, I told Jocelyn that I had finished a large section of writing that morning, but still had more to do. "I wish I knew when baby might come! I would be able to manage my time better," I told her.

"There's no magic way to tell when baby will arrive," said Jocelyn. "Even if I were to check to see if you were dilated, it wouldn't necessarily mean anything. Some women sit at 1 to 2 cm dilated for a week before labor begins."

I nodded. I sighed. "I'm so excited to meet this baby," I told her.

"Baby's heart sounds great. You are doing great. Now, just breathe and take some time to relax, ok?"

I left her office committed to relaxing. As I was driving away, I remembered that I had some articles with me to read for work, and thought it would be peaceful to consume them while having a pedicure. I drove to a salon not far from my house and enjoyed the peacefulness of working while the nail technicians doted on me—until I noticed that something had shifted and that some fluid seemed to be leaking from me. I attempted to wait patiently as my toenails dried, but I was fairly certain my water had broken while sitting in the pedicure chair. By the time I was walking out to my car, I was nervously aware that fluid was flowing out of me. "This is happening," I thought.

How Did I Get Here?

At the end of my first year of graduate study in 2003, I unexpectedly found myself pregnant for the first time. Despite constant nausea for more than the expected first trimester, I dedicated myself to completing coursework and educating myself about pregnancy, childbirth, and infant care. I also found myself needing to choose a new obstetric/gynecological provider, as prenatal and postnatal care were not provided by the student health center at the University. I didn't know where to begin looking for a provider, as all of my health care had been chosen by my parents or provided by student health services until this point. I was friendly with a woman I knew from the gym I attended, and I knew she had a baby. She referred me to Dr. Halloway, who she liked because he was an independent practitioner and that he had accurately identified reasons she had difficulty conceiving initially. In 2003, online sites for rating physicians were not common or well-trafficked, leaving few options for finding recommendations for physicians outside of references from social network members.

During childbirth education classes, my social network of individuals expecting and with children expanded, and I learned that Dr. Halloway did not come highly recommended. Our birth educator was diplomatic, but clearly did not favor him. A birth doula who came to visit our class to talk to us about her services took me aside after class and indicated that she had assisted at a couple of births at which he attended. "He sometimes makes executive decisions without consulting the mother," she said. "If you trust him and you're comfortable with that, I'm sure he's fine. But if you want other recommendations, let me know."

The comments from the doula were jarring, but I had established care with Dr. Halloway and had no complaints entering the third trimester. At this time, I had established a short and simple birth plan, indicating that I preferred a low-intervention birth, I understood pain management was available to me and I would ask for it if I desired, and that outside of an emergency medical procedure, no intervention or medical action, even what seemed routine, should be taken without my full consent. I documented that I gave permission to my husband to offer consent on my behalf if I was unable to voice it. I also asked that my baby not be separated from a parent after birth, and that in the case of emergency, decisions should be made to protect the life of the baby, even at risk to me as the mother.

When I gave the birth plan to Dr. Halloway at my appointment, he said, "With your history of vulvar vestibultis, let's plan on an epidural." "I understand that I might be at risk for increased pain during delivery, but that would come at the very end. I read that it shouldn't interfere." He interrupted, "No. It's just not a good idea." He set the birth plan aside and continued with the examination. I knew the conversation about pain medication was over.

That afternoon I made an appointment with the Center Medical and Associates midwife team that several of individuals in my birth class had recommended. They had expressed that they were pleased with the care from the midwives, and my research on the differences between obstetric and midwifery care had informed me that it would be a good fit for my preferences. I understood that the team of CNMs delivered at Mount Nittany Medical Center, the hospital that served the State College area, and that if intervention was needed, obstetric care was immediately available. My first visit with one of the nurse midwives, and each subsequent one, confirmed my decision: the midwives were committed to supporting a low-intervention approach to childbirth, informing me of options along the way as needs for intervention presented.

***

I arrived home from the salon and I called my husband at work. "I believe my water broke," I told Ryan. "Are you sure?" he asked. "I'm fairly certain. I'll call Jocelyn, I just had an appointment with her this afternoon." "What did she say at the appointment? Were you dilated? Were you in labor then?" "She didn't check to see if I was dilated. The midwives tend to minimize vaginal exams to decrease risk of infection. I wasn't in labor then. I'm not having contractions now, in fact. I believe this is referred to as premature rupture of membranes."

Ryan decided to come home from work, and I called Jocelyn. "It sounds like your membranes ruptured," Jocelyn indicated. "Congratulations! I'm so happy to hear that your baby is on the way. Given that you haven't had contractions yet, take some time to get ready to go to the hospital and labor at home for a bit. Aahna Peterson is the midwife on call tonight. I want you to give her a call around 6pm to check in, ok?"

"Of course. Ok!" I thanked her and hung up the phone. I nervously roamed around my home, packing what I needed for the hospital, intermittently reading about rupturing of membranes in the books I had accumulated about labor and delivery. I had trouble concentrating, and was nervous as I read about increased risk of infection after rupture. Ryan returned home, and we discussed what to do. "Once you get to the hospital, they probably won't let you eat, so we should eat before they ask you to go in," Ryan suggested. We did, and I began to experience contractions. I called Aahna precisely at 6 p.m.

Aahna was the only midwife in the practice I hadn't had an opportunity to visit during my pregnancy, but she was the longest practicing midwife in the area and had an exceptional reputation among the people in my social network. Despite my anxiety and uncertainty about next steps in labor in delivery, knowing that people I knew and trusted placed trust in her helped me to trust her, diminishing my anxiety and uncertainty. "Hi, Jennifer. I understand your water broke this afternoon around 3:45pm?" "Yes, that's right." "How are your contractions?" "Not very severe. Not very regular." "They'll probably start coming on stronger soon. That tends to happen after the membranes rupture. For now, have something to eat and rest. Call me in a few hours, ok?" Over the next two to three hours, mild, irregular contractions ensued. I called Aahna around 8:30 p.m. and let her know. "That's fine. Get some sleep. When the contractions are strong enough to wake you up, call me."

Throughout the night, I managed mild contractions. I couldn't sleep, but not because of the contractions, but because I was going to have a baby soon! I called Aahna at 6:45 a.m. "Hi, Aahna. Contractions are coming about 3 or 4 times an hour. They aren't particularly severe." All right. It's about time to come into the hospital." "I had hoped to labor at home until things had progressed a bit more." "Twelve hours have passed since the rupture of membranes and there's an increase of infection. It's important for you to come to the hospital." Her voice seemed more serious. I panicked. "I see. We'll leave right away." I went to the bedroom and gently tried to wake Ryan. "I talked to Aahna. She said we need to go to the hospital. It's been more than 12 hours since my water broke, and there's an increased risk of infection now."

We left quickly and arrived at Mount Nittany Medical Center just after 8 a.m. Aahna greeted me with an embrace. She led us into a delivery room and introduced us to Kerry, the nurse who would be assisting with labor and delivery. "How've you been feeling this morning? How are contractions?" asked Kerry. I paused. "I … I haven't had a severe contraction since around 5:30am, actually. They seem to have slowed down." I looked from Aahna to Kerry for information on how to interpret this. "Let's have you lay down and I'll take a look, ok?" said Aahna. After examining me, Aahna confirmed that my membranes had ruptured, and I was dilated about 3 cm. "I'm concerned that labor is not progressing as quickly as we would hope. About 16 hours have passed since your membranes ruptured, yes?"

I nodded. "I'd like to start you on an antibiotic drip to decrease risk of infection. I'd also like you to consider some options for speeding things up a bit. Pitocin is a common option that you might have read about that we would give you intravenously. Another is a Cytotec, which can be given intravaginally. This may be a good option that will help you efface, and we may be able to remove it before it is completely absorbed." I didn't know what to say or ask. I looked at Ryan, who also seemed at a loss. "Will either option limit me from being able to walk or move around?" "We will need to make sure to monitor you and baby regularly. With Cytotec, you will be able to move around just as much as you would otherwise. With Pitocin, we will need to keep you on fetal monitors, but you can get up to use the restroom." I nodded and Aahna looked to Ryan and me as if to see if we had other questions. "I'm going to order the IV drip and let you think about it, ok?" After Aahna left, I began to feel tearful. "I don't think things are going well. Things aren't progressing as they should. I'm so nervous." "What do you want to do?" "I don't know … I really don't want to go down the road of Pitocin if at all possible. I've heard it's rough. I don't know very much about Cytotec." "If Aahna says it's ok we should go with it."

When Aahna returned, we discussed Cytotec as an option with her and agreed it was the best course of action. She administered it just after 11 a.m. and indicated that she would check my progress at 4 p.m. In the meantime, I walked freely around the birth center, periodically receiving antibiotics and spending time on an external fetal monitor. The baby's heart rate was fine, and I seemed to be progressing appropriately. I walked throughout the birth center, drank water regularly, used the restroom, and felt more at ease with each contraction that rolled over my body. As they became more noticeable and more evenly spaced, I grew in confidence that labor was progressing as it should.

At 4 p.m., Aahna examined me, right on schedule. "I'm pleased. You're 4 cm dilated and completely effaced." "That's good?" She nodded. "That's good," I said with relief. "Do you think we need further intervention?" Ryan asked. "At present, I don't see need for anything else. Let's check you in a couple of hours." "Ok. I'm set. Now I just need to figure out how to manage," I thought to myself. I broke out one of the books I had brought with me and reminded myself of what I read about managing during labor and delivery. Kerry, the nurse, brought in a rocking chair and a birth ball for me, suggesting ways to find a manageable position.

At 6 p.m., Aahna returned to examine me and was pleased again to inform me that I was making progress. I was 6 cm dilated and doing well. The contractions became more severe and Kerry suggested I take a warm shower. Afterward, I changed and slipped into bed. Aahna returned and began to massage my feet with lavender oil and encouraged me to relax. I breathed in and another contraction washed over me. I rose from the bed and back to the rocking chair. "I can relax here. If I relax, and breathe, I can manage the contractions," I thought. Over the next hour, I managed very well. I figured out how to work with the pain of each contraction. At 8:45 p.m., Aahna said, "It's time to start pushing." "Pushing?" I thought. "But I've just figured this part out. How am I supposed to push?" I didn't argue, however; I complied.

I climbed into the bed and assumed a squatting position. Ryan supported my arm on the right, Kerry on my left. With Aahna guiding me, I began to try to push during contractions. "Perhaps try on your hands and knees," Aahna suggested. I tried bending forward, but the pain was excruciating in that position. I settled back into a half sitting, half squatting position. At each contraction, Aahna urged me to push. I tried, but I was resisting the pain. "Do something!" I screamed at Aahna. "What do you expect me to do?" Aahna asked. I considered that seriously. I had to do this, but I didn't know how, and I was giving up. I just stared at Aahna. She murmured to Kerry, who left the room. Another contraction overcame me. The next thing I knew, I heard a new, cheery voice. "How are you, dear? I'm Nancy, one of the nurses here. Let's get this baby moving, shall we?" A contraction mounted. "All right, hon. You've got this. Push. Push. Breath in. PUSH." I screamed. "Yes! You've got this! Ok! Take a breath. You are doing a great job! Ok. Another contraction is going to be coming. You feel it? Ok. Breathe. You've got this. Just like last one. Work with it. Push ... That's right! Great!! Push!" Nancy's calm, positive encouragement was what I needed. Two pushes later, and Ryan was able to see the baby's head. "Really?" "Yes! Full of brown hair!"

Aahna said, "Keep going. The worst is almost over. Soon the head will be out." I scoffed. "After the head comes shoulders!" I think I was beginning to dislike Aahna. Perhaps she knew it, but Aahna's faced remained steady. Kerry looked at Nancy, who chuckled. "All right. Come on now. Here we go." Another contraction came over me, and with Nancy's encouragement, I pushed and pushed with all I had. Every push brought my dear baby out further. One, the head. Next, the shoulders. Next, the rest of the body. Then I heard soft crying. Within a few moments, Aahna handed her to me, a healthy little girl as red as a tomato. "Congratulations," Aahna said, and she smiled.

She indicated that it would be recommended to add Pitocin to the IV I still had from the antibiotic drip, to assist in the delivery of the placenta. She asked my permission to do so. Hesitantly, I looked to Ryan, who was so in awe with our new baby that he wasn't paying attention. "Yes, that's ok, if you think so," I murmured. Despite my hesitation, I trusted Aahna.

I held my baby, later named Evey, for as long as I could before Ryan and the nurses took her for a bath. I dearly wanted to continue to hold her, but Aahna was making sure that I safely delivered the placenta. Eventually, I had my baby back in my arms to nurse and to hold. Forty-eight hours later, we were released home to start the adventure of parenting, a whole new area of uncertainty to behold.

Healthy Mother, Healthy Baby.

SECOND BIRTH: PAST-EXPERIENCE GUIDES UNCERTAINTY MANAGEMENT

On February 8, 2006, I awoke around 5:30 a.m. with cramping abdominal pain. I had been uncomfortable and a bit ill since the previous weekend with a fever and back pain, which I attributed to a cold. After not being able to get back to sleep, I rose as usual to take a shower and start the day. After a morning appointment with my midwife, I had plenty of work as a graduate student to accomplish. During the process of getting ready, I began to suspect that the cramping pain might signal something I ought check out.

At what seemed like a reasonable morning hour, I called a fellow graduate student friend, who had two children. "Hi, Beth. How are you? I have a question." "Sure, Jenn. What's up?" "I've not been feeling well this morning. I kind of felt off all week, really, but around 5:30 am, I woke up just feeling crampy. I just don't feel well," I said taking a breath. "Anyway. I remember that you had a UTI when you were pregnant. What are other symptoms of that?" "Has it been hurting when you urinate or anything like that?" "No. Just … cramping. What are Braxton Hicks contractions like?" "They feel like regular contractions, but they're not very regular. Have you been drinking enough water? Dehydration can contribute to Braxton Hicks contractions." "Yes, I have. I've been up since … Ohhh. It's just so uncomfortable, Beth … But. Anyway. Yes. I've been up since 5:30am and have made sure to drink lots of water." "Jenn. How close are you to your due date?" I took another breath to manage the discomfort. "I'm about 12 days away." "Jenn, is it possible you might be in labor? Because you sound like you're in labor." "Really? When I was in labor with Evey, I felt contractions up higher … But now that you mention it." Another wave of cramping pain washed over me. "Oh, Beth! I think you're right. This seems like labor."

We both laughed. "I have an appointment with my midwife this morning, so she'll check." We got off of the phone and I told Ryan that it seemed like I was in labor. We figured, after the long labor I had with Evey, that I had a long journey ahead. Although we knew that second births tend to progress more quickly than first ones, we went about our daily routine eating breakfast and getting Evey ready to go to nursery school. The waves of cramping pain became more regular, so I called the midwives' office to see if they wanted me to come into my scheduled appointment, or just go to the hospital. I spoke to Aahna on the phone, who asked me to come to the office as soon I could get there. Ryan and I arrived at the office around 9:15 a.m. Aahna saw me and confirmed I was in labor, dilated 6 cm. She encouraged me to go straight to the hospital to meet Daeja, the midwife on call that day. I was hesitant to go into the hospital. Labor with Evey lasted over thirty hours, and I was not interested in spending the entire labor in the hospital again. However, Aahna reminded us that labor had a tendency to progress more quickly during a second birth.

Because Ryan needed pick up a few things at home, he took me next door to the hospital and headed back to our house. I checked in at the hospital's labor and delivery division and I was in a birthing room before 10 a.m. I did my best to concentrate on relaxing and coping with the contractions that were becoming more and more severe. Daeja arrived at the birthing room and she and the nurse on call, Nicole began to monitor my progress with an external fetal monitor around 10:10 a.m. Everything seemed to be progressing normally, with contractions about 4.5 minutes apart. Around 10:30 a.m., Daeja checked my progress and found I was between 7 and 8 cm dilated and completely effaced. I was beginning to feel a bit more apprehensive about being at the hospital without Ryan at this point, but Daeja did not leave my side. Ryan arrived by 10:45 a.m. and with his presence I had more confidence.

After almost two hours had passed, the contractions seemed to be slowing down. Daeja checked on my progress around 12:45 p.m. and I was almost completely dilated. However, my membranes were still intact and seemed to be preventing the baby from descending any further. Daeja felt that if the membranes were ruptured that the labor would progress more rapidly. "Take some time to think about it. I'll be back to talk to you soon," Daeja said. I was beginning to feel tired and was ready for the baby to be born. Especially being so close to the end of the process, Ryan and I decided that if Daeja thought rupturing the membranes would be beneficial, we should. Daeja returned shortly after, and we asked her to rupture my membranes.

At 1:10 p.m., Daeja broke the membranes. After a few minutes without feeling a noticeable increase in the severity of the contractions or rapidness of progress, I was disheartened and felt as though the baby would never come. I looked at Ryan and Daeja and asked if the baby would be there soon. I felt despaired. Ryan responded, "Yes! Very soon!" I scowled at him. "How would you know? It could be hours." Daeja, who, like Aahna, seemed to have mastered a calm, minimally expressive demeanor while attending a birth, cracked a smile. "It won't be hours," she said. I took a deep breath and let it out. "Ok. I believe you."

After what seemed like an eternity (but couldn't have been more than twenty minutes) of sitting in the bed waiting for the baby, Daeja told me I needed to get up, use the toilet, and move around. I sighed. I was tired, and I had no interest in moving, but complied, knowing that moving around would help baby shift into place to be born, and trusting Daeja. In the middle of a contraction, as I neared the toilet, I began to tip forward toward it, feeling like I might have to push at the next contraction. I planned to tell Daeja and Ryan that I needed to go back over to the bed, but I did not have any words to utter anything. After the contraction ended, I could not find a voice to talk before the next contraction began. Daeja did not need to be told that I needed to push. With an increase in sternness in her tone, she told Ryan they needed to get me back to the bed. Each taking one of my arms to help me balance, then guided me over to the bed and I fell onto my hands and knees. I knew it was time to push. Pushing was the most difficult part of birthing Evey, thus, I had read up on effectively pushing and I felt prepared and in control. I pushed with confidence. At one point, Daeja told me to take it easy and go slowly, and for a moment I did. However, I was tired and wanted to hold my baby. So, I pushed with passion and to my amazement, Cate was born at 2:01 p.m.

HEALTHY MOTHER, HEALTHY BABY

Uncertainty Management, Trust, and Decisions during Labor and Delivery

My experience of having midwife-attended births in 2004 and 2006 resonates with research demonstrating that midwives support patients with low-intervention birth situations and preferences, provide education and information to help patients make informed decisions (e.g., Matthias, 2010; Parratt & Fahy, 2003) and are associated with overall positive patient satisfaction (Kozhimannil, Attanasio, Yang, Avery, & Declercq, 2015). Additionally, my experiences lend insight into the role of trust in one's provider during labor and delivery, particularly regarding uncertainty management and decision-making. I had trusted Aahna as a provider, which was essential in making decisions about interventions to help labor progress and then to use Pitocin to help stimulate delivery of the placenta after birth. Similarly, I trusted Daeja to guide me through labor and delivery. She never left my side when my husband was not present, and I trusted her word that labor would be over soon when I experienced despair, which helped me manage. Trust in one's medical provider is important and powerful; the connection between patient trust in physicians and improved health outcomes is well documented (e.g., Mollborn, Stepanikova, & Cook, 2005; Safran et al., 1998). When coupled with shared decision-making between patient and physicians, patients' trust in physicians has been found to be associated with a variety of positive clinical outcomes (e.g., Parchman, Zeber, & Palmer, 2010; Safran et al., 1998). Uncertainty management, trust in one's provider, and making quality medical decisions in labor and delivery appear to be intimately intertwined. Given that decisions during childbirth are made in times of urgency and anxiety, understanding how provider-patient interactions are shaped by trust and in turn influence uncertainty management and medical decisions is vital.

Using the ecological perspective as a lens for understanding the connections between trust, uncertainty management, and medical decisions also has utility. My experiences show the importance of one's personal social network in influencing health and health-related decisions, such as choice of providers and interpreting medical symptoms, as emphasized in past research (e.g., Cline, 2011). Beth helped me determine I was in labor. As such, I sought medical attention earlier than I would have otherwise. My experiences also demonstrate that one's trusted social network members can influence trust of providers. Had I not understood that Aahna was respected in the community as an exceptional midwife, my interactions with her during labor and delivery would have been impacted. I would have experienced a heightened sense of uncertainty during an already stressful labor experience. The culture of medical care and birthing in State College during the early 2000s, which supported a woman's choice of obstetric or midwife care at the community hospital, undoubtedly lent to these positive birth experiences, and lays in stark contrast to the culture of birthing I experienced subsequently.

THIRD BIRTH: A NEW MEDICAL ENVIRONMENT

In the late summer of 2007, my family moved from State College, PA to St. Louis, MO. I had been offered a tenure-track faculty position at St. Louis University (SLU), and my husband transferred his employment as well.

Before moving, I researched medical providers for our family's health-care needs. Moving from Centre County to the metropolitan area of St. Louis offered a very different health-care culture. To offer some context for the differences between the two locales, the population of St. Louis City in 2007 was 355,653, with the population of the surrounding metropolitan area at 2,806,368 (Federal Reserve Bank of St. Louis, 2018). The population in

State College, PA, in 2010 was around 42,034 (U.S. Census Bureau, 2018). In St. Louis, the largest employer is BJC Health Care, employing 28,351 individuals. Also, in the top five employers are SSM Health with almost 15,000 employees, and Mercy hospital with 14,195 (Keller, 2017). In State College, PSU is the largest single employer in the area (employing 26,353 individuals in 2015), followed by Mount Nittany Medical Center, employing 2,289 individuals. The proportions alone offer an interesting and very different health-care context.

The search for providers in St. Louis was daunting given the number of medical institutions in the area, and I had few local contacts. I talked to a local mother who seemed to have similar parenting values, who recommended a pediatrician covered by our new insurance, whose practice was only a fifteen-minute drive from our home. Sifting through reviews online was arduous, given the number of providers, many of whom were located 30 or more minutes from our home or not covered by our insurance. Once we arrived in Saint Louis, I gathered sound recommendations for most other providers my family needed. However, gynecological care was more challenging. Having positive experiences with CNM care in State College, I sought to transfer care to a similar midwife practice. Following a quick online search, which pulled only one midwife in the Saint Louis area practicing out of her home, I discovered the practice of midwifery in Missouri, until very recently, was not legal, and was presently being contested. In May 2007, a bill with provision to legalize the practice of Certified Professional Midwives (CPMs) in Missouri was passed. However, the Missouri State Medical Association and other opponents of midwifery in Missouri moved for a placement of injunction against the provision, which was made permanent in August of 2007. In 2008, the Missouri Supreme Court upheld the law legalizing the practice of CPMs to provide services related to pregnancy, including prenatal, delivery, and postpartum services.

Given the controversial state of midwifery practice in Missouri at the time I moved, I thought it best to establish care with a traditional obstetrician/gynecologist. So, I asked around. Everyone had an OB/GYN she loved. I was hopeful and asked why. The responses went something like this, "Why? Well. She's just great. I've never had a problem," or "She went to Washington University—great education." Thinking ahead to the possibility that I might have another child I asked mothers about labor and delivery. The responses were unsatisfying to me. "Ah. It was ok. My OB delivers out of Hospital X and it's kind of the baby factory." "I loved delivering out of Hospital Y! Great nurses and the food was wonderful!" I heard lukewarm stories of labor and delivery, not particularly good stories, or very difficult stories to hear that ended with, "After all was said and done, healthy baby, healthy mom, so I can't complain!" I delayed establishing OB/GYN care because I never heard a satisfying recommendation.

In fall of 2009, I became ill with what seemed like gastrointestinal issues. I went to my primary care physician (PCP), who referred me to OB/GYN. I ended up in a random gynecology practice of Dr. Folsom, was and could get me in the next day. After hearing my symptoms and without examining my body, Dr. Folsom diagnosed me with Pelvic Inflammatory Disease (PID). She gave me a prescription for a sexually transmitted disease, which she explained caused PID. After spending less than five minutes with me, she moved to leave the room. I stopped her, "Wait, please." She turned, cocked her head to the side and raised her eyebrows at me.

"I understand that this may be an appropriate diagnosis, but might we explore other possibilities? We haven't discussed my sexual history, but I have one partner—my husband. I know statistically that women may incur sexually transmitted infections from husbands who have other partners. However, the likelihood of this is rather low. What are other possible conditions associated with the symptoms I'm having?"

Dr. Folsom sighed. "I don't treat patients like you very often, so I don't know. If your test results come back negative, then we can discuss other possibilities." My jaw must have dropped and I thought, "Wait, what? Patients like me? What do you mean? She's turning to leave again. Focus on the important questions." I found my voice and asked, "So, should I wait to begin the medication until we get the test results?"

"Start taking the medication now." Dr. Folsom left and closed the door behind her.

I was dumbfounded. I was uncertain, anxious, and in pain. Without knowing what else to do, I began taking the medication. I called for test results several days later. The nurse indicated that my test results were negative. "So should I stop taking the medication?" I asked. "Of course. You're test results are negative," the nurse replied. "I'm still experiencing severe abdominal cramping constantly. Like labor contractions. I have for a couple weeks now. It's debilitating. What should I do?"

"Oh. You should come back in to see Dr. Folsom. I'll set you up an appointment."

Two days later, I sat in Dr. Folsom's office, still in pain. This time, Ryan came with me.

"I don't know why you are back. You haven't finished the medication I prescribed."

"I called your nurse."

"Yes, it's on record how often you've pestered my nurse."

I took a moment to breathe before responding, as calmly as I could. "I called for my test results, as no one had called me. Your nurse told me the test results were negative for any sexually transmitted infections and to stop taking the medication. I'm still in pain."

"Your test results were not negative. You should not have stopped the medication."

"Your nurse told me the test results were negative! She told me that there was no need to continue the medication! That is why I scheduled an appointment to see you!" I heard my voice raise with intensity as I spoke.

Dr. Folsom looked in her file and then uttered, "Excuse me," and left the visiting room.

My husband said, "Calm down. She's the doctor. You shouldn't raise your voice to her."

"She is not treating me well, Ryan! I asked you to come and support me!"

Dr. Folsom returned. "Your test results were negative. You do not have any STDs and thus the diagnosis of PID is not likely accurate. I suggest that we get you in for an exploratory laparoscopy on Thursday to see what's going on." She handed me a pamphlet explaining what would be done and said her nurse would be in to set up the time.

I said, "I'm going to have to think about it."

"Excuse me?" said Dr. Folsom. She sounded offended and shocked.

"I would like to think about this. I don't feel comfortable with this."

"If you say you're in pain, and you want to not be in pain, then we should find out what is going on," she said. I detected a hint of a patronizing tone in her voice. "If you do not schedule for Thursday, it could be a while before we can fit you in."

"I understand. I can call your office and let you know."

"Fine." Dr. Folsom left the office and slammed the door behind her.

"Jenn, what are you thinking? You're in pain, and she recommends this procedure. It's not a good idea to delay," Ryan insisted.

"I'm sorry, but I do not trust this doctor, Ryan. I don't want her touching my body!"

"Jenn, she's a doctor!"

The nurse came in at that moment with paperwork and numbers to call the office to schedule the laparoscopy. "Who do I talk to about transferring my files to a different practitioner?" I asked her.

"Jenn, what are you doing?" Ryan asked.

"I'm transferring care."

"To who???"

"Dr. Kildare. She's a parent at the kids' school. She works for Mosaic Health."

"Mosaic Health? Isn't that one of the centers for ... for the indigent?"

"Yes. Dr. Kildare has a heart of gold, which is probably why she works there. And there's no reason I can't be seen there."

That afternoon, I called to make an appointment with Dr. Kildare. However, by the time I was able to see her, my symptoms began to subside. The

condition that ailed me is still unclear. However, Dr. Kildare became my OB/
GYN. I decided she understood me as a patient. After all, we were working
women and mothers. Professionals.

Dr. Kildare recommended I not attempt to have children for six months in
order to observe my system and ensure all was in working order. By summer
2011, I unexpectedly found myself pregnant, with a due date of November
2011. I was overjoyed, but my life and the pregnancy were marked with a
high degree of uncertainty and stress. I had taken on a teaching assignment for
the fall semester for a forty-student graduate course in Public Health, outside
of my home department. I was excited about the class, but it would be a new
course preparation and a new audience. I had a new department chair entering
that summer, and I was uncertain how he would respond to my pregnancy. I
learned that other senior faculty members in my department suggested that
I had gotten pregnant to extend the tenure probationary period, which they
considered an unfair advantage for me. Meanwhile, I had been diagnosed
with partial placental praevia, a condition in which the placenta was partially
covering the opening of the cervix. As my pregnancy progressed, the placenta
stretched upward to the point that it was low lying and was not seen as an
interference with having a vaginal birth. However, Dr. Kildare insisted that I
not labor at home due to risks associated with a low-lying placenta. "I want
you in the hospital as soon as labor begins," she had told me.

On October 19, 2011, at 9:30 p.m. just after I had put my daughters to bed
that evening and breathed a sigh of relief that I too could sleep, my water
broke. "Oh God. It's just like Evey," I thought. I remembered how my water
broke without contractions and being in labor with Evey for over thirty hours.
I wanted to go to sleep before going to the hospital. However, Dr. Kildare's
insistence that I go to the hospital immediately upon labor rang in my ears. I
called a sitter. I packed a bag. I needed to follow Dr. Kildare's recommendations. I was a higher risk, given the low-lying placenta.

I arrived at the hospital and explained my water broke and that I was in
labor. The nurses said they would check the fluid to ensure it was amniotic
before they would admit me. After they collected a sample, Dr. Stehlen,
a resident fellow, confirmed I was in labor. "We'll be admitting you and
starting you on Pitocin. I've ordered it, so as soon as you're up in your
room, we'll start your IV and we should have a baby before long," she told
me, and smiled. "Oh. Why is it necessary to start Pitocin?" I didn't look at
my husband, who was with me, for fear he would say to respect the doctor, as he did with Dr. Folsom. "Your water has broken, and you haven't
begun contractions. It's important to get labor moving as quickly as possible as there is a high risk of infection. Pitocin is what we give you to get
labor moving," Dr. Stehlen said. The smile had left her face, and her tone
undercutting.

"My membranes ruptured before contractions started with my first birth as well. At that time, protocol was that as long as baby was term, amniotic fluid was clear, fetal heart rate was normal, and there was no evidence of infection or fever, laboring without intervention was fine. Is that not still the case?" Dr. Stehlen looked at me, her blue eyes considering me. "Are you refusing Pitocin?" "I'm asking if there is an indication that it is necessary at this time." "It is the recommended course of action." "Is it necessary? I prefer to labor naturally unless it is necessary." "I am going to place a call to your provider." She left the room and I heard her voice through the wall. "She says she doesn't want Pitocin … I'll put her down as non-compliant." A few minutes later, Dr. Stehlen returned. "Would you like to speak with Dr. Kildare?"

My heart began to beat more quickly as I was handed a phone. "Hello?" "Hi, Jennifer. Dr. Kildare. How are you? I understand your in labor." "Yes." "So, Pitocin is what I would also recommend when membranes rupture before contractions, but I have no problem with you waiting to start Pitocin if you want to. We can give you 12 hours to see how we're doing." "Ok. So if labor progresses and I begin to dilate and efface at an appropriate rate, there's no need to augment, correct?" "Correct. We'll give you some time." "All right. Thank you." I handed the phone back to Dr. Stehlen. "We'll move you up to a room," she said.

After I got into the room, I tried to sleep, but I was asked to constantly wear an external fetal monitor and I couldn't get comfortable. A resident performed a vaginal exam each hour. When morning came, I wanted to walk, but I wasn't permitted to leave the room. I longed for the space and hallway at Mount Nittany Medical Center, to be able to move freely. I hadn't realized what a luxury that had been. Slowly and surely, the contractions poured on, and I embraced. But I was tired. I was hungry. I wanted to move. I was nervous about making progress. Doctors continued to check me on the hour, which interrupted my ability to cope with contractions. The room seemed to get smaller and smaller as I walked the space, trying to manage. The presence of my husband in the room, a source of comfort during my previous birth experiences, was taking up space that I felt like I needed to move.

Around 9:30 a.m., I began to feel like I was making good progress. A new resident came in and checked me. I was dilated 8 cm. I believed I was beginning to get close. I spent the next hour trying to get into a position to give birth, but I was having trouble. The nurse came in to check on me and I said to her and my husband, "I need to find a good position to manage the contractions." I remember the nurse then went over to a tray covered with white blankets. She uncovered it, revealing sterile instruments for assisting with delivery, and left the room. "Hope!" I thought. "She knows that I'm getting close! I can do this." I thought.

About thirty minutes later, around 11 a.m., Dr. Kildare entered the room, the first time I'd seen her since beginning labor. "Hi, Jenn. Let me give you a check here." I made my way back to the bed to be checked again. "She's still at 8cm," she said. "She's not making progress." "What? No. No no no. Ask the nurse. She knows. She uncovered the tools. But no. No. I'm not making progress. Oh, God no," I moaned internally. "No!" I wailed. "Oh no. I can't do this." "You've been at this a long time. You're not making progress. Let's get you an epidural," said Dr. Kildare. "I can't do this. I'm so tired." Dr. Kildare left the room.

"Jenn, do you really want the epidural?" Ryan asked. "I've been up for DAYS. I am EXHAUSTED. I'M NOT MAKING ANY PROGRESS. I CAN'T DO THIS," I screamed at him. "Please, Jenn," he begged me. I believe that my husband was then at the receiving end of some words (shouted harshly) that are not appropriate for academic publication. Suffice to say that an anesthesiologist was at my bedside within ten minutes and an epidural was administered.

I collapsed on the bed free of pain. I closed my eyes. My husband said I laid down for at most seven minutes before I was up again and said firmly: "I need to push." The nurse who happened to be there said, "Ok ..." and did not come to me; did not seem to believe me. I then repeated, "I need to push." She checked me, and then shouted down the hall, "Get Dr. Kildare! Hurry!" "She headed back to Mosaic Health!" was the reply. "Baby's coming!" "She thought it would be another few hours!" "Baby is coming NOW!"

Dr. Kildare made it back in time to catch baby Ry, who was born less than forty-five minutes after I had been told I was not making progress; born less than twenty minutes after receiving an epidural, that I complied to only after I was told I was not making progress, *which I believed because my doctor told me so*, even though just moments before I thought I must have been close to giving birth. Nonetheless, baby Ry was born with health. He nursed vigorously. I held him and loved him. My husband took him for his first bath.

I was then left alone in the hospital room, praying, reflecting on what had happened. "Healthy mother. Healthy baby. Healthy mother. Healthy baby," I kept repeating in my head. I felt dizzy. I felt like I was fading. Something wasn't right. I pressed the call button for the nurse. Maybe I was just tired. I must just be tired. "Healthy mother. Healthy baby. Press the call button again. Oh God, something isn't right. I'm not well. Where' the nurse? Press the call button. Please. Someone answer. Where is the nurse? Please, God. Please," I prayed. I pressed the call button again. "Yes?" a voice finally answered. "I'm not well. I'm not feeling well." "Ok. Someone will be in in a minute." "Thank you," I murmured.

A nurse came in. "Hello! How are you?" "I'm dizzy. Something's not right." "You just had a baby! That's a normal feeling!" she said cheerfully.

"I'm not feeling right. Something's wrong." "Okay, sweetheart. Let's take a look at you." She felt my head. She looked at me. I began to pass out. "Something's wrong." She lifted the blanket across my stomach and I saw out of the corner of my eye that I was sitting in a pool of blood. I heard the nurse gasped and call for help. I faded out.

"Get her up to surgery," I heard. I opened my eyes. The room was filled with people. I saw my husband's face in the crowd. "What's happening?" "Do you trust me?" It was Dr. Stehlen. I looked into her steel blue eyes. The obstetrician who had checked me in the night before. The one who had, without discussing with me my options, ordered that I be given an IV of Pitocin to start contractions. The one who I had heard on the phone with my primary obstetrician in the next room, saying I was non-compliant. I took a breath and placed my lips together and looked into her eyes. I tried not to swallow evidently, not wanting her to know, not wanting to give away that I felt vulnerable, not wanting to answer that I did not know if I could trust her. "Am I at risk of losing my fertility?" She stared at me. I stared back. She looked down, so I couldn't see her eyes. "Please do what you need to do, but please protect my fertility if at all possible. This is my request, which I would like you to honor in whatever intervention you take." Without looking up at me, she ordered morphine. Then she breathed in and looked up at me again. "You're going to have to trust me. Can you do that?" "I don't have much of a choice," I thought. I breathed in, pursed lips. Within moments, the morphine coursed through my veins. My husband's head moved farther away as the nurses and assistants stepped in front of him; his concerned face ebbed back and back to the wall. "Go be with our baby," I remember saying and a nurse ushered him out.

A hand on my stomach. A hand between my legs. A critical look on her face. Dr. Stehlen plunged her hand into me. Her wrist. How far was her arm in me? Deep within my uterus. I felt her gloved fingers grasp once. Twice. Out. I gasped. And again, this time with even more determination. Out came a handful of blood clotted, dark red, which she dropped into a silver bowl, which appeared next to me in the hands of a nurse who seemed to appear out of nowhere. And a third time. I thought I might lose consciousness. And a fourth. The final, just small bits of bright red tissue. "That should do it," she said, and she stepped back, pulled the latex gloves off, and swaggered away, like she had just won a duel.

The nurse with the silver bowl continued to clean and care for me, while the other nurse, who I recognized as the one who had found me dizzy and had since pressed herself against the wall next to me, seemed to return to the present moment and tentatively began to attend to me again. When the nurse with the silver bowl was out of ear shot, she whispered to me, "DID YOU SEE THAT?!?" I looked at her. "DID YOU SEE WHAT JUST HAPPENED?" she whispered with excitement. "SHE JUST SAVED YOUR

LIFE. WITH HER BARE HANDS. YOU WERE SUPPOSED TO GO UP
TO SURGERY. OH MY GOD. THAT WAS ... WOW. I'VE NEVER
SEEN ANYTHING LIKE THAT BEFORE." I don't remember very much
for the rest of the day. I must have been reunited with my son. I must have
fed him. I must have slept. The next morning another obstetrician visited
me. She asked what I remembered. She talked about how nursing was
going, and all the normal things. Everything proceeded as per script, as
though all was normal.

According to Dr. Stehlen's notes, in my medical records:

"Called by nursing re increased blood loss over 1 hour and dizziness ...
   Uterus 2 cm above umbilicus, foggy. Bimanual performed & 1500 ml clot
expressed ...Most likely 2/2 atony. No further bleeding p meds given will
closely follow."

According to the RN Incidental Update:

"Patient found to be c/o dizziness ... Dr. (Stehlen) notified and into see patient
... Manual extraction of clots per Dr. (Stehlen) at bedside ... Patient remained
awake and cooperative. Tolerated procedure well."

I did not know at the time that I had experienced a massive postpartum
hemorrhage, nor did I know that the leading cause of pregnancy-related
death globally and in the United States is associated with postpartum hemorrhage (Say et al., 2014). The recovery from childbirth was difficult. I was
weak, and like so many women in the United States, I faced uncertainty not
only regarding my health and my baby, but about returning to work. I faced
the graduate class in the week following birth, feeling pressure not to leave
my senior level colleagues with undue work because I chose to have a baby.
I spent the next weeks nursing, feeling ill, bleeding, and grading papers,
all the while experiencing anxiety and uncertainty about my health. I took
care of my baby first, my students as best I could, and my body was faint-
ing under me, while my husband picked up the care of my older daughters.

At my postpartum visit with Dr. Kildare, I did not disclose very much
about how awful I was feeling or how much work I was doing. I remember
choosing her as a physician because she was a working mother and understood the demands on my time. I trusted she must have gone through similar
difficulties as a mother and obstetrician. This is the way we are mothers and
professionals. We don't complain. I remember hearing my colleagues, students, and relatives say, "Congratulations! Healthy mom! Healthy Baby!" I
smiled and agreed. After all, baby Ry and I were alive. However, I felt like
I was dying.

FOURTH BIRTH: PAST-EXPERIENCE
GUIDES UNCERTAINTY MANAGEMENT,
TRUST, AND DECISIONS

In early fall of 2013, I was overjoyed to find myself pregnant with my fourth baby. For the first time, I was due after the close of a semester and I was looking forward to finishing up the term and having my first real maternity leave. Having reflected on my birth experience with my son in 2011 and having learned more about the health-care system in St. Louis, I was better prepared to navigate my birth experience.

I decided not to return to the care of Dr. Kildare. She was a sound practitioner and I appreciated her as a professional, but decided it was best to move on. But to whom? Although midwifery had been legalized in Missouri by the time I was pregnant, the culture of birthing had not shifted much in the St. Louis area. At the time I was deciding on a new practitioner, I had the option of birthing at one of six major hospital systems in the St. Louis area and from all of the obstetricians therein, but no midwives. Over the past five years, I hadn't heard any additional encouraging stories about birth experiences in the area, and everyone I encountered was as lukewarm about their birth experiences as I had heard years ago. Healthy mom, healthy baby, unsatisfying experience. The obstetrician was phenomenal, though. Clearly, the obstetrician saved the day and made everything right at the end.

I went the route of choosing a practitioner based on religious affiliation. Dr. Barrett was part of a Catholic practice in the area. I found Dr. Barrett to be a gentle, soft spoken individual who, other than the relics of St. Gianna in his waiting room and other religious artifacts and literature about Catholic-endorsed reproductive practices, followed the script of other OB/GYNs pretty closely. I trusted him to follow the protocol and lean toward less intervention, but I also trusted him to act as an obstetrician would—not a midwife. I knew that I would need more support during birth than would be provided by him, the hospital staff, and my husband.

I remembered the doula who had visited my birth class in 2003 and decided to look into having one for labor and delivery support. A doula, according to DONA (2018), an international doula certifying agency, is a trained professional who provides physical, emotional, and informational support to a mother before, during, and shortly after childbirth with the aim of helping her to achieve a healthy, satisfying birth experience. I asked for recommendations for doulas from my social network and found very few. I looked online and many of the doula profiles did not resonate with me. Although I preferred a low-intervention birth, I was not interested in having a doula so slanted toward natural birth that I would be perceived a failure if something did not go as planned. I needed a support person who would support me regardless of how the birth progressed. Eventually, I found Milana Podderzhka, who seemed like a good match, so I requested an interview with her. During the interview, Milana exhibited terrific listening skills. She engaged in a recipro-cal interview, getting to know me, my values, preferences, my perception of my husband's role, how I hoped she could support me, how I thought I would perceive touch during the birth experience, and how my other births had proceeded. I learned about her birth experiences and her approach as a doula—one of support and respect. She communicated very clearly and calmly with me, acknowledging her role as one of service, helping me to get the information I need to make informed decisions during birth, and facilitat-ing communication between me and my care providers in order to ensure a healthy, positive birth experience. I was impressed with her approach and I trusted that she would serve me very well in the capacity as a doula.

Friday, May 30, 2014, started out much like the times I went into labor with my first daughter and my son. After dinner with my family that evening, I tucked my three children into bed, and slipped between the covers myself. Then my water broke. Instead of jumping up in panic, thinking I had to rush to the hospital, as with labor the previous birth, I breathed a sigh of relief. I had spoken with Dr. Barrett that day at my appointment and asked his recom-mendations for the amount of time I might labor at home if my membranes ruptured before contractions began. He had indicated that he was comfortable with about twelve hours. I relaxed. I sent a text message to Milana, letting her know labor was beginning and that I planned to rest until the next morning before going into the hospital. I slept lightly for the next two hours.

Contractions began more regularly about 11:30 p.m. and became more intense throughout the night. I sent Milana a message at 5 a.m. indicating that I would like her to come to the house. She arrived by 5:30 a.m. She watched and supported me at the house through the morning activities with my other children, as the contractions came in waves over me. We made the decision to go to the hospital around 7 a.m. Milana drove me, and my husband stayed behind to get the kids to school and arranged care for them afterward, agree-ing to meet us at the hospital. When examined initially after check-in, I was reported to be about 5–6 centimeters dilated and about 80 percent effaced.

I felt slightly discouraged, as I had hoped that I would be further along. I was tired and after having three prior childbirth experiences, I figured it would be afternoon before I would deliver, which seemed a long time away. "I'm so tired. I don't want to do this," I said to Milana. She encouraged me to find effective ways to cope and helped me find strength. Ryan arrived by 8:30 a.m. By 9 a.m., I felt extremely tired and discouraged. I told Ryan and Milana I wasn't sure I could manage. The feeling persisted for a few contrac-tions, and Ryan suggested I could be in transition to the final stage of labor, but I wasn't convinced that could be the case, given that I was expected only to progress about a centimeter each hour.

Not long after, I felt like I might vomit. Milana confidently indicated that I must be transitioning to the last stage and that I was making progress toward delivery. I believed her. Milana said to a nurse, "The baby will be here soon. Perhaps it's time to call the doctor?" "Ok," the nurse responded and continued typing at the computer in the delivery room. After a minute, Milana asked the nurse, "May I have a pair of latex gloves, please? Just in case." "Sure. Go right ahead," replied the nurse, gesturing toward the box, but still not leaving the computer. A contraction came over me, and I felt the need to bear down. Milana acknowledged a shift in my voice as I managed the contraction. "Ok," she murmured. "Let's get her to the bed, Ryan," she said to my husband. With their support, I managed to kneel on the bed as another contraction washed over me. "The baby is coming," I said. "I know," Milana calmly responded. "Nurse? A doctor?" I heard the nurse stop typing. She gasped, and I heard her shoes pad across the tile toward the door. Another contraction overcame me. I felt the need to push, which I did very gently, remembering instructions from previous births. The contraction released and Milana rubbed my back. I knew her hands were there to catch the baby, just in case.

Another contraction. Another gentle push. I heard steps and a male voice. "All right. Might I check your progress?" "NO," I responded as another contraction rolled in. Pushing was inevitable and I did, a moan escaping my throat. "Ahh. Let's get you in a different position, shall we?" said the male voice. Another contraction. "NO. The baby is coming," I said. And the baby came. The hands of the male person who had spoken to me with authority caught my baby. Ryan and Milana helped me turn onto my back and I was handed little Mari. After I looked into her beautiful little face and held her sweet little body, I looked up at the male stranger who "delivered" my baby. "Hi," he said. "Who are you?" I asked. "I'm just the janitor, actually." I stared. We all stared. "That was a joke. I'm Dr. Michael. I'm on call for Dr. Barrett this weekend. Nice to meet you!" We laughed, awkwardly. Healthy mother. Healthy baby.

DISCUSSION AND CONCLUSION

As outcomes associated with maternal and fetal health-care in the United States have declined in recent years (MacDorman et al., 2016), attention to what these concerning trends reflect about birth culture is necessary in order to address the issue. The culture of maternal health care, at the national and organizational level, is socially constructed by interactions (Hofstede, 2003), principally those between providers and patients. These interactions, particularly in the context of maternity care, can have important influences on health outcomes (Brown et al., 2003; Hunter et al., 2008) and overall health and well-being (Street, 2003). They may be marked by uncertainty for both the expectant mother (Matthias, 2009) and medical provider (Matthias, 2010), and carry with them the dominant view of childbirth as inherently high risk (Cahill, 2001; Hall et al., 2012). These interactions have the potential to impact medical decisions during labor and delivery, which can have consequences for outcomes (Cook & Loomis, 2012). To provide insight into the birth culture in the United States, I offered an authoethnographic account of my experiences as a birthing patient on four occasions. An ecological perspective on provider-patient communication is used to guide the exploration and highlight the influences on uncertainty management during labor and delivery. In doing so, the importance of challenging the dominant cultural narrative of birth as risk can be seen, as well as critical needs for future research with regard provider-patient communication in maternity care.

First, taking an ecological perspective emphasized that uncertainty and anxiety during the pregnancy experience go beyond concerns of the expectant mother's health and the health of her baby (Glazier et al., 2004). Such stressors can impact the health of a patient and her offspring before, during, and after birth, and a provider can encourage appropriate management of stress and anxiety. During my first pregnancy, I felt comfortable talking to Jocelyn, my midwife, about the work I was trying to finish prior to birth. When she encouraged relaxation, I embraced it as a directive. On the other hand, I decided not to disclose the stress I experienced postpartum or how physically exhausted I was to Dr. Kildare after my third birth. I knew she was a mother of three, and a fellow working professional. I expected that she had encountered similar difficulties during her experiences and thought that I ought not complain. In retrospect, I know that failure to do so potentially jeopardized my own health and might have compromised my ability to care for my infant. However, I accepted the dominant cultural narrative of independence as a woman and mother, which Dr. Kildare represented as a fellow working mother. As I faced returning to a tenure-track position following a life-threatening childbirth experience, I expect that neither Dr. Kildare nor I knew how to navigate conversations about how best to support myself and my child while managing a challenging work environment. Yet, given the implications for health, knowing how to manage such conversations is imperative, and a vital direction for health communication research.

Taking an ecological perspective also offered insight into the important social contexts that impacted trust in my providers. Clearly, interpersonal social contacts influenced my trust in providers during labor and delivery, such as when Aahna was the attending midwife during my first birth. I hadn't seen her prior to arriving at the hospital, but her reputation was strong in the community, which helped me trust her recommendations for care. Initially during my third birth experience, and for the entirety of my fourth, I was attended by a provider I did not know and trust had not been established. The initial encounter with Dr. Stehlen during my third birth experience negatively impacted my trust in her, as her talk with me was marked with the traditional power differential seen in physician-patient interactions (e.g., Beisecker, 1990; Fisher; 1993) and obstetric care (Pizzini, 1991): I was not part of a nonemergency decision to augment the labor process. When I questioned the decision, Dr. Stehlen asked if I was "refusing" treatment and noted that I was "non-compliant." The trust between Dr. Stehlen and I was damaged—not only that of mine in her, but her in me. This impacted our later encounter when I hemorrhaged. I will never forget that she asked, "Do you trust me?" I will never forget her hesitancy in following my request to do what she could to protect my fertility, as it wasn't the first course of action she recommended; I was supposed to go immediately for surgery.

Clearly, not just the trust of the patient in the provider is at stake during the medical encounter, but also the trust the provider has in the patient. Mutual trust is essential for the provider-patient relationship and has important consequences for care (e.g., Thom et al., 2011). Although some research has examined the provision of accurate information by a patient (Miller, 2007) as well as the impact of mutual trust on cooperation and minimizing the need for monitoring (Cook et al., 2004), little research has examined mutual trust between patients and providers and its impacts on patient care.

One outcome associated with a provider's trust in the patient and mutual trust may be that of a patient's trust in self, patient empowerment, among other important outcomes. My encounter with Dr. Folsom, for example, appeared to be marked with some degree of lack of trust in me as a patient. She did not entertain other possibilities for my diagnosis, which increased my sense of anxiety, uncertainty, and vulnerability. I took the medication prescribed, trusting her judgment and not my own sense of self or trust in my husband's fidelity. Test results indicated that the medication was not needed, but the mutual trust between Dr. Folsom and I had been damaged due to misdiagnoses and poor communication, and I switched care providers. Additionally, after my third childbirth experience and having difficult interactions with my providers that were not marked with mutual trust, when I was left alone and felt unwell, I wondered if I was just tired and did not trust my interpretation of my symptoms. The nurse who came to check on me did not seem to trust my assessment that something might be wrong either. Indeed, the nurses during my third and fourth childbirth experiences did not trust my or my doula's assessment that I needed to push. I am grateful that my doula served as a voice for me during my fourth birth experience, as articulating needs during labor can be difficult. Similarly, I am thankful that my midwives during my first two birth experiences listened to my voice during labor, even when I could not express with words what I was experiencing. Trust in providers and support persons, trust in the patient, and mutual trust between providers and patients appear to be powerful during labor and delivery experiences and can facilitate listening and action that can positively influence outcomes. Future research in these areas is essential for enhancing maternity care.

Improving maternity care in the United States, particularly during labor and delivery, will be a complicated and multifaceted endeavor that requires specialists from many areas of expertise, including health communication. Scholars in health communication are ideally positioned to examine and enhance the communication processes associated with the management of inevitable uncertainty associated with pregnancy, labor, and delivery, as well as the trust between providers and patients that can influence effective management of uncertainty. Considering the complex ecology within which the provider-patient encounter is situated, particularly regarding the social elements that expectant mothers and their providers bring to their interactions, will undoubtedly lend insight as to how to improve the encounters and help shift the dominant cultural narrative of birthing in the United States to one that empowers women and their providers toward birth experiences not marked by risk-aversion, but courage and confidence.*All person's names, except those of immediate family members, have been changed. The names of health-care organizations in the St. Louis region were changed. Those in the State College area were not, given that they would readily be identified due to the limited number of practices in the area.*

REFERENCES

Adam, B., & van Loon, J. (2000). Repositioning risk: The challenge for social theory. In B. Adam, U. Beck, & J. van Loon (Eds.), *The risk society and beyond: Critical issues for social theory* (pp. 1–23). London: Sage.

American Society of Clinical Oncology. (2017). The state of Cancer care in America, 2017: A report by the American Society of Clinical Oncology. *Journal of Oncology Practice, 13*(4), e353–e394. doi: 10.1200/JOP.2016.020743.

Beisecker, A. E. (1990). Patient power in doctor–patient communication: What do we know? *Health Communication, 2,* 105–122.

Bylund, C. L. (2005). Mothers' involvement in decision making during the birthing process: A quantitative analysis of women's online birth stories. *Health Communication, 18,* 23–39.

Brown, J. (2018). The fight for birth: The economic competition that determines birth options in the United States. *University of San Francisco Law Review, 52*(1), 1–30.

Brown, J. B., Stewart, M., & Ryan, B. L. (2003). Outcomes of patient provider interaction. In T. L. Thompson, A. M. Dorsey, K. I. Miller, & R. Parrot (Eds.), *Handbook of health communication* (pp. 141–162). Mahwah, NJ: Lawrence Erlbaum Associates.

Bush, G. (March 21, 2001). President Bush speaks at the American College of Cardiology Annual Convention [Transcript]. *The White House Archives.* Retrieved from https://georgewbush-whitehouse.archives.gov/news/releases/2001/03/2001 0321-2.html.

Cahill, M. (2001). Male appropriation and medicalization of childbirth: An historical analysis. *Journal of Advanced Nursing, 33*(3), 334–342. doi: 10.1046/j.1365-2648.2001.01669.x.

Casimir, L. (June 26, 2018). Why are so many of San Francisco's black mothers and babies dying? *The Guardian.* Retrieved from https://www.theguardian.com/world/2018/jun/26 /black-maternal-mortality-babies-san-francisco-crisis.

Cherniak, D., & Fisher, J. (2008). Explaining obstetric interventionism: Technical skills, common conceptualisations, or collective countertransference? *Women's Studies International Forum, 31*, 270–277. doi: 10.1016/j.wsif.2008.05.010.

Cline, R. J. (2011). Everyday interpersonal communication and health. In T. L. Thompson, R. Parrott, & J. Nussbaum (Eds.), *Routledge handbook of health communication, Second Edition* (pp. 377–396). New York, NY: Routledge.

Cohen, P. N. (2016). Maternal age and infant mortality for white, black, and Mexican mothers in the United States. *Sociological Science, 3*(2), 32–38. doi: 10.15195/v3.a2.

Cook, K., & Loomis, C. (2012). The impact of choice and control on women's childbirth experiences. *Journal of Perinatal Education, 21*(3), 158–168. doi: 10.1891/1058-1243.21.3.158.

Cook, K., Kramer, R., Thom, D., Stepanikova, I., Bailey, S., & Cooper, R. (2004). Trust and distrust in patient-physician relationships: Perceived determinants of high and low trust relationships in managed care settings. In R. Kramer & K. S. Cook (Eds.), *Trust and distrust in organizations: Dilemmas and approaches* (pp. 65–98). Thousand Oaks, CA: Russell Sage Foundation.

Davis, R. R., Hofferth, S. L., & Shenassa, E. D. (2014). Gestational weight gain and risk of infant death in the United States. *American Journal of Public Health, 104*(S1), S90–S95. doi: 10.2105/AJPH.2013.301425.

Davis-Floyd, R., & Davis, E. (1996). Intuition as authoritative knowledge in midwifery and home birth. *Medical Anthropology Quarterly, 10*, 237–269.

DONA. (2018). What is a doula? *DONA International.* Retrieved from https://www.dona.org/what-is-a-doula/.

Downe, S., Simpson, L., & Trafford, K. (2007). Expert intrapartum maternity care: A meta-synthesis. *Journal of Advanced Nursing, 57*(2), 127–140. doi: 10.1111/j.1365-2648.2006.04079.x.

Ellis, C. (1997). Evocative autoethnography: Writing emotionally about our lives. In W. G. Tierney & Y. S. Lincoln (Eds.), *Representation and the text: Re-framing the narrative voice* (pp. 115–139). Albany, NY: State University of New York Press.

Ellis, C., & Bochner, A. (2000). Autoethnography, personal narrative, reflectivity: Researcher as subject. In N. K. Denzin & Y. S. Lincoln (Eds.), *Handbook of qualitative research* (pp. 733–768). Thousand Oaks, CA: Sage.

Federal Reserve Bank of St. Louis. (2018). Resident population in St. Louis, MO-IL (MSA). *FRED Economic Data.* Retrieved from https://fred.stlouisfed.org/series/STLPOP.

Fisher, S. (1993). Doctor talk/patient talk: How treatment decisions are negotiated in doctor-patient communication. In A. D. Todd & S. Fisher (Eds.), *The social organization of doctor–patient communication* (pp. 161–182). Norwood, NJ: Ablex.

Foss, K. A., & Foss, S. K. (1994). Personal experience as evidence in feminist scholarship. *Western Journal of Communication, 58,* 39–43.

Gage, T. B., Fang, F., O'Neill, E., & DiRienzo, G. (2013). Maternal education, birth weight, and infant mortality in the United States. *Demography—Chicago Then Washington the Silver Spring, 50*(2), 615–635.

Gergen, K. J., & Gergen, M. M. (1997). Narratives of the self. In L. P. Hinchman & S. K. Hinchman (Eds.), *Memory, identity, community: The idea of narrative in the human sciences* (pp. 125–142). Albany, NY: State University of New York Press.

Glazier, R. H., Elgar, F. J., Goel, V., & Holzapfel, S. (2004). Stress, social support, and emotional distress in a community sample of pregnant women. *Journal of Psychosomatic Obstetrics and Gynecology, 25,* 247–255.

Gray, J. B. (2014). Social support communication in unplanned pregnancy: Support types, messages, sources, and timing. *Journal of Health Communication, 19*(10), 1196–1211. doi: 10.1080/10810730.2013.872722.

Hall, W. A., Tomkinson, J., & Klein, M. C. (2012). Canadian care providers' and pregnant women's approaches to managing birth: Minimizing risk while maximizing integrity. *Qualitative Health Research, 22*(5), 575. doi: 10.1177/1049732311424292.

Hofstede, G. (2003). *Culture's consequences: Comparing values, beliefs, institutions and organizations across nations* (2nd ed.). Thousand Oaks, CA: Sage.

Howard, J. (February 20, 2018). The least and most dangerous countries to be a newborn. *CNN.* Retrieved from https://www.cnn.com/2018/02/20/health/unicef-newbo rn-deaths-by-country-study/index.html.

Hunter, B., Berg, M., Lundgren, I., Olafsdottir, O. A., & Kirkham, M. (2008). Relationships: The hidden threads in the tapestry of maternity care. *Midwifery, 24,* 132–137.

Jackson, E. A. (January 5, 2017). NCDR cardiovascular care trends. *American College of Cardiology.* Retrieved from http://www.acc.org/latest-in-cardiology/ ten-points-to-remember/2017/01/05/14/21/trends-in-us-cardiovascular-care-20 16-report.

Jacobson, L. (July 5, 2012). John Boehner says U.S. health care system is best in the world. *PolitiFact.* Retrieved from http://www.politifact.com/truth-o-meter/state ments/20 12 /jul/05/john-boehner/john-boehner-says-us-health-care-system-best -world/.

Keller, K. (July 18, 2017). St. Louis' largest employers. *St. Louis Business Journal.* Retrieved from https://www.bizjournals.com/stlouis/subscriber-only/2017/06/16/ employers.html.

Kingdon, C., Neilson, J., Singleton, V., Gyte, G., Hart, A., Gabbay, M., & Lavender, T. (2009). Choice and birth method: Mixed-method study of caesarean delivery for maternal request. *British Journal of Obstetrics and Gynaecology, 116*(7), 886–895. doi: 10.1111/j.1471-0528.2009.02119.x.

Kirkham, M. (1989). Midwives and information-giving during labour. In S. Robinson & A. M. Thomson (Eds.), *Midwives, research and childbirth (Vol. 1)* (pp. 117–138). London: Chapman & Hall.

Kozhimannil, K. B., Attanasio, L. B., Yang, T., Avery, M., & Declercq, E. (2015). Midwifery care and patient-provider communication in maternity decisions. *Maternal Child Health Journal, 19*(7), 1608–1615. doi: 10.1007/s10995-015-1671-8.

MacDorman, M. F., Declercq, E., Cabral, H., & Morton, C. (2016). Is the United States maternal mortality rate increasing? Disentangling trends from measurement issues. *Obstetric Gynecology, 128*(3), 447–455. doi: 10.1097/AOG.0000000000001556.

Martin, N. (April 23, 2018). Redesigning maternal care: OB-GYNs are urged to see new mothers sooner and more often. *National Public Radio*. Retrieved from https://www.np r.org/2018/04/23/605006555/redesigning-maternal-care-ob-gyns -are-urged-to-see-new-mothers-sooner-and-more-o.

Martin, C. M., & Kasperski, J. (2010). Developing interdisciplinary maternity services policy in Canada: Evaluation of a consensus workshop. *Journal of Evaluation in Clinical Practice, 16*, 238–245. doi: 10.1111/j.1365-2753.2009.01326.x.

Matthias, M. S. (2009). Problematic integration in pregnancy and childbirth: Contrasting approaches to uncertainty and desire in obstetric and midwifery care. *Health Communication, 24*, 60–70.

Matthias, M. S. (2010). The impact of uncertainty on decision making in prenatal consultations: Obstetricians' and midwives' perspectives. *Health Communication, 25*(3), 199–211. doi: 10.1080/10410230903544977.

Matthias, M. S., & Babrow, A. S. (2007). Problematic integration of uncertainty and desire in pregnancy. *Qualitative Health Research, 17*, 786–798.

Miller, J. (2007). The other side of trust in healthcare: Prescribing drugs with the potential for abuse. *Bioethics, 21*(1), 51–60.

Mercy. (2018). *Mercy Birthing Center Midwifery Care—St. Louis*. Retrieved from https://www.mercy.net/practice/mercy-birthing-center-midwifery-care-st-louis/.

Mollborn, S., Stepanikova, I., & Cook, K. S. (2005). Delayed care and unmet needs among health care system users: When does fiduciary trust in a physician matter? *Health Services Research, 40*, 1898–1917.

National Academy of Sciences. (2013). Birth settings and health outcomes: State of the science. In Board on Children, Youth, and Families; Institute of Medicine; National Research Council (Eds.), *An update on research issues in the assessment of birth settings: Workshop summary*. Washington, DC: National Academies Press.

Parchman, M. L., Zeber, J. E., & Palmer, R. F. (2010). Participatory decision-making, patient activation, medication adherence, and intermediate clinical outcomes in type 2 diabetes: A STARNet study. *Annals of Family Medicine, 8*, 410–417.

Parratt, J., & Fahy, K. (2003). Trusting enough to be out of control: A pilot study of women's \sense of self during childbirth. *Australian Journal of Midwifery, 16*, 15–22.

PLOS. (March 20, 2018). State-by-state causes of infant mortality in the US: State-by-state analysis links sudden unexpected deaths of infants (SUDI) to high proportion of full-term infant mortality in the U.S. *Science Daily*. Retrieved from https://www.sciencedaily.com/ releases/2018/03/180320141337.htm.

Pinar, W. F. (1997). Regimes of reason and the male narrative voice. In W. G. Tierney & Y. S. Lincoln (Eds.), *Representation and the text: Re-framing the narrative voice* (pp. 81–113). Albany, NY: State University of New York Press.

Pizzini, F. (1991). Communication hierarchies in humor: Gender differences in the obstetrical/gynecological setting. *Discourse and Society, 2,* 477–488.

Rathert, C., Wyrwich, M. D., & Boren, S. A. (2012). Patient-centered care and outcomes: A systematic review of the literature. *Medical Care Research and Review, 70*(4), 351–379. doi: 10.1177/1077558712465774.

Reed-Danahay, D. E. (1997). Introduction. In D. E. Reed-Danahay (Ed.), *Auto/ethnography: Rewriting the self and the social* (pp. 1–20). New York: Berg.

Rothman, B. K. (1991). *In labor: Women and power in the birthplace.* New York: Norton.

Safran, D. G., Taira, D., Rogers, W. H., Kosinski, M., Ware, J. E., & Tarlov, A. R. (1998). Linking primary care performance to outcomes of care. *Journal of Family Practices, 47,* 213–220.

Say, L., Chou, D., Gemmill, A., Tuncalp, O., Moller, A., Daniels, J., Gulmezoglu, A. M., Temmerman, M., & Alkema, L. (2014). Global causes of maternal death: A WHO systematic analysis. *The Lancet Global Health, 2*(6), e323–e333. doi: 10.1016/S2214-109X(14)70227-X.

Street, R. L. (2003). Communication in medical encounters. In T. L. Thompson, A. Dorsey, K. I. Miller, & R. Parrott (Eds.), *Handbook of health communication* (pp. 63–82). Mahwah, NJ: Lawrence Erlbaum.

Street, R. J., Makoul, G., Arora, N. K., & Epstein, R. M. (2009). How does communication heal? Pathways linking clinician-patient communication to health outcomes. *Patient Education and Counseling, 74*(3), 295–301. doi: 10.1016/j.pec.2008.11.015.

Thom, D. H., Wong, S. T, Guzman, D., Wu, A., Penko, J., Miaskowski, C., & Kushel, M. (2011). Physician trust in the patient: Development and validation of a new measure. *Annals of Family Medicine, 9*(2), 148–154. doi: 10.1370/afm.1224.

U.S. Census Bureau. (2018). State College borough, Pennsylvania. *QuickFacts.* Retrieved from https://www.census.gov/quickfacts/fact/table/statecollegeboroughp ennsylvania/POP010210#viewtop.

Walsh, D., & Newburn, M. (2002a). Towards a social model of childbirth: Part one. *British Journal of Midwifery, 10,* 476–481.

Walsh, D., & Newburn, M. (2002b). Towards a social model of childbirth: Part two. *British Journal of Midwifery, 10,* 540–544.

WHO, UNICEF, UNFPA, World Bank Group, and United Nations Population Division Maternal Mortality Estimation Inter-Agency Group. (2015). United States of America. *Maternal Mortality in 1990–2015.* Retrieved from http://www.who. int/gho/maternal_health/countries/usa.pdf.

World Health Organization. (2015). *Trends in maternal mortality: 1990 to 2015: Estimates by WHO, UNICEF, UNFPA, World Bank Group, and the United Nations Population Division.* Geneva, Switzerland: World Health Organization. Retrieved from http://www.afro.who.int/ sites/default/files/2017-05/trends-in-maternal-mor tality-1990-to-2015.pdf.

World Health Organization. (2015). *Department of Reproductive Health and Research (1997) Care in Normal Birth: A Practical Guide.* Geneva: WHO.

Chapter 15

Ableist Biases

*A Tale of Three Lives**

Joyeeta G. Dastidar

DAX

As the result of a propane leak that lit on fire, at the ripe age of twenty-six, Dax Cowart suffered not only from third-degree burns across 68 percent of his body (ears, face, upper extremities, trunk, legs), but was also blinded (from corneal damage) and had to have the distal parts of his hands amputated, with the remnants marred by contractures. He did not wish to continue living under these conditions, and his desire to die was twofold: first, he did not receive adequate analgesia for the daily baths in the Hubbard tank required to keep infection of his wounds at bay (White & Engelhardt, 1975, p. 9). Second, he was previously a good looking able-bodied outdoorsy young male, and he did not wish to live the rest of his life as someone who suddenly found himself blind and crippled (Dax's Case). While the physical suffering Dax was experiencing as a direct consequence of the medical therapies he was being treated with were an important factor in his decision, another primary driver in Dax's decisions was his emotional suffering from knowing that it was impossible for him to return to being the able-bodied person he was before the accident. One question that occurs to me in pondering Dax's case is, how much does ableism affect Dax's bleak outlook on his life? To be fair, I could imagine feeling as he did immediately afterwards had I been through something similar, and I can only guess how I would have fared beyond that period. Perhaps it would have been different if Dax was born with his disabilities as he'd have a lifetime to get used to them, and he'd know

* Acknowledgement: The author would like to thank Danielle Spencer for her helpful comments on the first draft of this chapter.

no other life. Dax had been able-bodied, and he felt that a drastic reduction in his prior physical capabilities would result in a life he would not want to live. But how much of this was due to biases he had internalized, that many of us have, about being disabled?

Dax's case brings to the forefront the matter of principlism, in which two or more principles are applicable and only one can prevail. In Dax's case, the two ethical principles that were at odds with one another were those of beneficence and respect for autonomy. There was no question that what Dax's physicians wanted to do was in the best interest of prolonging his life, and it is also quite possible they did not want the burden of his death weighing down on them even if that is what Dax wished for himself. However, whether his life *should* be prolonged was up for debate per Dax, and perhaps he should have had the right to have his wishes not only taken into consideration, but—after adequate psychological evaluation to ensure Dax was competent and consistent in expressing his wishes—implemented as well.

Dax's physicians exerted their will over him by having him undergo psychiatric evaluation to deem him incompetent, thereby leaving the decision-making to his mother. Even though the psychiatrist's evaluation found Dax to have capacity, his physicians still overrode Dax's wishes. Dax's mother was a woman who was inclined to follow the recommendations of Dax's physicians for many reasons: a desire to not lose her son, a fear of losing her son before he reaccepted her Christian faith (White & Engelhardt, 1975, p. 9) and trusting that her son's physicians would do right by him (Dax's Case). In other words, his providers took advantage of his physical disabilities to have their duty toward beneficence trump Dax's right to autonomy. Dax was understandably displeased with this course of action.

What stood out about Dax's case was that his desire to die was not due to a terminal diagnosis, but due to an inability to accept the limitations of the disabled life he would live if he was to receive the recommended treatments and survive (White & Engelhardt, 1975, p. 10). Dax had strong feelings against continuing treatment due to the impact his new disabilities would have on his life, stating, "I know that there's no way that I want to go on as a blind and a cripple" (Cowart & Burt, 1998, p. 15). At the heart of this sentiment was ableism, discrimination against the disabled in favor of the able-bodied, or in Dax's case, discrimination against his current self in favor of his former self, combined with his physical suffering: "I am enjoying life now ... but I still would not want to be forced to undergo the pain and agony I underwent to be alive now. I would want that choice to lie entirely with myself and no others."

Robert Burt's conversations with Dax seemed to center around how much Dax was devaluing his capacity to improve and achieve things that remained within his realm of possibility (Cowart & Burt, 1998, pp. 15–16). Burt asks himself, "How can I as a helper, someone who wants to be useful and helpful to him, communicate in a way that is fully understandable and believable what the real range of options are to him, disabled, that he, formerly able-bodied and now still able-bodied in his image of himself, is not able to see." We learn of all that Dax would ultimately go on to do. In his interview with Burt, Dax rattles off an impressive list of accomplishments: climbing a fifty-foot utility pole via belaying in a ropes course, writing poetry, studying, and practicing law (Cowart & Burt, 1998, p. 17). Dax was twice married. The first marriage ended in divorce. His second marriage to a high school acquaintance in February of 1983 survived, indicating that his previously spoken and understandable fear of being alone was not borne out (Engel, 1983).

SHUVO

My brother Shuvo had a similar life story in that he became gravely ill early in adulthood and was left with a significant chronic illness that would be with him for the rest of his life. It was there that the similarities ended. Less than six months after his college graduation, at the age of twenty, Shuvo became sick with viral symptoms in late October. My father picked him up one Friday after work to have him recuperate at my parents' place for the weekend. By Saturday morning, my brother was comatose from a severe case of viral meningoencephalitis. He was not awake in the initial days while hospitalized in the intensive care unit (ICU) and many decisions were made on his behalf by his physicians and my parents. Even after Shuvo woke up, unlike with Dax, there was no debate about going full-court press with maximal medical therapies. Once Shuvo was ready to leave the ICU and later the hospital, he agreed with pursuing the recommended rehabilitation strategies as his goal was the same as his family's and medical team's goal: to get better and leave the hospital.

While Dax's disabilities were clear from the beginning, Shuvo's degree of residual chronic illness (refractory epilepsy with a decreased level of function primarily manifest as moderate and progressive memory loss and milder speech impairments) was not as apparent at the outset, or even for years to follow. The progression of Shuvo's disability was not something that my family and I realized could happen until it became obvious that the decline was already taking place. It seemed even his providers were not aware of this, or at least this possibility was not clearly communicated to us. Perhaps it was uncommon or even more so difficult to predict the course of the disability.

In all societies, the disabled must grapple with issues of autonomy and dependence, but in more sociocentric cultures, dependence can be managed through love and a feeling of mutuality (Whyte & Ingstad, 1995, p. 11). Consequences of one's epilepsy depend on the individual's social background (including protectiveness), personality, severity of illness, as well as cultural beliefs and opportunities in their society. The single most important framework for the lives of individuals with epilepsy is often being part of a family (Whyte, 1995, pp. 237–238). Dax Cowart did have a family, though he lost his father in the fire, and his relationship with his mother seemed strained and distant much of the time, possibly due to the stress of the repercussions of the accident. Reading the various articles and papers about the Cowart case, one got the sense that Dax was living in a world of his own, with a "me against the world" approach. Shuvo has a family, and we were always around both while he was in the hospital, and later when he returned home. I do think Shuvo's strong family support helps him cope with his dependence on others through love, though he understandably wishes he did not have to be dependent. One hopes that through his marriages Dax has found a similar supportive mutuality.

One important factor in Dax and Shuvo's cases was the age at the time the disability occurred. The disability was neither congenital, where either of them grew up not knowing any other life, nor late in life, after his identity had already been established. Dax and Shuvo had neither a lifetime to adjust and adapt, nor a well-established pre-illness identity to fall back on. One study in the United States shows that lifelong disability can be a "master status" for an individual, but if it occurs after one's economic and social position is well established, disability in an elderly person plays more of a subordinate role (Whyte & Ingstad, 1995, p. 17). For both Dax and Shuvo, their disability became their "master status": the blind cripple for Dax, the epileptic for Shuvo. The terms themselves conflate disability and identity.

CULTURAL CONTEXT

Disability is culturally relative, that is, the definition of disability depends on capacities valued in a setting, for example, vision loss in a beautiful area, cognitive impairment in a society that values educational achievement, being physically handicapped where people earn their income through manual labor. The ideas of disability, handicap, and rehabilitation emerged in Europe and spread to the rest of the West but are only now coming to surface in developing countries. Disability is differentiated from inability in that it is a capability that was lost and could potentially be rehabilitated to its original condition (Whyte & Ingstad, 1995, pp. 7–8), though for both Dax and Shuvo, the likelihood of rehabilitation to their pre-illness condition was zero.

The parallels between Dax and Shuvo seemed to be limited to both being struck with a tragic illness in their youth leaving them with significant residual chronic illness. I came to realize the important role ableism played in both their stories, but the ways in which ableism impacted their lives were quite different. For Dax, as detailed above, the ableism came about through a set of introjected values and was an internal drive so strong it made him wish he could die. For Shuvo, the ableism was largely external, and imposed upon him by his health-care providers and his loved ones. Ultimately, both sets of ableist attitudes were borne out of the burden of societal expectations.

Like Dax's case, people were prioritizing their duty toward beneficence over Shuvo's autonomy in that they were insisting what they wanted for Shuvo was more important than what he might have in mind related to what he knew he would be capable of doing. The people who were trying to help Shuvo (myself included) could have harmed him by defining him as a patient with epilepsy which was an illness that had to be treated and overcome. Perhaps if complete seizure control—ideally through a minimal number of medications and interventions—was attainable, our goal of a "cure" would not have been so dangerous. However, as we eventually learned through years of accompanying Shuvo on his health journey, no amount of invasive testing, surgery, or medications would cure him of his epilepsy. Over time, we came to understand that having an unattainable goal ultimately seemed futile and damaging to the psyche.

In *Constructing Normalcy*, Lennard J Davis writes that the "problem" is not the person with the disability, but the way in which normalcy is constructed such that the disability is the problem (Davis, 2013, p. 3). In societies where there is a norm, bodies that deviate from the norm such as those with disabilities can be seen as deviants, versus in societies where there is an ideal, and no individual attains that ideal, everyone has a non-ideal status (Davis, 2013, p. 6). Problems with the idea of the norm include creating the idea of a deviant body, forcing the idea of a normal body to fit into stricter parameters than the bell curve of reality, and the revision of the normal distribution into quartiles creating a new kind of a eugenic ideal with an imperative to strive to become that (Davis, 2013, p. 8). In problematizing Shuvo's seizures, we were identifying Shuvo's brain with its abnormal electrical impulses as deviant and making it impossible for Shuvo to fit into average society as a normal person. Instead of controlling Shuvo's seizures as much as possible with the help of modern medicine and accepting the residual seizures as a unique part of Shuvo who was integrated into society, we were forced to metaphorically alienate Shuvo as sick and not belonging to healthy society.

LIA

That's not to say that Shuvo's uncontrolled seizures were not problematic, for they certainly were, especially the ones resulting in bodily harm. One sees in the story of the Lee family in *The Spirit Catches You and You Fall*

Down: A Hmong Child, Her American Doctors, and the Collision of Two Cultures how much excess injury arose in part from a family who didn't understand the life-threatening nature of their daughter Lia Lee's epilepsy. Lia's epilepsy was diagnosed in infancy after a couple of hospitalizations and missed diagnoses due to the lack of a Hmong interpreter. Due to miscommunications and misunderstandings both on the immigrant Hmong family's part and the American providers' part, Lia Lee's parents, Foua and Nao Kao, not only disliked fully treating her seizures, but they also didn't understand the doctors' recommendations: Lia's parents believed seizures were a desirable quality that heightened Lia's perception and uniquely qualified her with the blessed opportunity to become a shaman (Fadiman, 1997, p. 22). Her medications were changed twenty-three times in less than four years, and there was no way to remember all the changes as Lia's parents were illiterate in both Hmong and English (Fadiman, 1997, p. 46).

Before she was three years old, Lia was even legally removed from her home and temporarily placed in foster care for a year before returning her to her parents due to concerns about Foua and Nao Kao's unwillingness to administer her medications. A constellation of factors led to a nearly two-hour seizure when Lia was four years old. The prolonged insult to her brain was complicated by a persistent vegetative state, which she remained in until her death when she was thirty years old (Fox, 2012). While it seems up for debate whether the seizures during the prolonged seizure episode when Lia was four were caused by medication nonadherence or an overwhelming *Pseudomonas* bacterial infection, the consensus was that Lia could have lived close to a normal life had her parents administered her anti-seizure medications as prescribed since her infancy (Fadiman, 1997, pp. 255–258).

Clearly the nonadherence to medications was not from a lack of love or caring on behalf of the Lee family. Lia's local family practice clinic marveled at this, noting her has a "clean, sweet-smelling, well-groomed child" during Lia's medical appointments (Fadiman, 1997, pl. 253). One could say Lia's survival for over two decades in her persistent vegetative state was testament to the quality care she received from her family at home. Nonetheless, in the Lee family's case, we see what harm can come from the other extreme, in not seeing the disease as something to be treated and seeing it through rose-colored glasses, a reverse ableism of sorts. It seems the goal should be more of a balance, treating what can be managed through modern medicine while accepting the natural limitations of the illness.

DEHUMANIZATION THROUGH EXPECTATIONS

Irving Zola notes that being disabled leads to the invalidation and infantilization of a person, indicating that what makes them different makes them less.

Finn Carling takes this a step further by discussing not only devaluation but also dehumanization of the disabled. If personhood is seen as being human in a way that is helpful and meaningful, individuals can be seen as being of lesser or greater value (Whyte & Ingstad, 1995, p. 10). Dax Cowart internalized this belief by seeing the postaccident version of himself as inferior and not having a life worth living. I got the sense that like Dax, when unable to work after a lifetime of productivity, that Shuvo felt lesser. I hoped it was not the case, and never had the courage to ask him due to a fear that asking him reinforced the notion in his mind, but I suspected that this feeling of inadequacy stemmed from his difficulty in being helpful to society in the traditional pre-chronic illness sense. Knowing Shuvo so well for so long and accompanying him on his journey, I don't think we as his family dehumanized Shuvo, but I do think that for his providers, he soon became "the case of refractory epilepsy on multiple antiepileptics status post Vagal Nerve Stimulator, status post stereotactically placed depth electrode EEG, status post Responsive Nerve Stimulator, and with overinvolved parents and physician sister."

In *Touch, Ethics and Disability*, Janet Price and Margrit Shildrick point out the dualism of encouraging seeing disabled people as distinctly other while holding them to attain the same norms as able-bodied people. In parallel, there is the medical model where disabled bodies are seen as targets for repair. While rehabilitation has therapeutic value, it cannot make an irreversibly disabled body "normal" (Price & Shildrick, 2002, pp. 66–67). Rehabilitation could not restore Dax's vision or his hands, nor could it make Shuvo seizure-free. I will say that following rehabilitation, Dax was able to accomplish remarkable things, including going to law school, practicing as a lawyer, and getting married. While Shuvo was able to find love and marriage, he was not as lucky as Dax in his postaccident educational and career success. It was not for lack of trying. Over time, Shuvo's medications (a very sedating cocktail of various antiepileptic drugs) and seizures themselves had effects on his brain, making him slower than usual. Classes and tasks he would previously have breezed through became challenging projects requiring significant amounts of time. It is helpful here to discuss the philosopher Susan Wendell's distinction between the healthy versus the unhealthy disabled. Healthy disabled are those whose medical condition is predictable and stable, like that of Dax's. Unhealthy disabled are people whose condition needs active treatment to maintain stability, like that of Shuvo's and Lia's (prior to her entering her Persistent Vegetative State). Without the treatment, the unhealthy disabled person can become medically unstable, as Shuvo was with a seizure leading to a fall complicated by an intracranial hemorrhage and Lia was during her prolonged hospitalization following her hours-long-grand mal seizure with concurrent bacterial sepsis. Being unhealthy disabled also limits the educational and work opportunities for an unhealthy disabled individual as compared with someone without the disabled's condition (Goering, 2015, p. 135).

Employment is a valuable personal and social goal and is often the primary means to financial security and access to health insurance. Unemployment for eligible workers maintaining an active job search ranges from 13 to 25 percent among those with epilepsy. Unemployment is higher among those with more severe, that is, tonic-clonic seizures. Reasons for the increased rate of unemployment include social isolation, lack of social skills, lack of family support, lack of information about employment opportunities, and fears based on past negative perceptions toward epilepsy on behalf of employers (Bishop & Allen, 2007, p. 251). Shuvo continues to try to participate in job training programs and the like, but given the number done to his brain and cognition, first through his meningoencephalitis, then through diagnostic and theoretically therapeutic surgeries, and with the superimposed side effects of his ongoing with his medication regimen, I wonder if the pressure for him as an unhealthy disabled to have a "normal life with a normal job" like the rest of us is unrealistic and unfair, setting him up for repeat failure.

The flip side to that is there are healthy disabled people like Dax who can do amazing things like go through law school and practice law and advocate for self-determination, and we would not want the disabled to miss out on reaching their full potential. I think the danger comes when one has a one-size-fits-all approach where we presume that the capabilities and goals of every disabled person is the same as the temporarily able-bodied population. Western societies simultaneously impose a social identity for the disabled, as citizens who have the same rights as others and should be integrated into society, and as workers like everyone else. "Paradoxically, they are designated so as to disappear, they are named so as to go unmentioned."

The problem is pretending everyone is equal doesn't make it so, while confining the disabled individual's goals to the common and familiar (Whyte & Ingstad, 1995, p. 9). For me, the goal has been to encourage and support Shuvo to do as much as he can achieve, but without setting unattainable goals for what that might be. The uncertainty of where that line lays has led to much confusion and mixed messaging among the members of our family. At one point, I suggested neuropsychiatric testing to better determine what was within the realm of possibility for Shuvo. The not knowing his boundaries was a struggle, and I thought some objective data could be helpful. In the end, I'm not sure how much practically useful information such testing would provide beyond what we can see ourselves in Shuvo's day-to-day activities and events.

In lieu of the medical model of disability, where the disability is focused on the physical impairment, perhaps as something to be treated and overcome, the social model of disability looks at the social factors affecting disability, including the exclusion of the disabled from full social participation. The social model of disability points out the way in which disabled people can be treated unfairly and become subject to medicalization of their problems. Other people's expectations of a disabled person's ability to work and quality of life can create further disability by making the disabled person feel badly about themselves. Often, the impairment is not so much the physical disability as the social disadvantages of negative attitudes and insistence on able-bodied norms and goals (Goering, 2015, pp. 135–137).

The key principle in Shawn Achor's TED article *What's the worst kind of praise you can give?* is that comparing an individual to others and concluding that they were "the best" does not enhance the other person, but rather indicates that your appreciation and support of that person is predicated on their superior position to others. Thus, he advocates for eliminating superlatives such as smartest or strongest or most handsome from our vocabulary. He concludes his talk with the saying "Comparison is the thief of joy." In other words, to truly enhance others, we need to stop with the comparisons. I feel we would do well to apply this principle to the disabled in the sense that our appreciation and love for them is not predicated on them having the same aspirations and goals as compared to that of an able-bodied person. We can appreciate and support them based on them being their unique selves with their unique hopes for themselves framed within the real restrictions their disability creates for them.

French disability scholar Henri-Jacques Stiker notes that in earlier times, the disabled were seen as different, but current norms dictate that they are ordinary and should be integrated into ordinary life and ordinary work (Whyte, 1995, p. 270). "Infirmities do not raise metaphysical problems so much as technical ones, to be taken in hand and administered by social workers, vocational trainers, and medical and legal specialists. The assumption is that we master all the outcomes; every condition can be treated and adjusted, though not all can be cured."

The realization of how ableism affects perceptions of the disabled is eye-opening, and this epiphany can be mutually freeing. Under ableism, there is failure on two fronts: with the provider/family feeling inadequate if unable to get their patient or family member back to a prior baseline level of functioning, and the sense of failure of the individual him or herself given unrealistic expectations of what they can attain. This is reminiscent of part of the response of one of Lia Lee's pediatricians, Dr. Neil Ernst, to the question of what he'd learned from taking care of Lia, "Lia taught me that when there is a very dense cultural barrier, you do the best you can, and if something happens despite that, you have to be satisfied with little successes instead of total successes. You have to give up total control." The same could be applied to diseases that cannot be cured despite the best levels of care and adherence. There is danger in expecting every person's illness narrative to be a triumph narrative, or perhaps more so in chronic illness (vs. terminal illness), the problem is in misidentifying what that triumph might be: Maybe just surviving and being around to spend time with your loved ones is enough. That might be one of the many lessons learned from Lia Lee's life in her persistent vegetative state. Maybe being a father, husband, son, and brother is enough to ask, hope, and aspire to for my brother Shuvo. What could be an approach that balances unnecessarily limiting a disabled individual while not setting them up for failure by having unrealistic expectations? One such approach could be a modified version both of Dr. Ernst's views on what could be learned from Lia's case as well as of the old adage "hope for the best but expect the worst." In other words, temper your expectations and be happy with whatever recovery is attained, and encourage and view any additional gains as a bonus if they happen, not as a failure if they don't.

REFERENCES

Achor, Shawn. What's the worst kind of praise you can give? https://ideas.ted.com/whats-the-worst-kind-of-praise-you-can-give/ Accessed March 12, 2018.

Bishop, Malachy, & Allen, Chase. (2007). Coping with epilepsy: Research and interventions. In Erin Martz & Hanoch Livneh (Eds.), *Coping with chronic illness and disability: Theoretical, empirical, and clinical aspects* (pp. 241–266). New York, NY: Springer.

Burton, Keith (Producer) & Pasquella, Donald. (1984). *Dax's case*. United States: Filmakers Library, Inc.

Cowart, Dax, & Burt, Robert. (1998). Confronting death: Who chooses, who controls? A conversation between Dax Coward and Robert Burt. *Hastings Center Report 28*, no. 1: 14–24.

Davis, Lennard J. (2013). Constructing normalcy: The bell curve, the novel, and the invention of the disabled body in the nineteenth century. In L. J. Davis (Ed.), *The disability studies reader – second edition* (pp. 3–16). New York, NY: Routledge.

Engel, Margaret. (June 26, 1983). A happy life afterward doesn't make up for torture. *The Washington Post*. Accessed August 8, 2018.

Fox, Margalit. (September 14, 2012). Lia Lee dies; life went on around her, redefining care. *The New York Times*. Accessed August 23, 2018.

Fadiman, Anne. (1997). *The spirit catches you and you fall down: A Hmong child, her American doctors, and the collision of two cultures*. New York, NY: Farrar, Straus and Giroux.

Goering, Sara. (2015). Rethinking disability: The social model of disability and chronic disease. *Curr Rev Musculoskelet Med 8*: 134–138.

Price, Janet, & Shildrick, Margrit. (2002). Bodies together: Touch, ethics, and disability. In M. Corker & T. Shakespeare (Eds.), *Disability/postmodernity: Embodying disability theory* (pp. 167–183). New York, NY: Continuum.

White, Robert B., & Engelhardt Jr., H. Tristaram. (June, 1975). A demand to die. *Hastings Center Report 5*: 9–10, 47.

Whyte, Susan Reynolds, & Ingstad, Benedicte. (1995). Disability and culture: An overview. In B. Ingstad & S. R. Whyte (Eds.), *Disability and culture* (pp. 3–34). Berkeley, CA: University of California Press.

Whyte, Susan Reynolds. (1995). Constructing epilepsy: Images and contexts in East Africa. In B. Ingstad & S. R. Whyte (Eds.), *Disability and culture* (pp. 226–245). Berkeley, CA: University of California Press.

Whyte, Susan Reynolds. (1995). Disability between discourse and experience. In B. Ingstad & S. R. Whyte (Eds.), *Disability and culture* (pp. 267–292). Berkeley, CA: University of California Press.

Index

About the Contributors

Ashley M. Archiopoli (PhD, University of New Mexico) is assistant professor of communication at the University of Houston–Downtown. Dr. Archiopoli's scholarly work explores issues of health-related quality of life with emphasis on health-related stigma, storytelling, and narrative medicine as well as patient-provider communication.

Ann D. Bagchi (PhD, University of Wisconsin–Madison; DNP, Rutgers University) is assistant professor in the School of Nursing at Rutgers University. Her research focuses on developing interventions to address HIV-related stigma and improving rates of routine HIV testing in non-HIV primary care settings.

Ambar Basu (PhD, Purdue University) is associate professor and director of graduate studies in the Department of Communication at the University of South Florida. Dr. Basu's research explores how communities living at the margins of society communicate about health, illness, and living. With an emphasis on theorizing culture as a site of social change, Dr. Basu's interest is in locating health disparities in the context of cultural, political, economic, and development agendas in marginalized spaces.

Russell A. Brewer (DrPH, University of Oklahoma) focuses his HIV research and programmatic efforts on addressing the socio-structural barriers (e.g., incarceration, stigma) to HIV prevention and care among black men who have sex with men (BMSM), persons living with HIV infection, and criminal justice-involved populations in Chicago and the southern United States.

Laura Brown (PhD, University of Texas at Austin) is Post-Doctoral Fellow in The Center for Health Communication at the University of Texas at Austin. She researches the ways that people communicatively manage their health information and identities in the context of illness and wellness. Foci include patient-provider interaction, disclosure processes, uncertainty, stigma, and decision-making. Dr. Brown's work appears in *Communication Monographs*, *Health Communication*, and *Journal of Applied Communication Research*.

Gina M. Brown (MSW, Southern University at New Orleans) was the PLHIV Stigma Index Coordinator in New Orleans, Louisiana. Brown is currently the community organizer at the Southern AIDS Coalition. She provides anti-stigma trainings to address HIV in the Deep South.

Barb Cardell (BA, Grinnell College) is board chair of Positive Women's Network-USA and the vice-chair of the US People Living with HIV Caucus. She works to develop meaningful involvement of people living with HIV in programs and policies that impact their lives and has been a trainer for the US Stigma Index.

Katherine M. Castle (PhD, University of Nebraska–Lincoln) is assistant professor of practice at the University of Nebraska–Lincoln. Her research focuses on understanding how people with chronic illness communicate to make sense of their illness experience, the implications of this process for physical, mental, and relational health and well-being.

Joyeeta G. Dastidar (MD, Vanderbilt University School of Medicine) is assistant professor of medicine at Columbia University Medical Center where she practices internal medicine.

Crystal D. Daugherty (MA, Abilene Christian University) is a doctoral student in communication at the University of Memphis. Daugherty researches narrative and the patient experience. A health communication researcher using multiple methods, she is a frequent international traveller who participates in humanitarian aid and academic research. She is currently writing her dissertation, which explores family health legacies, health narratives, and spiritually in rural Liberia.

Patrick J. Dillon (PhD, University of South Florida) is assistant professor of communication studies at Kent State University at Stark. Dr. Dillon uses ethnographic research methods to examine how people's day-to-day health experiences are impacted by macro-level social forces, such as health policy, economic inequality, and racism. He focuses on advancing health communication scholarship in three primary areas: end-of-life care, HIV/ AIDS, and substance abuse.

Ari Hampton has been working in the HIV field on the prevention and advocacy side for almost six years. He's also an HIV activist, where he works closely and strategically with state, national, and international agencies to provide youth living with HIV the best possible care and services.

Adam Hayden (MA, IUPUI) is a philosopher of science, a champion of narrative medicine, and a person living with brain cancer (glioblastoma). A graduate from the MA program at the Indiana University School of Liberal Arts at IUPUI, Adam was selected in 2018 as a distinguished alumnus. Following his diagnosis, he has delivered several invited lectures and presented work at academic conferences, on themes related to narrative practices in medicine.

Elizabeth A. Hintz (MA, Purdue University) is a PhD student in the Department of Communication at the University of South Florida, where she studies interpersonal health communication. Her research focuses on the effects of interpersonal interactions on health outcomes, particularly in the contexts of chronic pain and reproductive health.

Alexis Zoe Waters Johnson (PhD, University of Nebraska–Lincoln) is assistant professor of communication at Arkansas Tech University. Her research centers on how people cope with and make sense of narratives involving difficulty and trauma within families, health (e.g., cancer, end-of-life, mental health, chronic illness, terminal illness), and marginalized groups.

Vanessa Johnson (JD, Temple University) focuses in public health on empowerment via peer engagement, behavioral health practices; services for chronic health conditions; and harm reduction principles. She is the co-founder of the Ribbon Consulting Group, LLC, a national consulting firm whose mission is to improve community and resident health especially for individuals with hidden disabilities and chronic health conditions.

Krista Hoffmann-Longtin (PhD, Indiana University) is assistant professor of communication studies in the Indiana University School of Liberal Arts at IUPUI, and assistant dean in the Indiana University School of Medicine Office of Faculty Affairs and Professional Development. Her research focuses on communication education in the sciences and health professions, faculty development, and organizational/professional identity.

Jody Koenig Kellas (PhD, University of Washington) is professor of communication at the University of Nebraska. She studies how people communicate to make sense of identity, difficulty, health, and relationships. She is author of *Communicated Narrative Sense-making Theory* (2018) founder of Narrative Nebraska, dedicated to understanding the ways in which communicated sense-making, narratives, storytelling content, process, and functions can be translated to enhance individuals' and families' health well-being. She has published more than forty-five articles and chapters and received national awards for her scholarship.

Peter M. Kellett (PhD, Southern Illinois University at Carbondale) is associate professor of communication studies at University of North Carolina at Greensboro. His scholarship centers on how narrative methods can inform and transform our understanding of health and illness, as well as disability. He also has an enduring interest in narrative approaches to conflict analysis and transformation/peacebuilding. Thematic to his scholarship is the desire to see a more just and fair world through communication.

Andrea L. Meluch (PhD, Kent State University) is assistant professor of health communication at Indiana University, South Bend. Her research interests are at the intersections of health and organizational communication. Her most recent projects examine patient experiences of social support and stigma within healthcare settings.

Jennifer E. Ohs (PhD, Pennsylvania State University) is associate professor of communication, and graduate program coordinator in the Department of Communication, at Saint Louis University. Her scholarly interests lie at the intersection of interpersonal and health communication, with an emphasis on aging, lifespan, and intergenerational communication. Her research has examined medical decisions in older adulthood and healthcare decisions in families.

Mark P. Orbe (PhD, Ohio University) is professor of communication and diversity in the School of Communication at Western Michigan University where he holds a joint appointment in gender and women's studies. His research, teaching, and service efforts engage the inextricable relationship between culture, power, and communication.

Dwight Peavy has worked in the HIV/AIDS arena for more than twenty years. Peavy was the project manager for the New Jersey Statewide Stigma Index Project. Dwight currently serves as the coordinator/facilitator for the New Jersey Coalition to End Discrimination. He was the executive director for the Newark EMA HIV Health Services Planning Council for twelve years.

Rachel M. Reznik (PhD, Northwestern University) is professor of communication arts and sciences at Elmhurst College. She researches interpersonal communication with an emphasis on the ways in which relational processes influence health and well-being.

Meta Smith-Davis is assistant director of prevention at HAART and co-chair of PWN-Louisiana. She is living with HIV which has deepened her sense of responsibility to others living with HIV, specifically women of color.

Andrew R. Spieldenner (PhD, Howard University) is assistant professor in the Department of Communication at California State University–San Marcos. Dr. Spieldenner examines health and culture in three areas: the body, HIV, and the LGBTQ community. A longtime HIV activist, Dr. Spieldenner serves as chair of the US People living with HIV Caucus.

Laurel Sprague (PhD, Wayne State University) specializes in the areas of human rights, political participation, gender, and HIV. She currently leads community mobilization for the Joint United Nations Programme on HIV-AIDS (UNAIDS) and has supported community-based participatory research and action projects on HIV-related stigma, discrimination, and criminalization with networks of people living with HIV in the United States and across multiple regions of the world.

Maria K. Venetis (PhD, Rutgers University) is associate professor of interpersonal health communication at Purdue University. Her research examines the effects of provider-patient communication on patient psychosocial outcomes such as coping and satisfaction. She also studies how patients discuss or avoid talking about health-related concerns with close others.

Jill Yamasaki (PhD, Texas A&M University) is associate professor of health communication in the Jack J. Valenti School of Communication at the University of Houston. Her research focuses on narrative inquiry and practice in the contexts of lived difference, healthy aging, creative engagement in healthcare, and community connectedness.

Amanda J. Young (PhD, Carnegie Mellon University) is associate professor of communication at the University of Memphis. Her research interests are in patient/provider interactions, focusing on the ways that agency is produced in patient narratives through rhetorical choices and strategies. She is particularly interested in chronic illness narratives, with recent work focusing on cystic fibrosis and ICU care.